A Complete Guide to Nursing

Volume I

A Complete Guide to Nursing
Volume I

Edited by **Cynthia Wison**

FOSTER ACADEMICS
New Jersey

Published by Foster Academics,
61 Van Reypen Street,
Jersey City, NJ 07306, USA
www.fosteracademics.com

A Complete Guide to Nursing: Volume I
Edited by Cynthia Wison

International Standard Book Number: 978-1-63242-006-0 (Hardback)

Printed in China.

Contents

Preface

There are few professions deemed as important or given as much reverence as one in the medical profession. Though the hallowed halls of medicine have many specialties that branch off into different directions, nursing makes up a huge bulk of medicine and its practice, and rightfully so. Focussed on a different approach from other healthcare professionals in caring for patients, as well as training, a nurse is an essentiality on most medical situations. It is an emotionally fulfilling career that tends to take care of people in the long term. A respected profession, nursing also soothes the soul. One can also say that it has job security and forms a good foundation for those who want to pursue further medical opportunities. As a career, nursing offers specialties of its own that one can choose from on the basis of one's own motivation and vocation. Assisting doctors and taking care of the sick is no easy task and nurses usually have strong wills and empathy as well.

I wish to thank all those hardworking and tireless men and women who took up this vocation and helped to make medicine more comfortable for others. As almost everyone has experienced the hand of a nurse's work, except for those few who never fall sick, it is a privilege to both work with and fall under their care. One can only thank them for their work and for their support. Alongside those of the nursing profession, I would also thank my family and friends for their support.

Editor

1

The Efficacy of Optimism: Benefit Finding in the Treatment of Diabetes in Iranian Patients

Hossein Karimi Moonaghi,[1] Hossein Namdar Areshtanab,[2] and Leila Jouybari[3]

[1] *Department of Medical-Surgical Nursing, Faculty of Nursing and Midwifery, Mashhad University of Medical Sciences, Mashhad 9137913199, Iran*
[2] *Department of Postgraduate, Faculty of Nursing and Midwifery, Mashhad University of Medical Sciences, Mashhad 9137913199, Iran*
[3] *Faculty of Nursing and Midwifery, Golestan University of Medical Sciences, Gorgan 49155568, Iran*

Correspondence should be addressed to Hossein Namdar Areshtanab; namdarah871@mums.ac.ir

Academic Editors: S. Chan and M. Funnell

The incidence of diabetes mellitus is on the rise around the world. Middle Eastern countries will be facing a vast increase in the number of diabetes mellitus cases by 2030. Diagnosis of a chronic disease such as diabetes mellitus can be a shocking and life-altering event. Conversely, a diagnosis of a chronic illness can also offer the patient opportunities to change unhealthy behaviors such as poor diet, smoking, and lack of exercise, making them healthier than before their diagnosis. This is referred to as "benefit finding". This study reveals the many benefit findings of Iranian patients who have been diagnosed with diabetes mellitus and illustrates how benefit finding can be an integral part of long-term patient care.

1. Introduction

Diabetes mellitus is one of the most challenging and burdensome chronic diseases of the 21st century, and it is a growing threat to the world's public health [1]. Diabetes mellitus currently affects about 285 million adults worldwide and this figure is expected to rise to over 400 million adults by 2030 [2]. Type 2 diabetes mellitus is responsible for over 90% of all cases of diabetes [3]. Most new patients with diabetes are from developing countries and it seems that the Middle East is among the regions that will have the largest increase in the prevalence of diabetes by 2030. According to the research results, the prevalence of diabetes is about 8.7% in Iranians aged 25–64 years (9.2% in women and 7.5% in men). More than 1% of the Iranian urban population older than 20 years develops diabetes mellitus each year [4]. Diabetes mellitus can lead to serious complications and premature death [5]. Consequences of chronic diabetes include eye disease, circulatory problems and kidney failure, decreased quality of life, and increased use of health services [6]. The diagnosis of a life-threatening illness, such as diabetes, can be an extremely stressful and traumatic experience [7]. Studies have showed that living with diabetes has a negative impact on many aspects of daily life and the quality of life for people with diabetes [8].

Although negative outcomes of having an acute or chronic illness have received the most attention, studies can be found elucidating possible positive effects of serious illness [9]. However, some emerging evidence has shown that experience with life-threatening adversity can be an accelerator for personal growth and transformation. For example, research has found that patients may change the way they view themselves, their priorities, and their interactions with others in response to a health-related trauma [10].

The manner in which patients perceive positive of negative implications of their illness can influence various psychological consequences [11]. Posttraumatic growth could be one of the cognitive strategies used to deflect the negative effects of illness. When diagnosed, individuals may change their internal standards of what constitutes good health or other aspects of quality of life (recalibration), adjust their values and priorities (reprioritization), or redefine what they think is important (reconceptualization) to maintain an acceptable quality of life in the face of declining health [12]. Benefit finding has been associated with better psychosocial well-being and lower affective distress in numerous chronic illness populations. A review of the literature showed that the benefit findings are typically investigated in diseases such as cancers, spinal cord injuries, multiple sclerosis, and rheumatoid arthritis with only a few studies conducted among myocardial infarction and HIV/AIDS patients [13, 14]. On the other hand, several studies have been conducted on type 2 diabetes patients [15]. Available literature is based on studies conducted in western societies that differ in terms of cultural and social backgrounds from the Iranian society. Moreover, the studies have shown that sociocultural context could influence illness and outcome of the process of adaptation to disease [16, 17].

An understanding of benefit finding is significant in the proper provision of health care, such as nursing, as it appears that benefit finding aids in dealing effectively with illness and plays a prominent role in the cognitive process that facilitates adjustments to adversity [18]. The aim of this study is to explore positive change experiences of patients with diabetes in the Iranian population.

2. Materials and Methods

A purposive sample of fifteen patients was recruited. Patients were selected on the basis of the following inclusion criteria: a confirmed diagnosis of type 2 diabetes mellitus for at least two years; awareness of their diagnosis; cognitive and physical ability to participate; and a willingness to participate. Data were collected via in-depth, semistructured, and face to face interviews conducted between September 2011 and August 2012. All interviews were private and conducted at the participant's discretion with regard to place and time by the Diabetes Association of Iran, Tabriz branch. The interviews were conducted in Persian by corresponding author. Each participant was interviewed only once. The analysis was conducted in Persian and, for the purposes of this paper, translated into English. The interviewer asked the participants about their experiences of living with diabetes. The interviews were tape-recorded and transcribed verbatim. The first set of interviews lasted 60–80 minutes and the next set of interviews lasted 40–50 minutes (mean time of each interview is 45 minutes). Data collection continued until data saturation was achieved. That is, data collection had gone on up to when no new code emerged from analysis of the data. The analysis of the interview texts began once the first interview had been conducted and transcribed. Data were analyzed using qualitative content analysis techniques inspired by Graneheim and Lundman [19]. The analysis began by reading through each interview several times to obtain a sense of the whole of the participants' experiences. Then, the meaning units, which were words, sentences, or paragraphs that depicted important aspects of participants' experiences, were highlighted. These meaning units were then condensed to shorten the text but retain the content. In the next stage, these condensed meaning units, or codes, were abstracted from each interview transcript. Finally, using comparison, reflection, and interpretation, these codes were grouped into categories and subcategories by the first three authors. Criteria for enhancing the rigor of qualitative studies have been proposed by Lincoln and Guba and include credibility, transferability, dependability, and confirmability [20]. In the research process, researchers allocated sufficient time for data collection and retained close communication with study participants. The interviews were returned to the participants for verification of the accuracy of the results and to validate the congruity of the interpretive findings with their experiences. This ensured that researchers were correctly representing the ideas of the patients.

The data were coded and categorized independently by the authors and emergent themes were compared. Opinions of experts and also three Ph.D. candidates of nursing in data analysis as peer reviewers were used and cases were discussed over a two-week period. Regarding rigor, the research team discussed and interpreted the findings until an agreement was reached, wherein one author collected and analyzed the data (Hossein Namdar Areshtanab) and two researchers (Hossein Karimi Moonaghi, Leila Jouybari), who had expertise and were interested in conducting qualitative research, discussed, checked, and verified the meanings which were being emerged. These reviews enhanced the credibility of the data. To increase the dependability, one of the researchers collected and analyzed the data and other researchers checked and verified the results. Based on data collected from participants and memos taken after reading each of the interviews, participants were selected by considering maximum variation in terms of age, gender, previous experience with illness, family economic status, educational level, job background, and requirement of daily injectable insulin to provide transferability. Following the approval by the Ethics Committee of the Mashhad University of Medical Sciences, informed consents were obtained from all participants who met inclusion criteria for the study. All participants were assured that their personal data would remain confidential. Time and location were chosen by the agreement of the participants. Examples of interview questions are as follows.

(1) Can you tell us about your experiences of living with diabetes mellitus?

(2) Can you describe some things you did or experienced that were helpful in the management of your disease?

(3) What positive effects/changes do you feel may have occurred in your life due to diabetes mellitus?

3. Finding

Of the participants, 9 (60%) were males and the average age was 47.8 ± 12.0 years and 13 (86.7%) were married. Six (40%) had a lower educational background (illiterate to high school) and 6 (40%) had higher education backgrounds (college graduates). Females had a lower educational background than males. Most females were unemployed while most males were employed and three of them were retired. Participants

Table 1: Sociodemographic and clinical characteristics of participants.

Gender	Mean (SD) or number (%)
Male	9 (60%)
Female	6 (40%)
Age	47.86 ± 12
Marital status, number (%)	
Married	13 (86.6%)
Single	1 (6.7%)
Widowed	1 (6.7%)
Employment, number (%)	
Unemployed	3 (20%)
Employed	7 (46.7%)
Retired	5 (33.3%)
Education level, number (%)	
Illiterate to under diploma	6 (40%)
diploma	3 (20%)
Graduate	6 (40%)
Type of treatment, number (%)	
Oral medication	9 (60%)
Insulin	8 (53/3%)
Both medications	6 (40%)
Insurance, number (%)	
Covered	15 (100%)
Not covered	0
Income	
Low	5 (40%)
Medium	6 (33.3%)
High	4 (26.7%)
Duration of diabetes, mean (S.D)	8.7 ± 5.07 (1–25)
Family history	
Yes	9 (60%)
No	6 (40%)
Member of the Diabetes Association	
Yes	9 (60%)
No	6 (40%)

averaged 8.7 years living with a diagnosis of diabetes and 8 (53.3%) participants required daily insulin injection. Most of the participants (60%) were not members of the Diabetes Association (Table 1).

During the data analysis, three main themes emerged as the positive experiences of Iranian patients with diabetes: lifestyle modification; promotion of interpersonal interactions; and appreciating health (Table 2).

3.1. Lifestyle Modification. The participants considered their diseases as an agent in changing unhealthy lifestyle behaviors. This refers to positive changes in knowledge, behavior, self, and spiritual dimensions of participants. The category has four subcategories: promotion of knowledge; modification of behaviors; promotion of self; and promotion of spiritual aspects.

Table 2

Them	Subtheme/frequency and percentage
lifestyle modification	Promotion of knowledge ($n = 13$, 86.6%)
	Modification of behaviors ($n = 12$, 80%)
	Promotion of self ($n = 10$, 66.6%)
	Promotion of spiritual aspects ($n = 14$, 93.3%)
Promotion of interpersonal interactions	Promotion relationships between family members ($n = 11$, 73.3%)
	Participation in group activities ($n = 10$, 66.6%)
	Empathy with other patients with diabetes ($n = 10$, 66.6%)
Appreciating life	Taking advantage of opportunities in life ($n = 12$, 80%)
	Worthy of health ($n = 13$, 86.6%)

3.1.1. Promotion of Knowledge. Diabetes was seen as an agent in increasing personal knowledge and information about this disease and the proper functioning of organs of the body. The participants had not been aware of the disease but they had relative knowledge.

> *I thought that eating too much sugar causes diabetes or if my doctor says that I need to start using insulin, it means I failed to take care of my diabetes properly. However, now I know that type 2 diabetes mellitus is cause by genetics and lifestyle factors such as stress and lack of mobility... Or over time, the body gradually produces less and less of its own insulin and eventually oral medications may not be enough to keep blood glucose levels normal. Using insulin to get blood glucose levels to a healthy level is a good thing, not a bad one. (Man, aged 54)*

3.1.2. Modification of Behaviors. This subcategory presents statements of participants that diabetes gave them an opportunity to change their unhealthy habits, which they perceive as ruining their health but did not previously have enough willpower or incentive to stop. Also it provided an opportunity for patients who were sensitive to their health to adjust their life goals and expectations.

> *I already had a low physical activity level and I ate fatty and fried foods. Now I try to walk every day for at least one half hour and I eat more low-fat and low cholesterol foods such as vegetables and fruits. (Woman, aged 50)*

> *I was already overweight and smoking. I was not able to reduce my weight or stop smoking. I realized after diabetes that if I wanted to continue living, I should quit smoking and lose weight and I got it. (Man, aged 45)*

Following my illness, I regularly check my blood glucose, cholesterol, triglycerides and blood pressure. (Man, aged 52)

Before my illness, I wanted to work after retirement. Now I want to retire earlier so that I may buy a garden where I can plant trees and get relaxation. (Man, aged 57)

3.1.3. Promotion of Self. Diabetes mellitus was seen as an agent in modifying coping styles, identification with successful people, and an increase in empathy (feeling more compassionate to others).

Now, I prepare to participate in scientific studies about diabetes mellitus in order to progress in the treatment of it, while previously I had no such intention (meaning based coping). (Man, aged 43)

For forty-eight years my aunt has had type 2 diabetes mellitus and she lives comfortably with it. I always use her as a model on life with diabetes and I use her guidance in diabetes control." (Identification). (Woman, aged 61)

Before becoming ill, some of behaviors in diabetes such as stated discomfort of repeated injections of insulin or rigid diet were pointless for me. Now, I'm less judgmental because I realize that diabetics may have many reasons for their behaviors (Empathy). (Man, aged 50)

3.1.4. Promotion of Spirituality. Diabetes mellitus was seen as an agent in devoting more attention to spiritual issues. The participants were paying more attention to their spirituality following their illnesses. They believed that a closer relationship with God and greater spirituality could help them better tolerate the illness.

After I prayed and read the Koran, I feel inner peace and I better cope with the problems of life and diabetes. (Man, aged 49)

I begin my life with God's name every day. God is my real helper. (Woman, aged 41)

3.2. Promotion of Interpersonal Interactions. The participants considered this disease as the agent in changing interpersonal relations. It refers to positive changes in relationships between family members, participation in group activities, and empathy with other patients with diabetes.

Following my illness and over time, my wife has learned to comfort me and in the family nutrition programs, she is also considering my nutritional circumstances. The children understand my situation now and they support me. (Man, aged 62)

Following my illness, I am participating in educational classes of the Diabetes Association where I share my experiences with other patients. I have become familiar with the newest treatments for diabetes mellitus. I am participating in the group exercises with other patients. (Man, aged 38)

Before having diabetes mellitus, when I saw a patient with diabetes, I told myself that this is a very minor illness, but now when I see someone with diabetes mellitus I am very sad and upset. I tell myself it isn't a wound that you can open and close easily, nor is it a dislocation of a joint. It is really painful and hard to tolerate. (Man, aged 55)

3.3. Appreciating Health. Participants believed that the illness has helped them appreciate things that previously were not important to them. It refers to positive changes in using opportunities in life and realizing the value of health.

Following my illness, I realized that life is short and every moment of life is precious. (Woman, aged 65)

After this illness, I understood that good health is a great blessing and it is the most valuable thing in my life. (Man, aged 39)

The study was affected by duration of illness, family support, severity of illness, educational level, economic status, beliefs, and underlying diseases of the participants.

I know nothing will happen to me except God willing. Maybe my illness is a kind of test from God in my life. When I think deeply, I find out that this illness has got some benefits for me. (Woman, aged 62)

The research findings are shown in Table 2.

4. Discussion and Conclusion

Until now, there have been no studies conducted in Iran on posttraumatic growth following type 2 diabetes mellitus. This study shows that the participants have realized positive changes following type 2 diabetes mellitus depending on what meaning they ascribe to it. Studies have shown that how the individual cognitively processes information plays an essential role in coping with illness [21].

In this study, one of the positive changes after a diagnosis of type 2 diabetes mellitus was promotion of lifestyle. It was evidenced in knowledge, behavior, self-, and spiritual dimensions of participants. The present study found promotion of spiritual aspects as the most significant dimension of benefit finding. Considering the dominant religious culture in Iran and special role of religion and spirituality in facing stressful events, predominance of the spiritual promotion subtheme is quite justified. Thus, taking into account existing studies, it seems that promotion of lifestyle is one of the positive outcomes to chronic illness [15, 22–25].

In this study, the illness may not only influence the patients to change their lifestyles, but also affect the interpersonal interactions in relation to positive changes in relationships between family members, participation in group activities, and empathy with other patients with diabetes.

Thus, taking into account existing studies, it seems that positive changes in relationships are one of the positive outcomes to chronic illness [15, 18, 26–28].

Another positive change in the aftermath of the illness was appreciation of life. Thus, taking into account existing studies, it seems that appreciation of health is one of the positive outcomes to chronic illness [18, 23, 29]. In this study, length of time with the disease, high family support, low severity of illness, high educational level, high economic status, religious beliefs, and no underlying disease had positive impacts on posttraumatic growth in diabetes. Thus, taking into account existing studies, it seems that these factors have a positive effect on diabetes mellitus [30].

It can be concluded that, despite the difficulties of having diabetes, it may also have positive effects for those diagnosed. Consideration of the effects of the disease on patients' life experiences and understanding of their thoughts about the disease as well as the disease's impact on adaptation to disease are important elements in nursing care and education.

5. Limitations and Recommendations

In this study, the sample size is small and was carried out in one national context. Also, the findings reflect only the view of patients regarding positive effects of type 2 diabetes mellitus. Thus, as with other such qualitative studies, caution is needed in generalizing the findings to either Iran as a country or other countries around the world. Also, future study requires input from both health care providers and families. We believe that it is necessary to conduct a population-based survey to confirm these findings.

Conflict of Interests

The authors declare that they have no conflict of interests.

Acknowledgments

This paper is the result of an approved thesis in MUMS (no. 900603), funded by MUMS vice presidency for research purposes. The authors wish to thank the vice chancellor on research in Mashhad University of Medical Sciences who supported this study and also thank all participants and excellent cooperation of Tabriz branch Diabetes Association for their great help in conducting this research.

References

[1] T. Tuncay, I. Musabak, D. E. Gok, and M. Kutlu, "The relationship between anxiety, coping strategies and characteristics of patients with diabetes," *Health and Quality of Life Outcomes*, vol. 6, article 79, 2008.

[2] M. Donald, J. Dower, R. Ware, B. Mukandi, S. Parekh, and C. Bain, "Living with diabetes: rationale, study design and baseline characteristics for an Australian prospective cohort study," *BMC Public Health*, vol. 12, no. 1, article 8, pp. 1–10, 2012.

[3] E. Olshansky, D. Sacco, K. Fitzgerald et al., "Living with diabetes: normalizing the process of managing diabetes," *Diabetes Educator*, vol. 34, no. 6, pp. 1004–1012, 2008.

[4] H. Harati, F. Hadaegh, N. Saadat, and F. Azizi, "Population-based incidence of type 2 diabetes and its associated risk factors: results from a six-year cohort study in Iran," *BMC Public Health*, vol. 9, article 186, 2009.

[5] J. Oliva, A. Fernandez-Bolanos, and A. Hidalgo, "Health-related quality of life in diabetic people with different vascular risk," *BMC Public Health*, vol. 12, article 812, 2012.

[6] K. C. Sikdar, P. P. Wang, D. MacDonald, and V. G. Gadag, "Diabetes and its impact on health-related quality of life: a life table analysis," *Quality of Life Research*, vol. 19, no. 6, pp. 781–787, 2010.

[7] T. Barskova and R. Oesterreich, "Post-traumatic growth in people living with a serious medical condition and its relations to physical and mental health: a systematic review," *Disability and Rehabilitation*, vol. 31, no. 21, pp. 1709–1733, 2009.

[8] A. Nicolucci, K. Kovacs Burns, R. I. Holt et al., "Diabetes Attitudes, Wishes and Needs: Second Study (DAWN2): cross-national benchmarking of diabetes-related psychosocial outcomes for people with diabetes," *Diabetic Medicine*, vol. 30, no. 7, pp. 767–777, 2013.

[9] T. M. Norekvål, P. Moons, B. R. Hanestad, J. E. Nordrehaug, T. Wentzel-Larsen, and B. Fridlund, "The other side of the coin: perceived positive effects of illness in women following acute myocardial infarction," *European Journal of Cardiovascular Nursing*, vol. 7, no. 1, pp. 80–87, 2008.

[10] Y. W. Leung, D. A. Alter, P. L. Prior, D. E. Stewart, J. Irvine, and S. L. Grace, "Posttraumatic growth in coronary artery disease outpatients: relationship to degree of trauma and health service use," *Journal of Psychosomatic Research*, vol. 72, no. 4, pp. 293–299, 2012.

[11] J. M. Currier, S. Hermes, and S. Phipps, "Brief report: childrens response to serious illness: perceptions of benefit and burden in a pediatric cancer population," *Journal of Pediatric Psychology*, vol. 34, no. 10, pp. 1129–1134, 2009.

[12] D. de Ridder, R. Geenen, R. Kuijer, and H. van Middendorp, "Psychological adjustment to chronic disease," *The Lancet*, vol. 372, no. 9634, pp. 246–255, 2008.

[13] V. S. Helgeson, K. A. Reynolds, and P. L. Tomich, "A meta-analytic review of benefit finding and growth," *Journal of Consulting and Clinical Psychology*, vol. 74, no. 5, pp. 797–816, 2006.

[14] V. Tran, D. J. Wiebe, K. T. Fortenberry, J. M. Butler, and C. A. Berg, "Benefit finding, affective reactions to diabetes stress, and diabetes management among early adolescents," *Health Psychology*, vol. 30, no. 2, pp. 212–219, 2011.

[15] M. Yamakawa and K. Makimoto, "Positive experiences of type 2 diabetes in Japanese patients: an exploratory qualitative study," *International Journal of Nursing Studies*, vol. 45, no. 7, pp. 1032–1041, 2008.

[16] T. Z. Habib and M. D. S. Rahman, "Psycho-social aspects of AIDS as a chronic illness: social worker role perspective," *Antrocom*, vol. 6, no. 1, pp. 79–89, 2010.

[17] T. Gomersall, A. Madill, and L. K. M. Summers, "A metasynthesis of the self-management of type 2 diabetes," *Qualitative Health Research*, vol. 21, no. 6, pp. 853–871, 2011.

[18] M. Sato, Y. Yamazaki, M. Sakita, and T. J. Bryce, "Benefit-finding among people with rheumatoid arthritis in Japan," *Nursing and Health Sciences*, vol. 10, no. 1, pp. 51–58, 2008.

[19] U. H. Graneheim and B. Lundman, "Qualitative content analysis in nursing research: concepts, procedures and measures to achieve trustworthiness," *Nurse Education Today*, vol. 24, no. 2, pp. 105–112, 2004.

[20] N. K. Denzin and Y. S. Lincoln, *The Sage Hanbook of Qualitative Research*, Sage, Washigton, DC, USA, 4th edition, 2011.

[21] T. B. Kashdan and J. Q. Kane, "Post-traumatic distress and the presence of post-traumatic growth and meaning in life: experiential avoidance as a moderator," *Personality and Individual Differences*, vol. 50, no. 1, pp. 84–89, 2011.

[22] I. C. V. Thuné-Boyle, J. Stygall, M. R. S. Keshtgar, T. I. Davidson, and S. P. Newman, "Religious/spiritual coping resources and their relationship with adjustment in patients newly diagnosed with breast cancer in the UK," *Psycho-Oncology*, vol. 22, no. 3, pp. 646–658, 2013.

[23] P. A. A. Hassani, M. F. Koshknab, and F. Yaqhmaei, "Perceived positive effects of illness following acute myocardial infarction," *International Journal of Nursing and Midwifery*, vol. 1, no. 1, pp. 1–5, 2009.

[24] K. A. Walker, *A bittersweet existence: the lived experiences of four young women with diabetes mellitus [M.S. thesis]*, Queens Space Library: Education, Queen's University, 2008.

[25] E. C. Salick and C. F. Auerbach, "From devastation to integration: adjusting to and growing from medical trauma," *Qualitative Health Research*, vol. 16, no. 8, pp. 1021–1037, 2006.

[26] K. I. Pakenham, "The nature of benefit finding in multiple sclerosis (MS)," *Psychology, Health and Medicine*, vol. 12, no. 2, pp. 190–196, 2007.

[27] K. J. Petrie, D. L. Buick, J. Weinman, and R. J. Booth, "Positive effects of illness reported by myocardial infarction and breast cancer patients," *Journal of Psychosomatic Research*, vol. 47, no. 6, pp. 537–543, 1999.

[28] M.-A. Choe, G. V. Padilla, Y. R. Chae, and S. Kim, "Quality of life for patients with diabetes in Korea—I: the meaning of health-related quality of life," *International Journal of Nursing Studies*, vol. 38, no. 6, pp. 673–682, 2001.

[29] R. Fallah, F. Keshmir, F. Lotfi Kashani, E. Azargashb, and M. E. Akbari, "Post-traumatic growth in breast cancer patients: a qualitative phenomenological study," *Middle East Journal of Cancer*, vol. 3, no. 2-3, pp. 35–44, 2012.

[30] S. C. Lechner, S. G. Zakowski, M. H. Antoni, M. Greenhawt, K. Block, and P. Block, "Do sociodemographic and disease-related variables influence benefit-finding in cancer patients?" *Psycho-Oncology*, vol. 12, no. 5, pp. 491–499, 2003.

2

Job Burnout, Mood State, and Cardiovascular Variable Changes of Doctors and Nurses in a Children's Hospital in China

Shuchang He,[1] Yan Chen,[1,2] Junya Zhan,[1] Johnna Wu,[3] and Mark Opler[3]

[1] *Department of Psychology, Peking University, No. 5 Yiheyuan Road, Haidian District, Beijing 100871, China*
[2] *Capital Institute of Pediatrics, Beijing 100020, China*
[3] *Department of Psychiatry, New York University School of Medicine, New York City, NY 10016, USA*

Correspondence should be addressed to Shuchang He; shuchangh@pku.edu.cn

Academic Editors: A. Green and A. Kenny

Aims. This study examines mood and cardiovascular variables related to job stress and burnout in hospital personnel. *Main Methods.* 400 nurses and physicians from a children's hospital in China were recruited. Participants completed job stress, burnout, and mood state questionnaires. Cardiovascular variables such as body mass index (BMI), triglyceride (TG), and high density lipoprotein (HDL) were measured. *Key Findings.* Job stress and burnout were significantly associated with mood state. Statistically significant correlations were found between triglyceride levels and job stress scores ($r = 0.175$, $P < 0.01$), BMI and job stress scores ($r = 0.121$, $P < 0.05$), and HDL levels and job stress scores ($r = -0.117$, $P < 0.05$). *Significance.* Mood state changes may be related to job stress and job burnout, in turn, associated with triglycerides and HDL levels. Public health implications and interventions are discussed.

1. Introduction

Burnout is a psychosomatic syndrome characterized by the three core dimensions of emotional exhaustion (EE), feelings of depersonalization (DP), and reduced personal accomplishment (PA) along with mental weariness. Its etiology is generally thought to be long-standing stress at work or elsewhere [1]. Burnout is an important occupational problem in doctors and nurses [2] since they have continuous and constant contact with patient morbidities and mortalities [3]. Burnout affects nearly one in two salaried physicians and pharmacists in France [4]. A survey in a German university hospital found that more than half of the physicians/psychologists, a quarter of the nursing staff, and 10% of the remaining employees suffered from work-related mental stress disorders. Physicians and psychologists were especially affected by psychosomatic symptoms [5]. A three-hospital survey in China showed that surgeons and physicians had the highest scores of job burnout [6].

Among the three dimensions, emotion exhaustion is regarded as the principal dimension associated with the correlates and consequence of burnout [7]. It is important to study mood states because they not only influence the individuals in their work condition but they also have a work-family interface and are related to their behavior in their families as well [8]. Negative emotions are regarded as a plausible dispositional factor responsible for job satisfaction and influence the way people perceive their working environments [9]. The people with more positive mood states are more optimistic, are more likely to give higher quality services, and are more likely to have a greater sense of accomplishment, while negative moods are associated with giving poor service and increased absenteeism and turnover [10, 11]. More frequent negative moods are expected to contribute to tendencies to depersonalize patients [12].

Many published studies focus on emotional experiences at work [13]; they are not only associated with the performance and attitude of the individuals at work but are also related to their cardiovascular system activation [14]. Stress can influence the cardiovascular system via activated hypothalamic-pituitary-adrenocortical (HPA) and sympathoadrenomedullary (SAM) axes. Many documents demonstrate the possible association of job stress and cardiovascular heart disease [15]. High strain and active jobs are related to increased cardiovascular risk among women [16]. In a recent review on the autonomic nervous system and cardiovascular risk factors, Thayer and colleagues found that decreased vagal function is a risk factor for all-cause mortality and that work stress is associated with decreased HRV [17].

2. Methods

Participant. This study was conducted in Beijing, including doctors (132) and nurses (184) from a children's hospital. 400 questionnaires were distributed and a total of 316 questionnaires were completed and collected (the response rate was 79%). This study was approved by the Human Subject Ethics Committee of Department of Psychology at Peking University. The ethics committees of the hospital also approved the study. The demographic variable characteristic of the participants is listed in Table 1.

3. Questionnaire

The questionnaires included four parts. Part one was a demographic and general condition information section (e.g., age, gender, education year, department, marriage, etc.). General medical variables for each participant such as body avoirdupois, stature, blood pressure, blood lipid level, and blood glucose levels were obtained from their physical examinations within the last 12 months.

Part two was a job stress questionnaire, developed by Wang Lei and collaborators (Wang et al.). Wang's instrument includes 16 items scored on a Likert scale, ranging from 1 (never) to 7 (always); total scores reflect overall job stress. Job stress was divided into four levels according to the Lei scale total score: relaxed (<40), normal (40–64), overload (65–75), and much overload (>75).

Part three was comprised of the Profile of Mood States (POMS) from the Neurobehavioral Core Test Battery (NCTB) recommended by the World Health Organization, including 65 questions focusing on six domains; anger-hostility (POMSA), confusion-bewilderment (POMSC), depression-dejection (POMSD), fatigue-inertia (POMSF), tension-anxiety (POMST), and vigor-activity (POMSV). Participants responded to each item on a 5-point scale, ranging from 1 (never) to 5 (always) using the past week as a reference.

Part four involved assessment of job burnout. A Chinese version of the 15-item Maslach Burnout Inventory (MBI) [18] was utilized. This instrument includes three subscales that measured emotional exhaustion (EE), depersonalization (DP), and lack of personal accomplishment (PA). Responses to each MBI item ranged from never (0) to every day (6). Subscale scores were computed as the sum of the responses made to each item in a given subscale. Burnout was defined by high scores on the EE and DP subscales and low scores on the PA subscale [18]. A relative absence of burnout was characterized by the opposite pattern.

Table 1: The general condition of participants.

Item	Number	Percentage
Male	38	12.0
Female	278	88.0
Physician	132	41.8
Nurse	184	58.2
No position	82	25.9
Primary	124	39.2
Middle	77	24.4
Pre-high	23	7.3
High	10	3.2
High school and/or below	128	40.5
University	107	33.9
Graduate school	81	25.6
Medicine	129	40.8
Surgery	87	27.5
Emergency	52	16.5
Others	48	15.2
Unmarried	100	31.6
Married	213	67.4
Divorced	2	0.6
Widowed	1	0.3

Table 2: Job stress scores of participants.

Item	Relax	Normal	Much stress	Overload
Number	39	145	75	57
Percentage	12.3	45.9	23.7	18.0

4. Statistics

Student's t-test, variance analysis, and Chi-square test were used to make comparisons. Pearson correlations were computed to examine the association among scores in three main dimensions, job stress, mood state scores, and cardiovascular variables.

5. Results

5.1. Job Stress. The total scores of job stress in the 316 participants were from 21 to 103.

The mean value was 60.81 ± 16.31 (see Table 2).

5.2. Job Burnout. Our data showed that the mean scores on the job burnout subscales were 22.04 ± 8.34 for emotional exhaustion (EE), 13.47 ± 6.52 for feelings of depersonalization (DP), and 15.72 ± 6.40 for reduced personal accomplishment (PA) (see Table 3). These values indicated a moderate to higher level of emotion exhaustion, a moderate level of depersonalization, and a much higher level of personal accomplishments in the nurses and doctors.

T-test showed that the scores of the three dimensions of job burnout had no significant difference between male and female participants (see Table 3).

TABLE 3: Job burnout scores of different demographic variables.

Demographic characteristics	n	EE	DP	PA
Sex				
Male	38	4.2 ± 1.5	3.2 ± 1.5	2.5 ± 1.0
Female	278	4.4 ± 1.7	3.4 ± 1.7	2.6 ± 1.1
t		−0.781	−0.69	−1.015
P		0.435	0.491	0.311
Age				
20–29	152	4.1 ± 0.1	3.1 ± 0.1	2.7 ± 0.1
30–39	108	4.6 ± 0.2	3.7 ± 0.2	2.8 ± 0.1
≥40	56	4.8 ± 0.2	3.4 ± 0.2	2.2 ± 0.1
F		5.622	4.049	5.706
P		0.004	0.018	0.004
Education				
High school or below	128	4.5 ± 0.1	3.4 ± 0.1	2.6 ± 0.1
University	107	4.6 ± 0.2	3.5 ± 0.2	2.7 ± 0.1
Graduate school	81	4.0 ± 0.2	3.0 ± 0.2	2.5 ± 0.1
F		3.867	2.254	1.102
P		0.022	0.107	0.334
Department				
Medicine	129	4.6 ± 0.1	3.3 ± 0.1	2.6 ± 0.1
Surgery	87	4.5 ± 0.2	3.6 ± 0.2	2.6 ± 0.1
Emergency	52	4.6 ± 0.3	3.5 ± 0.2	2.9 ± 0.1
Others	48	3.7 ± 0.2	2.9 ± 0.2	2.3 ± 0.2
F		3.348	2.057	2.607
P		0.02	0.11	0.05
Is married[A]				
Unmarried	100	3.8 ± 1.7	2.8 ± 1.6	2.6 ± 1.1
Married	213	4.7 ± 1.6	3.6 ± 1.6	2.7 ± 1.1
t		−4.224	−4.497	−0.664
P		<0.001	<0.001	0.507

[A]There are also two divorced and one widowed.

Comparing the scores of the three dimensions regarding the age, sex, marriage, years of education, and the department, results showed that no significant difference was observed between men and women with regard to the scores of three dimensions of job burnout. The participants >40 years old showed slightly higher scores on the EE scale. Participants 30–39 years old showed higher scores on the DP and PA scales. Married individuals had higher scores on EE and DP compared with unmarried ones. Participants from different departments also showed significantly different EE scores among medicine, surgery, and others (see Table 3).

5.3. Mood State. No significant differences were observed when comparing scores of mood state between men and women. However, there were significant differences among age groups with regard to the six mood factors. There were also significant differences by years of education in mood state scores. Comparison between married participants and unmarried ones showed that there were significant differences with regard to the six mood factors ($P < 0.001$). Comparing the mood scores of participants in different departments, we observed that the scores of POMST, POMSA, POMSF, and POMSC significantly differed between different departments (see Table 4).

Correlational analyses demonstrated that job stress scores were statistically significant and positively related to scores of emotion exhaustion, depersonalization, and reduced personal accomplishment ($P < 0.01$) (see Table 5).

A statistically significant positive correlation emerged between scores of the three dimensions of job burnout and scores of negative mood state (POMSA, POMSC, POMSD, POMSF, and POMST), and negative correlations were seen between scores of the three dimensions of job burnout and POMSV scores ($P < 0.01$) (see Table 6). Statistically significant positive correlations were found between blood triglyceride level and job stress scores ($r = 0.175$, $P < 0.01$) and BMI and job stress ($r = 0.121$, $P < 0.05$). A statistically significant negative correlation was found between blood HDL level and job stress scores ($r = -0.117$, $P < 0.05$). No statistically significant correlations were found between

TABLE 4: POMS scores of different demographic variables.

Demographic characteristic	n	POMST	POMSD	POMSA	POMSV	POMSF	POMSC
Sex							
Male	38	11.7 ± 7.6	16.1 ± 14.6	14.7 ± 11.0	17.0 ± 5.9	9.9 ± 7.0	9.7 ± 5.3
Female	278	12.1 ± 6.5	16.7 ± 11.9	15.0 ± 9.9	15.7 ± 6.1	10.8 ± 6.1	9.8 ± 4.5
t		−0.349	−0.267	−0.188	1.187	−0.864	−0.136
P		0.727	0.789	0.851	0.236	0.388	0.892
Age							
20–29	152	11.0 ± 0.5	14.0 ± 1.0	13.3 ± 0.8	17.3 ± 0.5	9.2 ± 0.5	9.0 ± 0.4
30–39	108	13.0 ± 0.6	19.0 ± 1.2	16.7 ± 1.0	14.1 ± 0.6	12.0 ± 0.6	10.8 ± 0.4
≥40	56	12.7 ± 0.9	19.2 ± 1.6	16.1 ± 1.3	15.5 ± 0.8	12.2 ± 0.8	10.4 ± 0.6
F		3.304	7.068	4.068	9.362	8.871	5.342
P		0.038	0.001	0.018	<0.001	<0.001	0.005
Education							
High school or below	128	11.5 ± 0.6	15.3 ± 1.1	14.5 ± 0.9	16.6 ± 0.5	10.4 ± 0.6	9.3 ± 0.4
University	107	12.5 ± 0.6	18.9 ± 1.2	16.6 ± 1.0	14.7 ± 0.6	11.7 ± 0.6	10.6 ± 0.4
Graduate school	81	12.2 ± 0.7	15.7 ± 1.4	13.6 ± 1.1	16.3 ± 0.7	9.8 ± 0.7	9.6 ± 0.5
F		0.746	2.843	2.414	3.182	2.288	2.272
P		0.475	0.06	0.091	0.043	0.103	0.105
Department							
Medicine	129	12.7 ± 0.6	17.4 ± 1.1	15.2 ± 0.9	15.7 ± 0.5	11.3 ± 0.5	10.2 ± 0.4
Surgery	87	11.3 ± 0.7	16.2 ± 1.3	15.4 ± 1.1	16.4 ± 0.7	10.4 ± 0.7	9.9 ± 0.5
Emergency	52	13.4 ± 0.9	18.2 ± 1.7	17.3 ± 1.4	15.2 ± 0.8	11.8 ± 0.9	10.2 ± 0.6
Others	48	10.1 ± 1.0	13.5 ± 1.8	11.0 ± 1.4	16.4 ± 0.9	8.4 ± 0.9	8.1 ± 0.7
F		2.924	1.533	3.519	0.571	3.216	2.646
P		0.034	0.206	0.015	0.634	0.023	0.049
Is married[A]							
Unmarried	100	10.2 ± 6.3	12.2 ± 10.8	11.8 ± 9.9	18.2 ± 5.4	8.2 ± 5.8	8.4 ± 4.4
Married	213	12.9 ± 6.6	18.6 ± 12.3	16.4 ± 9.7	14.8 ± 6.1	11.8 ± 6.1	10.5 ± 4.5
t		−3.459	−4.48	−3.931	4.861	−4.934	−3.713
P		0.001	<0.001	<0.001	<0.001	<0.001	<0.001

[A]There are also two divorced and one widowed.

TABLE 5: Coefficient of correlation (r) of job stress and job burnout ($n = 316$).

	Job stress	EE	DP	PA
Job stress	1			
EE	0.562**	1		
DP	0.474**	0.699**	1	
RP	0.287**	0.68**	0.358**	1

**$P < 0.01$.

blood glucose and job stress, diastolic pressure and job stress, and systolic pressure and job stress (see Table 7).

6. Discussion

This study examined associations between job stress, job burnout, mood state, and cardiovascular variables in doctors and nurses from a children's hospital in Beijing. Results show that approximately 18% of the participants experience significant job stress. Job stress and associated job burnout was in turn related to mood changes. Increasing job stress may be related to higher negative moods and reduced positive moods. Participants with higher scores of job stress and job burnout may require further evaluation, considering that negative mood not only influenced health but also influenced job performance.

There were no differences between men and women in mood scores on the three dimensions of job burnout. A study from Sweden found differences in working conditions and social networks between women and men with burnout [19]. Patients with burnout differ from the general population with respect to individual and social factors as well.

One of the more intriguing findings from our study was the positive correlation between job stress scores and serum triglyceride levels. The negative correlation between job stress and HDL levels suggests that job stress might increase triglycerides and decrease HDL. Prior studies in Beijing have demonstrated changes in coronary heart disease and cholesterol levels over time [20]. High blood HDL level is regarded as a protective factor for the cardiovascular system. Consequently, the decreased blood HDL levels related to

TABLE 6: Coefficient of correlation (r) of job burnout and mood states ($n = 316$).

	POMST	POMSD	POMSA	POMSV	POMSF	POMSC
EE	0.516**	0.551**	0.480**	−0.425**	0.603**	0.481**
DP	0.503**	0.550**	0.510**	−0.314**	0.521**	0.486**
PA	0.331**	0.351**	0.278**	−0.283**	0.320**	0.305**

**$P < 0.01$.

TABLE 7: Coefficient of correlation (r) of job stress and cardiovascular variables ($n = 316$).

	Blood glucose	Diastolic pressure	Systolic pressure	TG	HDL	BMI	Job stress
Blood glucose	1						
Diastolic pressure	0.126*	1					
Systolic pressure	0.037	0.239**	1				
TG	0.332**	0.448**	0.099	1			
HDL	−0.458**	−0.328**	−0.076	−0.716**	1		
BMI	0.167**	0.474**	0.220**	0.403**	−0.332**	1	
Job stress	−0.002	0.081	0.061	0.175**	−0.117*	0.121*	1

HDL: high density lipoprotein. TG: triglyceride. *$P < 0.05$; **$P < 0.01$.

job stress may be a useful risk marker for patients in occupational settings. Prior findings suggest that job strain may be a modifiable risk factor for metabolic syndrome and subsequent cardiovascular disease [21]. A survey in China by Xu et al. found that high levels of effort, overcommitment, and low reward increased the risk of dyslipidemia among Chinese workers, and they were significantly associated with triglycerides and LDL rather than HDL or other factors. Changes in blood lipids may be the possible link between job stress and coronary heart disease [22], although prior findings are equivocal [23].

The negative correlations between BMI and job stress scores indicate that BMI may also be a potentially useful biomarker. A previous study showed that increases in BMI (1 kg/m^2) raised the risk for diabetes mellitus by approximately 26% in nonobese male Japanese [24]. Increased BMI may be a possible risk factor for diabetes in workplaces. A study found that increased BMI may occur because workers feeling stressed are prone to change their eating behavior and eat too much, which results in obesity [25].

Our study builds on the prior lines of evidence for the role of job strain as burnout syndrome seems to be a real independent cardiovascular risk factor. Training to manage emotions may increase cardiac vagal tone and may be cardioprotective [26]. Learning to control mood states and increasing positive mood may be an important intervention strategy to reduce job stress related to cardiovascular health.

7. Conclusion

This study concludes that job stress is related to three dimensions of job burnout, mood states, and cardiovascular variables in the doctors and nurses in a hospital setting in Beijing. High job stress and negative mood states appear to be associated with increased risk of developing cardiovascular diseases. We conclude that reduction of job stress is critical for prevention of cardiovascular diseases in the work place in order to foster a higher quality of life.

Conflict of Interests

The authors declare that there is no conflict of interests regarding the publication of this paper.

Acknowledgments

This research was supported by research projects (Key Projects in the National Science and Technology Pillar Program of China (no. 2009BAI77B04) and Natural Science Foundation of China, Grant no. 81271491/H0920).

References

[1] C. Maslach, W. B. Schaufeli, and M. P. Leiter, "Job burnout," *Annual Review of Psychology*, vol. 52, pp. 397–422, 2001.

[2] H. J. Freudenberger, "Staff burn-out," *Journal of Social Issues*, vol. 30, pp. 159–165, 1974.

[3] A. Caruso, C. Vigna, V. Bigazzi, I. Sperduti, L. Bongiorno, and A. Allocca, "Burnout among physicians and nurses working in oncology," *La Medicina del Lavoro*, vol. 103, pp. 96–105, 2012.

[4] M.-A. Doppia, M. Estryn-Béhar, C. Fry, K. Guetarni, and T. Lieutaud, "Burnout in French doctors: a comparative study among anaesthesiologists and other specialists in French hospitals (SESMAT study)," *Annales Francaises d'Anesthesie et de Reanimation*, vol. 30, no. 11, pp. 782–794, 2011.

[5] A. Hiemisch, W. Kiess, and E. Brähler, "Mental job strain in a University children's hospital a study on stress experience and the resulting employee health," *Klinische Padiatrie*, vol. 223, no. 4, pp. 236–241, 2011.

[6] S. Wu, W. Zhu, H. Li, Z. Wang, and M. Wang, "Relationship between job burnout and occupational stress among doctors in China," *Stress and Health*, vol. 24, no. 2, pp. 143–149, 2008.

[7] D. C. Glass and J. D. Mcknight, "Perceived control, depressive symptomatology, and professional burnout: a review of the evidence," *Psychology and Health*, vol. 11, no. 1, pp. 23–48, 1996.

[8] L. N. Dyrbye, J. Freischlag, K. L. Kaups et al., "Work-home conflicts have a substantial impact on career decisions that affect the adequacy of the surgical workforce," *Archives of Surgery*, vol. 147, pp. 933–939, 2012.

[9] B. M. Staw, N. E. Bell, and J. A. Clausen, "The dispositional approach to job attitudes: a lifetime longitudinal test," *Administrative Science Quarterly*, vol. 31, no. 1, pp. 56–77, 1986.

[10] J. M. George and K. Bettenhausen, "Understanding prosocial behavior, sales performance, and turnover: a group-level analysis in a service context," *Journal of Applied Psychology*, vol. 75, no. 6, pp. 698–709, 1990.

[11] L. H. Pelled and K. R. Xin, "Down and out: an investigation of the relationship between mood and employee withdrawal behavior," *Journal of Management*, vol. 25, no. 6, pp. 875–895, 1999.

[12] K. L. Zellars, W. A. Hochwarter, P. L. Perrewé, N. Hoffman, and E. W. Ford, "Experiencing job burnout: the roles of positive and negative traits and states," *Journal of Applied Social Psychology*, vol. 34, no. 5, pp. 887–911, 2004.

[13] A. P. Brief and H. M. Weiss, "Organizational behavior: affect in the workplace," *Annual Review of Psychology*, vol. 53, pp. 279–307, 2002.

[14] A. Erez and A. M. Isen, "The influence of positive affect on the components of expectancy motivation," *Journal of Applied Psychology*, vol. 87, no. 6, pp. 1055–1067, 2002.

[15] A. Steptoe and M. Kivimäki, "Stress and cardiovascular disease," *Nature Reviews Cardiology*, vol. 9, pp. 360–370, 2012.

[16] N. Slopen, R. J. Glynn, J. E. Buring, T. T. Lewis, D. R. Williams, and M. A. Albert, "Job strain, job insecurity, and incident cardiovascular disease in the women's health study: results from a 10-year prospective study," *PLoS ONE*, vol. 7, Article ID e40512, 2012.

[17] J. F. Thayer, S. S. Yamamoto, and J. F. Brosschot, "The relationship of autonomic imbalance, heart rate variability and cardiovascular disease risk factors," *International Journal of Cardiology*, vol. 141, no. 2, pp. 122–131, 2010.

[18] C. Maslach and S. E. Jackson, *MBI: Maslach Burnout Inventory*, University of California, Palo Alto, Calif, USA, 1986.

[19] T. Stenlund, C. Ahlgren, B. Lindahl et al., "Patients with burnout in relation to gender and a general population," *Scandinavian Journal of Public Health*, vol. 35, no. 5, pp. 516–523, 2007.

[20] J. Critchley, J. Liu, D. Zhao, W. Wei, and S. Capewell, "Explaining the increase in coronary heart disease mortality in Beijing between 1984 and 1999," *Circulation*, vol. 110, no. 10, pp. 1236–1244, 2004.

[21] E. M. Edwards, S. O. Stuver, T. C. Heeren, and L. Fredman, "Job strain and incident metabolic syndrome over 5 years of follow-up: the coronary artery risk development in young adults study," *Journal of Occupational and Environmental Medicine*, vol. 54, pp. 1447–1452, 2012.

[22] W. Xu, J. Hang, W. Gao, Y. Zhao, T. Cao, and L. Guo, "Association between job stress and newly detected combined dyslipidemia among Chinese workers: findings from the SHISO study," *Journal of Occupational Health*, vol. 53, no. 5, pp. 334–342, 2011.

[23] Y. Demiral, A. Soysal, A. Can Bilgin et al., "The association of job strain with coronary heart disease and metabolic syndrome in municipal workers in Turkey," *Journal of Occupational Health*, vol. 48, no. 5, pp. 332–338, 2006.

[24] T. Nagaya, H. Yoshida, H. Takahashi, and M. Kawai, "Increases in body mass index, even within non-obese levels, raise the risk for Type 2 diabetes mellitus: a follow-up study in a Japanese population," *Diabetic Medicine*, vol. 22, no. 8, pp. 1107–1111, 2005.

[25] N. Nishitani and H. Sakakibara, "Relationship of BMI increase to eating behavior and job stress in a 2-year cohort study of non-obese male Japanese workers," *Obesity Research and Clinical Practice*, vol. 1, no. 3, pp. 179–185, 2007.

[26] P. Cursoux, M.-P. Lehucher-Michel, H. Marchetti, G. Chaumet, and S. Delliaux, "Burnout syndrome: a "true" cardiovascular risk factor," *Presse Medicale*, vol. 41, pp. 1056–1063, 2012.

Challenges of Introducing Participant Observation to Community Health Research

Meng Zhao[1] **and Yingchun Ji**[2]

[1] *College of Nursing and Health Sciences, Texas A&M University Corpus Christi, Island Hall 350E, 6300 Ocean Drive, Unit 5805, Corpus Christi, TX 78412, USA*
[2] *Asia Research Institute, National University of Singapore, 21 Lower Kent Ridge Road, Singapore 119077*

Correspondence should be addressed to Meng Zhao; meng.zhao@tamucc.edu

Academic Editors: P. Di Giulio, R. Griffiths, and S. Keeney

Participant observation elicits unique observation data from both an insider's and an outsider's perspectives. Despite the growing tendency to adopt participant observation strategies in health care research regarding health-related beliefs and types of behavior, the use of participant observation in current research is mostly limited to structured clinical settings rather than community settings. In this paper, we describe how we use participant observation in a community health research study with Chinese-born immigrant women. We document discrepancies between these women's beliefs and types of behavior regarding health and health promotion. We further discuss the ethnical, time, and setting challenges in community health research using participant observation. Possible solutions are also discussed.

1. Introduction

Derived from cultural anthropology, participant observation (PO) is a qualitative research methodology that is widely used by sociologists and anthropologists [1]. The objective of PO is to offer researchers a method to investigate the perspectives of a group in a given community [2]. What makes the PO method distinctive is that PO emphasizes the role of the researcher as a participant in a community [2]. Researchers do not merely observe their study informants distantly and objectively but actively participate in the informants' daily activities to understand the informants' daily dynamics from both an insider's and an outsider's perspectives [2]. The research setting for PO is the study informants' own daily environment rather than a setting assigned by researchers [2]. Therefore, as an exploratory qualitative approach, PO is particularly appropriate for any community health research [2, 3].

Data elicited from PO strategies are unique, offering a different perspective from the self-reported data retrieved from interviews, focused groups, or quantitative research methods [2]. Therefore PO complements other approaches for data collection [2]. The PO strategies can help researchers to gain an understanding about the sociocultural context where the study informants' daily activities occur [2]. It provides researchers with unique opportunities to explore the study informants' unanticipated types of behavior or activities [2]. It further allows researchers to investigate these types of behavior or activities and reframe the research questions with a deeper understanding of the research problem [2].

Despite the growing tendency to adopt PO strategies in health care research regarding health-related beliefs and behavior [4], the use of PO in current research is mostly limited to structured clinical settings, such as hospitals or nursing homes rather than real, open community settings [5, 6]. This can be due to the challenges that researchers encounter in community health research. If researchers are not familiar with their informants' neighborhoods, arranging an observation in a community can be very time consuming [2]. Moreover, there can be more unexpected issues occurring in a real community setting than in a structured clinical setting [7]. These issues are difficult to handle. Therefore, applying PO to community health research is highly challenging and expensive regarding the researchers' energy, time, and financial resources [7]. However, considering that PO's unique combination of both an insider's and an outsider's perspectives can elicit data that cannot be retrieved by other research methods [2]. PO strategies should be more considered for community health research.

In this paper, we outline challenges that we encountered when conducting a community health research study with a group of Chinese-born immigrant women using the PO approach. Possible solutions to these challenges are also discussed.

2. Methods

To understand how culture influences health beliefs and types of health promotion behavior among Chinese-born immigrant women, we conducted a community health research study at the research triangle area in North Carolina between April 2009 and July 2010. We recruited a total of fifteen informants aged between 40 and 68 for the study. Applying ethnography, the primary data collection methods were semistructured interview with open-ended questions and PO. We first conducted semistructured interviews with each informant and arranged follow-up interviews when needed. Then we managed to spend time with the thirteen informants who agreed to do PO and participated in their daily activities.

2.1. Data Collection. Using a flexible interview guide, we conducted the semistructured interviews in Chinese. Examples of the interview questions were "What is health?" "What does it mean to you to have good health (or be healthy)?" "What is poor health?" "How does someone get good health?" and "How does someone maintain good health?" All the interviews were one-on-one and were digitally recorded. If ongoing analysis indicates the necessity for data clarification or deeper depth of the data, we would arrange follow-up interviews. Therefore, follow-up interview questions varied from one informant to another.

To observe the informants' everyday activities, we arranged PO with them at their convenient time when they usually went on some health-related activities. We paid special attention to their conversations and types of behavior related to health and health promotion during the observation. Following the observation data sheet (Appendix A) proposed by Spradley [2], our observation allowed a casual, relaxed, and friendly interaction between the informants and the researcher. We spent time with the informants when their regular daily activities went on without interruption. We used the observation data sheet to document what we observed such as the informants' appearances, facial expression, and their types of behavior or gestures. We also documented the informants' interactions and verbal communications with us and any other people on the observation sites. In addition, we took field notes through the entire observation and wrote down reflections about the observation and about ourselves.

For example, when going grocery shopping with one informant, we noticed that she kept comparing the food we bought to what she bought. After the comparison, she tried to convince us why the food she bought was good for her health. To this scenario, we reflected the potential reason underlying her behavior. It is likely that our role as a researcher with doctoral training in health care at a prestige university placed certain pressure on her grocery shopping. It is inevitable that informants may respond or modify their types of behavior when interacting with the researchers during the PO [8]. However, this type of modification also provides a unique opportunity to understand the informants' deeper motivations behind certain types of behavior [8]. As researchers, we should constantly be aware of the influences of interactions on informants' types of behavior and try hard to participate in the informants' daily activities with minimal intervention in their decision making [7].

The reflection and reflexivity were important regarding adjusting our interaction with the informants and our interpretation of the observation data. We are the tool for the data collection and data analysis in our study [2]. Our sociocultural background has impacts on the way how we observed our informants, how we interacted with them, and how we interpreted our observation data [7]. We need to maintain a constant balance between our professional and educational role, which carries a distant researcher's bias and our involvement in the informants' community, which offers an insider's perspectives [7].

2.2. Data Analysis. For data analysis, we entered our data in a commonly used qualitative data analysis software—Nvivo 8. The software helped us with both data organization and data analysis. In our study, we coded the interview data (interview transcripts and field notes for interviews) and the observation data (field notes for observation and observation data sheets) separately. Then we compared the interview data with the observation data.

Under the qualitative data analysis guideline of Miles et al. [9], the coding process was ongoing and iterative but mainly involved four stages. Firstly, we elicited the descriptive codes, which labeled the details in the data straight forwardly with little interpretation [9]. Examples were name, gender, location, and actions [9]. These descriptive codes usually served as first-order codes [9, 10]. Secondly, based upon the better understanding of the data and the elicited descriptive codes, we developed more general pattern codes. These pattern codes represent broader categories than descriptive codes and usually served as the higher-level codes [9, 10]. The development of the pattern codes was to figure out the themes or categories in the data [9]. Thirdly, after we elicited descriptive codes and patterns codes, we eventually established a provisional list of a large number of codes. It was necessary to sort the codes into some sort of order or into groups. We then adopted tree codes, a function in Nvivo 8 to achieve this objective [11]. With tree codes, lower-order codes were nested into higher-order codes, and, eventually, all the codes were grouped in a hierarchical order [11]. The rule for the ordering process was that the higher-order codes should be more inclusive and more general; lower-order codes, on the contrary, should be more exclusive and more specific [10]. Fourthly, we organized the codes using a within-case or cross-case display proposed by Miles et al. [9] to make data more comparable for interpretation in one case or cross cases. A matrix or a network provides a visual way to reorganize the codes systematically so that the relationships among the main themes were to some extent visually straight forward and therefore easier to be figured out [9]. Throughout the coding process, we wrote memos and kept journals to document our ideas about the codes and track the changes that we had made to the coding process as Miles et al. [9] recommended.

To protect the informants' privacy and confidentiality, the study had gone through the Institutional Review Board (IRB) procedure at the University of North Carolina at Chapel Hill before fieldwork. To be eligible for the study, the informants should be capable and willing to discuss their health beliefs. If PO is required, the informants should agree to do PO. Before being enrolled in the study, all the informants are needed to sign an informed consent form which outlined the research purpose, design, procedure, potential benefits, and risks of the study. We explained clearly the questions and concerns beforehand. We considered data before, during, and after data collection and data analysis. Only people in our research team had access to the consent forms, interview digital records, transcriptions, and field notes. The data cannot be disclosed to other people without the informant's consent. The personally identified data were no longer retained when the research study was finished.

3. Results

3.1. Community's Impacts on Belief and Behavior. Observation data that we elicited from our study helped us to gain a better understanding of the sociocultural context of our informants from a more holistic perspective. As we observed during PO, the majority of the informants were connected with the local Chinese community in one way or another. Most of them went to the local Chinese grocery stores regularly for grocery shopping. Moreover, most of them read Chinese newsletters and spoke Chinese at home. In addition, most of their close friends were Chinese. The local Chinese community therefore had great impacts on these women's daily lives. Their health beliefs were heavily shaped by the Chinese community such as whom to rely on for health information, where to go grocery shopping, how to cook, what to eat, and where to do exercises.

3.2. Discrepancies between Beliefs and Types of Behavior. The comparison of PO data with interview data indicates discrepancies between the informants' beliefs and their actual types of behavior. The findings from the study illustrate how people say may be incongruent with what they do. Food and exercise were two major themes in our study for health promotion among Chinese-born immigrant women. When comparing what these women said to what they actually did concerning food and exercise, seven of the thirteen (54%) participants demonstrated some types of behavior that were inconsistent with what they said.

3.2.1. Food Choices. Most informants believed that eating "healthy" food can benefit them from getting sick. This is consistent with the Chinese cultural belief that food therapy is parallel to medicine therapy for daily health [12]. Some participants believed that only "natural" food can be "healthy." Any food that has additives is considered as "unnatural" and "unhealthy." This again matches the Chinese cultural belief that human beings are a part of the nature and a harmony should be established between human beings and the nature [12]. The following excerpts from their interviews clearly demonstrate the importance of "natural" food. One woman said that

> *...even if the product is labeled as "natural", I do not consider it as natural. Natural food by definition is the food that I can cook. It's real food, not something that has been labeled as natural product, but is actually processed. That's why I never eat processed food or take those health supplements. The natural food I am referring to is those grown by themselves, not artificially synthesized...I don't buy semi-finished or finished food, since I don't know what they are made of...*

Another woman had very similar comments about food and additives. She said that

> *...natural food is better. I mean the food that I can see and touch and grow in the nature...I worry about those semi-finished or finished food, since I don't know what additives they (the makers) might put in the food...(that's why) I rarely go out for eating...*

However, during PO, these two women did not always act according to what they claimed about "natural food." When going out with the first woman for grocery shopping, she bought prepared food such as cake which she bought for her breakfast because she had to finish the breakfast quickly to catch up the bus for work. When visiting the other woman at her home, we noticed that she had some opened and unopened canned fruits and vegetables in her refrigerator. She explained that she did not always have time for grocery shopping and had to buy some canned food.

Regarding food, the majority of the informants also claimed that the balanced diet contributed to good health. The idea of balanced diet was similarly reported in previous studies for Chinese-born immigrant women [13] and was a unique health belief among Chinese-born immigrant women compared with other Asian groups [12]. One woman who had stayed in the United States for more than six years said

> *...balanced diet is important...At our home, we usually eat some vegetables, fruits, rice, and flour. We also eat some meat and eggs each day...*

Another woman who had stayed in the United States for more than nineteen years said that

> *...for good health, we need to balance what we eat for the three meals per day. We should eat a lot of vegetables and fruits, but we also need to eat some meat or eggs. It is not healthy to eat only some particular food. Every kind of food is beneficial in some way to our health...*

Despite these words, these same two women, who we observed on separate occasions, upon entering a grocery store, picked up advertisement flyers and went directly to the food on sale. The first thing they looked for was the price tag. The food they selected were not only based upon their idea of "natural food" or "balanced diet" but also heavily influenced by the price of the food.

3.2.2. Exercise. Most informants explained during the interviews that exercise was beneficial and should be done regularly to maintain good health. The idea of exercise for health promotion is widely accepted in Chinese-born immigrant women [13]. It is also widely accepted in other Asian immigrant groups such as Filipino, Korean, and Vietnamese [12]. One woman clearly described her exercise habits during the interviews. She said

> *There is a standard in the United States. (That is) at least twenty minutes a day, with a moderate amount of exercises, even just walking is good to health.*

Regarding herself, she said

> *I usually walk the stairs every day for exercise... More than one hundred stairs each day. Sometimes I also use the treadmill for exercise. I usually spend more than thirty to forty minutes on the treadmill...I also love to do stretch exercise, if I choose to do so, I might spend one to two hours on it.*

However, when going out with her for a speed walking at a public garden, we observed that, after only fifteen minutes of walking, she was panting, sweating, and looked very tired. It seemed unlikely that she was doing the amount of exercises that she had described in the interview. It is likely that if she had done regular exercise as she described, she would not find the speed walking so hard to finish. In conversation with her friend, who also went with us for the walking, we learned that this was only the second time this informant went to the garden, while her friend went walking there four to five times a week.

4. Discussion

4.1. Benefits to Apply PO. The PO data depicted a dynamic picture of what the sociocultural context meant to the Chinese-born immigrant women and how the community influenced their health beliefs and types of behavior. Ho [14] similarly documented the impacts of China town on Chinese immigrant patients' enrollment in a therapy program in New York city in an ethnographic study. Ethnographic studies about other immigrant groups such as Latinos, Haitians, and Puerto Ricans also documented the influence of sociocultural context on the immigrants' health beliefs [15–17]. All these studies considered PO as a highly valued and unique research method to explore the sociocultural context in community health research.

The investigation of why the inconsistency occurs between beliefs and types of behavior can further give researchers more insights in the research questions examined [2]. These insights will help researchers to reframe their research questions from the informants' perspective rather than to impose structured questions on informants from the researchers' perspective. However, previous health research studies using an ethnographic approach rarely discussed this kind of inconsistency and therefore failed to take full advantage of using PO in their studies.

Based upon our findings, the realistic restrictions such as the cost of the food, the time to prepare or cook the food, the time to go grocery shopping, and availability of and accessibility to Asian grocery shops all contributed to the discrepancies in our study. These restrictions intertwined with Chinese-born immigrant women's beliefs in "natural food" and "balanced diet" when they made their food choices. During our fieldwork, we found that the women in the study who preferred buying Asian food had to depend on American grocery stores for grocery shopping because there were few Asian grocery stores close to where these women lived. These realistic barriers were not unique among Chinese immigrants but were similarly reported in Latino immigrants [18]. Addressing these discrepancies can elicit more data to help researchers better understand the community they studied.

It is also usual for people to exaggerate the amount of exercise or expected activity that they actually would do [19]. Research informants may also want to present a more positive image of themselves [19]. To obtain a realistic picture of the informants' cultural beliefs and types of behavior regarding health promotion, PO is a valuable approach for community health research. Without PO, we would have to depend on interview data alone in our study. Therefore, we may have the impression that people did what they claim or what may be ideal in their belief and would not have acquired such a deep understanding of the restrains that people have to face in their daily life.

Using PO in community health research also allows researchers to get familiar with the research setting and the research informants [2]. When researchers become more involved in the informants' community, the informants are more likely to disclose their real beliefs and perspectives rather than the ideal or positively tuned stories to the researchers [7, 8]. From our experience in the study, when we got along well with the informants, they felt more relaxed during their interactions with us and tended to disclose more information. For example, one woman began to complain about her stress from her new job when we jogged together three months after our first meeting, which she had not mentioned in the interviews. PO enabled us to build up trust relationships with the informants and opened the window to their real life.

4.2. Challenges with PO. Despite the benefits of using PO in community health research, there are challenges that researchers have to face. These challenges can impede researchers from using PO and should be taken into full consideration when designing a community health research project. In the following sections, we will focus on two types of challenges emerging in our study.

4.2.1. Ethical Challenges. To protect human subjects, any research project involving humans conducted in the United

States should be monitored and reviewed under the Institutional Review Board (IRB) procedure [20]. IRB procedure requires and regulates a planned research project to notify research participants as clear as possible what they will be asked to do if involved in the project [20]. All the benefits and potential risks should also be notified to protect the rights of research participants [20]. As a result, IRB procedure raises an ethical challenge for any health researchers who plan to use PO in community health research.

Potential problems with using PO can be both ethical and methodological. In our study, the IRB procedure required us to inform the informants about the kinds of activities that we were likely to observe in the consent form. However, when conducting PO, it is unlikely to predict all types of behavior and actions that may occur in an unfamiliar community setting [7]. It is methodologically unrealistic to provide a fully informed consent form. Moreover, as the study is exploratory in nature, we aimed to investigate what kinds of activities are relevant to these Chinese-born immigrant women's health and health promotion. All these were waiting for exploring in the field after the research began. However, the IRB procedure had already set limits to what activities would be observed before conducting PO in the field because it required us to inform our informants with the specific activities that would be observed. Therefore, we were restricted to observe only certain activities without further investigation of other activities that potentially influence Chinese-born immigrant women's health and health promotion. Furthermore, due to IRB procedure, informants can stop data collection at any time, which is reassuring to the informants but can affect the data richness and depth.

Another challenge is how much or how little the researchers should impose themselves into the informant's life. We, as researchers, always keep ourselves open enough to the informants. We observed and participated to a certain degree in their daily lives as an insider; however, on the other hand, we had to try our best not to interrupt their daily norms as an outsider [2].

Finally, when doing PO in a real field, researchers may have to interact with people other than their study informants [7]. Although this kind of interaction is usually informal, these people's identity and human rights should also be protected according to the IRB rules [20]. In our study, when observing the informants' activities such as grocery shopping or exercise, we sometimes inevitably had some interactions with other people, such as the participants' friends or family members. The problem then becomes whether we should disclose our study to these people and how many details we should disclose to them. Considering the fact that the informants in our study were reluctant to let these people know what they were doing in the study, we had to face the challenge to meet both sides' ethical requirements. Therefore, we had to find the balance between sufficiently informing these people to protect their ethical needs and at the same time protecting the research informants' privacy.

4.2.2. Time and Setting Challenges. In addition to the ethical challenges, researchers also face time and setting challenges. Unlike research conducted in a semicontrolled clinical setting, research in a community setting has unique challenges. Compared with a clinical setting which is restricted to a ward, a hospital, or a clinic, a community setting has a geographically larger and open space and is much harder to handle [7]. Conducting PO in a community setting usually requires researchers to spend more time with the informants on their regular activities [7]. It can be more time consuming than collecting the same depth and amount of data in a structured clinical setting. These time and setting challenges, however, may not be practical for the majority of applied health research studies, which usually have very limited timeframe [7].

In our study, we spent almost fifteen months for PO data collection, which was much longer than we had expected. Because PO strategies required us to go out with the study informants for observation in their local community settings, we had to arrange our time to match the informants' time schedules. Making these arrangements can be harder and more time consuming than arranging a visit to a clinical setting such as a hospital unit or waiting room. In a clinical setting, researchers usually wait in the clinic for the informants to come [5], while in a community setting, researchers have to approach the informants in various communities [7]. We had to meet informants at their convenience wherever their local communities were for observations. In addition, activities in the community setting were less predictable and less controllable than a structured and well-protected clinical setting where daily routines and geographic boundaries are more established [7]. These time and setting challenges make PO more challenging than interviews or focus groups alone.

4.3. Strategies with Participant Observation. Considering the advantages of using PO in community health research, we propose some solutions to the challenges discussed above.

4.3.1. Solutions to Ethical Challenges. Compared to the IRB procedure in other disciplines, the IRB process in health care is stricter. Deceptive or covert PO strategies that have been used in some traditional ethnographic studies cannot be applied in a community health research study [20]. The description of how to implement PO in a study should be as detailed as possible and avoid any vagueness while maintaining the flexibility to be open to unanticipated situations [20]. Given the fact that the data collection process involving PO can be improvisational and context-driven [2], health researchers should describe and anticipate the potential benefits and risks that may arise from PO in the study proposal. Moreover, researchers should also develop appropriate strategies to enable themselves to be flexible during observation without violating the informants' privacy or ethical rights.

Based upon our experience with IRB application, approval to use PO in a community health research study is likely but there is no universal solution to all research projects. Health researchers should develop their own strategies according to their research questions and research designs. Researchers should also constantly consult with the IRB as their plan develops. In the IRB application, the following aspects should be highlighted if planning to use PO: (a) have a clear statement of why PO should be used in the study with a focus on the difficulty in eliciting data from other research approaches; (b) anticipate as fully as possible the activities that might be observed and the settings in the community that the activities would occur; (c) describe the strategies as clearly as possible how the researchers get access to the settings where the observation occurs; (d) develop a detailed plan of what should be observed and documented during PO.

After balancing the benefits and risks, the IRB reviewers may require or waive researchers to fully describe the PO process in the written consent for the informants. If a detailed description is required, researchers should clearly explain what an informant may be asked to do if joining the study. For those people who interact with the informants or the researchers during the observation, researchers can request a possible waiver of consent from the IRB. If a waiver is not likely, a verbal consent may be requested to meet the IRB requirements. In this verbal consent, the purpose of the study should be stated without disclosing too much information about the research participants. The one we used in our study is attached as an example (Appendix B). A plan to document the observation data should also be developed. In our study, we followed the observation data sheet (Appendix A) proposed by Spradley [2].

4.3.2. Solutions to Time and Setting Challenges. To handle the time and setting challenges during the fieldwork for PO in community health research, researchers should develop appropriate outreach strategies to arrange their observation timeframe more reasonably. Furthermore, because a community setting is harder to handle for observation [7], researchers should be clear about what data should be documented before conducting the observation in the field. Having a detailed observation plan to focus on the data needed is a useful strategy to conduct PO in a community setting.

However, real life is not running in a warded clinic. Unexpected things occur all the time. If handled in an appropriate and strategic way, they can be a plus to PO [7]. It is always helpful to keep an open mind and be well prepared for all the surprises in the field.

5. Conclusions

Researchers encounter ethical, time, and setting challenges when conducting PO in community health research. Despite these challenges, PO has irreplaceable advantages over other qualitative research methods to elicit unique contextually rich data that are not able to be fully elicited from self-reported strategies [2, 7]. We learn from our study with Chinese-born immigrant women that there are no uniform solutions to PO in a community setting. Researchers should have a clear data collection plan when doing PO. Researchers should also evaluate potential benefits and challenges to determine how PO can be applied in a specific community health research study.

Appendices

A. The Observation Data Sheet

(This is an example of types of information that can be observed during participant observation for the research. The participant observation approach will be casual, relaxed, and friendly as the observer spends time with the participant when the participant goes about her normal activities. During the observation, focus should be put on the participant. Only those individuals who interact with the participant or the PI will be observed.)

Observer:

Participant (dummy number used only):

Date and Time:

Site:

Actors (who interact with the participant or the PI):

Activity:

The following aspects should be observed.

(1) The participant and the actors' appearance: clothing, physical appearance, and anything that might indicate the participant or the actors' membership in a group or a subgroup such as possible profession, socioeconomic class, and ethnicity.

(2) The participant and the actors' verbal behavior and interactions: who speaks to whom and for how long; who initiates interactions; languages or dialects spoken; tone of voice; how they use their voices to communicate different emotions.

(3) The participant's physical behavior and gestures: what the participant does; whom the participant interacts with; how the participant uses her body (eye contact? gestures?) to communicate different emotions.

(4) The actors' physical behavior and gestures during their interaction with the participant or the PI: what the actors do; who does what; who interacts with whom; how actors use their bodies (eye contact? gestures?) to communicate different emotions.

(5) The participant and the actors' personal space during the interaction: how close the participant and the actors stand to one another; what the participant and the actors' preferences regarding personal space suggest about their relationships.

(6) Human traffic for the actors: during the observation time, actors who enter, leave, and spend time at the observation site (where actors enter and exit; how long they stay; whether they are alone or accompanied; number of people).

(7) Actors who stand out: identification of actors who receive a lot of attention from others (the characteristics of these individuals; what differentiate them from others; whether others consult them or they approach others; whether they seem to be strangers or well known by others who are present).

B. Verbal Consent Script

Hello, My name is__________. I'm doing a research that requires looking at interaction. I'm here observing today. Do you mind if I include you in the observation? The observation is voluntary, of course.

(if consented) Great! Thank you for your cooperation!

(if not consented) That's fine. Have a good day!

Conflict of Interests

The authors declare that there is no conflict of interests regarding the publication of this paper.

Acknowledgment

The authors would like to thank the Sigma Theta Tau International Nursing Society Alpha Chapter in the University of North Carolina at Chapel Hill for its financial support to make this study possible.

References

[1] B. L. Berg and H. Lune, *Qualitative Research Methods for the Social Sciences*, Pearson, Boston, Mass, USA, 8th edition, 2011.

[2] J. P. Spradley, *Participant Observation*, Holt, Rinehart and Winston, New York, NY, USA, 1st edition, 1980.

[3] D. L. Jorgenson, *Participant Observation: A Methodology for Human Studies*, Sage, Thousand Oaks, Calif, USA, 1989.

[4] J. H. Watts, "Ethical and practical challenges of participant observation in sensitive health research," *International Journal of Social Research Methodology*, vol. 14, no. 4, pp. 301–312, 2011.

[5] M. McKnight, "The information seeking of on-duty critical care nurses: evidence from participant observation and in-context interviews," *Journal of the Medical Library Association*, vol. 94, no. 2, pp. 145–151, 2006.

[6] A. J. Browne, C. M. Varcoe, S. T. Wong et al., "Closing the health equity gap: evidence-based strategies for primary health care organizations," *International Journal of Equity Health*, vol. 11, p. 59, 2012.

[7] K. M. DeWalt and B. R. DeWalt, *Participant Observation: A Guide for Fieldworkers*, AltaMira Press, Walnut Creek, Calif, USA, 2nd edition, 2010.

[8] H. Johnson, J. Douglas, C. Bigby, and T. Iacono, "The challenges and benefits of using participant observation to understand the social interaction of adults with intellectual disabilities," *Augmentative and Alternative Communication*, vol. 27, no. 4, pp. 267–278, 2011.

[9] M. B. Miles, A. M. Huberman, and J. Saldaña, *Qualitative Data Analysis: An Expanded Sourcebook*, Sage, Thousand Oaks, Calif, USA, 3rd edition, 2013.

[10] M. Q. Patton, *Qualitative Research & Evaluation Methods*, Sage, Thousand Oaks, Calif, USA, 3rd edition, 2001.

[11] QSR International, NVivo8 tutorials, 2013, http://www.qsrinternational.com/support_tutorials.aspx?productid=18.

[12] M. Zhao, N. Esposito, and K. Wang, "Cultural beliefs and attitudes toward health and health care among asian-born women in the United States," *Journal of Obstetric, Gynecologic, and Neonatal Nursing*, vol. 39, no. 4, pp. 370–385, 2010.

[13] W. Liang, E. Yuan, J. S. Mandelblatt, and R. J. Pasick, "How do older Chinese women view health and cancer screening? Results from focus groups and implications for interventions," *Ethnicity and Health*, vol. 9, no. 3, pp. 283–304, 2004.

[14] M.-J. Ho, "Health-seeking patterns among Chinese immigrant patients enrolled in the directly observed therapy program in New York City," *International Journal of Tuberculosis and Lung Disease*, vol. 8, no. 11, pp. 1355–1359, 2004.

[15] R. L. Bowen and C. M. Devine, "'Watching a person who knows how to cook, you'll learn a lot' Linked lives, cultural transmission, and the food choices of Puerto Rican girls," *Appetite*, vol. 56, no. 2, pp. 290–298, 2011.

[16] S. M. Holmes, "An ethnographic study of the social context of migrant health in the United States," *PLoS Medicine*, vol. 3, no. 10, article e448, pp. 1776–1793, 2006.

[17] J. Menard, E. Kobetz, J. Diem, M. Lifleur, J. Blanco, and B. Barton, "The sociocultural context of gynecological health among Haitian immigrant women in Florida: applying ethnographic methods to public health inquiry," *Ethnicity and Health*, vol. 15, no. 3, pp. 253–267, 2010.

[18] J. F. Kilanowski, "Migrant farmworker mothers talk about the meaning of food," *MCN The American Journal of Maternal/Child Nursing*, vol. 35, no. 6, pp. 330–335, 2010.

[19] W. Bleek, "Lying informants: a fieldwork experience from Ghana," *Population and Development Review*, vol. 13, no. 2, pp. 314–324, 1987.

[20] Food and Drug Administration, Code of federal regulations-Title 21: food and drugs, 2013, http://www.accessdata.fda.gov/scripts/cdrh/cfdocs/cfcfr/CFRSearch.cfm?CFRPart=101.

4

"Negotiating, Navigating, and Networking": Three Strategies Used by Nursing Leaders to Shape the Adoption and Incorporation of Simulation into Nursing Curricula—A Grounded Theory Study

Karyn Taplay,[1] Susan M. Jack,[2] Pamela Baxter,[2] Kevin Eva,[3] and Lynn Martin[1]

[1] *Department of Nursing, Faculty of Applied Health Sciences, Brock University, 500 Glenridge Drive, St. Catharines, ON, Canada L2S 3A1*

[2] *School of Nursing, Faculty of Health Sciences, McMaster University, 1280 Main Street West, Hamilton, ON, Canada L8S 4K1*

[3] *Centre for Health Education Scholarship, Faculty of Medicine, University of British Columbia, 950 West 10th Avenue, Vancouver, BC, Canada V5Z 1M9*

Correspondence should be addressed to Karyn Taplay; ktaplay@brocku.ca

Academic Editors: S. Keeney, S. Kennerly, and A. B. Wakefield

Background. Implementing simulation requires a substantial commitment of human and financial resources. Despite this, little is known about the strategies used by academic nursing leaders to facilitate the implementation of a simulation program in nursing curricula. *Methods.* A constructivist grounded theory study was conducted within 13 nursing programs in Ontario, Canada. Perspectives of key stakeholders ($n = 27$) including nursing administrators ($n = 6$), simulation leaders ($n = 9$), and nursing faculty ($n = 12$) were analyzed using the constant comparison method. *Results.* Nursing leaders, specifically nursing administrators and simulation leaders who successfully led the adoption and incorporation of simulation into nursing curricula, worked together and utilized negotiating, navigating, and networking strategies that impacted the adoption and incorporation of simulation into nursing curricula. *Conclusions.* Strategies that were found to be useful when planning and executing the adoption and incorporation of an innovation, specifically simulation, into nursing curricula provide practical approaches that may be helpful to nurse leaders when embarking upon an organizational change.

1. Introduction

The use of simulation as a teaching strategy in nursing education has developed significantly within the past decade [1–3]. Despite the increased use of simulation and the attention received [3], the integration of simulation into nursing curricula has been inconsistent. In 2004/05, the Ontario Government provided each nursing program in the province with approximately $500,000 in funding to purchase simulation equipment [4]. Prior to this time, the use of mid- to high-fidelity simulation equipment as a teaching strategy was uncommon in most programs of nursing. Mid- to high-fidelity equipment is defined as life-like equipment that can imitate real-life responses to medical conditions [5, 6]. What followed was a time of dynamic change in nursing curricula as nursing programs started the process of incorporating simulation which provided an opportune time to examine how organizational culture shapes the adoption and incorporation of simulation.

Taplay and colleagues [7] discovered key organizational elements that shape a common process of adoption and incorporation of simulation into nursing curricula. Institutions that were able to navigate this process and integrate simulation into all levels of curricula in which nursing content was taught were classified as high uptake. The key organizational factor that was identified in high uptake sites was the shared leadership among nursing leaders. This paper represents an effort to delve more deeply into the shared leadership among nursing administrators and simulation leaders and to explain the three leadership strategies (negotiating, navigating, and networking) that played a key role in the adoption and incorporation of simulation into nursing curricula in Ontario, Canada. While the focus of this study was mid- to high-level fidelity equipment, the common term "simulation" will be used throughout this paper.

Leaders engage in processes that bring value to an organization by influencing change [8] thereby shaping organizational culture [9, 10]. Now more than ever, academic nursing leaders are expected to be innovative and facilitate change because nursing education is undergoing a period of great change with the incorporation of new technologies, including simulation. Young and colleagues [11] conducted a phenomenology study exploring the experiences of becoming a nurse faculty leader among a group of 21 nurse educators. The participants in this study often reported that they felt unprepared to assume leadership roles and lacked the skills or strategies needed to manage change. Horton-Deutsch and colleagues [12] identified three strategies used by nurse educators when faced with leadership challenges: "reflecting," "persevering through difficulties," and "learning to relate to others in new ways" (page 487). Pearsall and colleagues [13] suggest an additional strategy of "doing your homework" (page 1) as a way to manage change. The researchers found that learning about a subject and weighing the positives and negatives before making decisions lessened their concerns about change when taking risks. They suggested that risk taking is a key factor in academic leadership since it involves trying something different or innovative. Although these researchers identified general strategies used by nursing leaders when they were met with challenges, there remains a gap in the literature related to strategies that academic nurse leaders use when trying to adopt and incorporate new technology. Further insight is needed to understand the processes and strategies nurse leaders use to facilitate the integration of simulation into nursing programs.

2. Method

2.1. Design. The principles of grounded theory [14] guided all methodological decisions related to sampling, data collection, and analysis. This approach was used to guide this research because it provided an opportunity to examine how nursing leaders managed the complex process of adopting and incorporating simulation into nursing curricula. A review of institutional mission and vision statements served to provide organizational context and insight into the cultures in which this simulation initiative was occurring [10, 14].

2.2. Sampling. Participants from 13 of 34 provincial nursing programs were included in this study. Participants included nursing administrators, simulation leaders, and nursing faculty members. Maximum variation, a method of purposeful sampling, was used to capture the differences in nursing programs by geography and structure of program [14]. All geographic regions of the province were represented as were both college and university nursing programs and the collaborations between them. In addition, maximum variation sampling was used to enhance the degree of representation among the participants themselves.

Theoretical sampling, a hallmark of grounded theory research, helps to explore, define, and recognize attributes of themes as they emerged. This type of sampling continued until no new properties emerged which indicated that theoretical sufficiency was achieved [15].

2.3. Data Collection. Data were collected using two rounds of audio-recorded face to face or telephone semistructured interviews. Initial interviews focused on the process of adoption and incorporation of simulation and were approximately 60–75 minutes. Second interviews, focused on emerging categories, in particular the leadership roles which facilitated the process, were approximately 30–60 minutes. NVivo 9 software [16] was used to organize and manage all data.

2.4. Data Analysis. All interviews were transcribed verbatim and then analyzed line-by-line and incident-by-incident by the primary investigator (KT). The ensuing codes were developed and defined through the use of the constant comparative method of analysis comparing data within and across sites [14]. The codes were then condensed into categories. Concurrent data collection and analysis, a feature of grounded theory research, was used to aid in the process of developing the categories and in defining the properties and characteristics which led to the nascent structure of the developing theory. To stay true to the participants' perspectives, *in vivo* codes were used and "will be highlighted in quotations throughout the paper".

2.5. Ethics. Two research ethics boards approved this study. Consent was obtained from all participants who were informed that their participation was voluntary. Anonymity and confidentiality were maintained by removing all identifiers and numerically coding the data.

3. Results

3.1. Demographic Data. Participants included simulation leaders ($n = 9$), nursing administrators ($n = 6$), and nursing faculty ($n = 12$). All participants were female and registered nurses. All had a baccalaureate degree with the majority having a master's degree (85.1%); 14.8% had a PhD. They ranged in age from 20 to 70 years. The majority (75%) were between the ages of 41 and 60 years. The primary place of employment was almost evenly divided between universities (55.5%) and colleges (44.4%). Participants (37.5%) had an average of 3–5 years (range 1–20 plus years) of experience using mid- to high-fidelity simulators.

Among the sites in this study there was variability in the uptake of simulation ranging from high to low. The cause can be understood in part by considering the leadership differences which presented in this study. The most apparent difference between the high uptake sites and the mid and low uptake sites was the consistent leadership shared between the nursing administrators and the simulation leaders. This shared leadership was the key element that shaped the adoption and incorporation of simulation into nursing curricula.

3.2. Nursing Leaders. Nursing administrators were identified as a chair, dean, or director of nursing within their respective nursing programs. In their administrative roles, they were instrumental in the development of the new simulation leader role. Nursing administrators in the high uptake sites realized that the workload would need to be shared and had the insight to create a new role to facilitate the integration of simulation. They also recognized that the simulation initiative required an individual who was willing to take the lead. This was highlighted by one simulation leader who stated:

> *The Dean approached me to spearhead the (simulation) initiative and ... plan for the acquisition of equipment and facilities. It was considered a special project that I was asked to lead ... my job description was altered to accommodate additional responsibilities (002).*

This represented the significant level of responsibility and decision-making power bestowed upon the simulation leaders.

This change in work responsibilities also came with a change in title. The people who took on the role of simulation leader were identified by such titles as simulationists, simulation champions, simulation specialists, or simulation coordinators. The simulation leader role differed considerably across organizations with respect to title, responsibility, and expectations. However, despite the differences, most identified having some if not all of the following responsibilities: developing and sharing expertise about all aspects of simulation; developing or designing simulations; supporting nursing faculty members and clinical instructors in the development of the knowledge and skills to enable their understanding of the equipment's capacity and utilization; providing technological support; managing the facilities; and organizing simulation experiences for students. Some simulation leaders also had the responsibilities of managing simulation committees, creating simulation templates, and motivating people to incorporate simulation into the curriculum.

The diversity of role expectations and responsibilities among the simulation leaders was institutionally driven and based on what worked best at the time for the institution and the nursing program, that is, what was the most feasible and what was the most expeditious to implement. This was highlighted by two simulation leaders describing their role. The first stated: "what I do is design and write out the scenarios and facilitate every simulation that happens in the lab and ... get more faculty and staff trained to feel comfortable doing (simulation)" (007). The second stated that her role consists of "primarily overseeing the simulation activities, the physical space, and the logistics of it. Not so much creating the actual simulation or the learning plan objectives, but taking the faculty's vision and bringing it to life" (001). The diversity within this role was further emphasized by organizational classification; some simulation leaders were classified as nursing faculty while others were classified as staff. The inconsistencies in title, responsibility, and work expectations among simulation leaders highlight the challenges associated with a newly developing role.

In the high uptake sites where nursing administrators and simulation leaders shared power, decision-making, and responsibilities related to the integration of simulation, three key strategies emerged that nursing leaders engaged in to facilitate the adoption and incorporation of simulation into their nursing curricula. These included "negotiating," "navigating," and "networking" that both nursing administrators and simulation leaders employed either jointly or independently.

3.3. Negotiating. The negotiations that leaders engaged in when developing goals and action plans included coming to an agreement regarding the resources and personnel needed to incorporate simulation into the curriculum. While the nursing administrators and simulation leaders were both required to negotiate with individuals, the process started with the administrators. Nursing administrators were involved in negotiations with upper level administration within the institution where they emphasized the importance of the simulation initiative and created awareness of what would be needed to be in place to support this initiative. This was an essential first step, since resources, space, and support from the institution were required to develop the simulation labs, particularly because the funding received from the province was earmarked for the purchase of simulation equipment only. The second step was to convey the need for a lead simulation person. Nursing administrators, particularly those from the high uptake sites, used three strategies during these initial negotiations: education to heighten awareness about the needs of the nursing department, followed by persistence and persuasion. One nursing administrator provided an example of how she had articulated the needs of the nursing program by stating that she had to "educate the Dean about what a nursing lab is, and introduce (simulation) into a culture where there's absolutely no knowledge of it" (005). Another administrator discussed the persistence she used to secure resources by stating "it took a lot of dialogue with senior administration, negotiations around space and the proposals for a simulation coordinator ... we were kind of persistent in making the argument" (025). She stated that she approached these negotiations with the philosophy "that you cannot get what you require unless you communicate your needs" (025).

The final negotiating strategy used was persuasion. Persuasion in this context involved emphasizing the institutional benefits that could result from the nursing program adopting and incorporating simulation into the curricula. Nursing administrators typically highlighted three institutional benefits when negotiating with upper level administration. First, integrating simulation was a way to become, or stay, competitive with other nursing programs. Second, having simulation integrated into the curricula could aid in the recruitment of potential students. Third, the accomplishments related to simulation (e.g., securing grants, conducting research, or the lab itself) could be used to publicly promote the nursing program and, in turn, promote the institution as a whole. These strategies used by nursing administrators helped to acquire the necessary resources and personnel for simulation.

Once resources were allocated for space and a new position was created, the nursing administrators were then able to share the negotiating responsibilities with the simulation leaders. The focus turned to increasing buy-in and the use of simulation among nursing faculty members which required different negotiating tactics by the nursing administrator and simulation leader. Nursing administrators created opportunities for faculty to learn about the potential for simulation and encouraged them to consider where simulation fits into courses or curricula. This was done by sharing information at meetings or by supporting the faculty members' attendance at conferences, whereas simulation leaders provided opportunities for nursing faculty members to gain hands-on experience with the equipment thereby enhancing their comfort level and providing opportunities to offer suggestions on how simulation could be incorporated into their specific courses. The institutions took a tandem approach to negotiations. Both types of leaders interacted with faculty members but used different negotiating strategies to implement simulation into the nursing curriculum.

3.4. Navigating. Navigating requires finding a way, creating a path, or setting a specific course of action through uncharted territory. It often involves using specific instruments or means. It requires direction or a plan and can be challenging [17, 18]. Participants in this study identified two strategies used to direct the pathway for simulation to be integrated into the curriculum. The first was the leadership style(s) used by the nursing administrators during the adoption and initial incorporation of simulation into the curriculum. The second was the development of the simulation leader's role.

Participants discussed three unique leadership styles employed by nursing administrators when navigating through the adoption and incorporation of simulation into the curriculum: (a) "participatory," (b) "delegative," and (c) "laissez-faire." The first two leadership styles were found in the high uptake sites and were accompanied by a vision or an idea of how an innovation could fit within the current curriculum consistent with charting a path or a course of action when navigating. Participatory leadership encouraged input from all members of the nursing department about the uses for simulation. Leaders who used this strategy presented simulation as a solution that could address challenges with gaps in the curriculum or augment clinical experiences offered to students. This type of leadership encouraged shared decision-making within the nursing department and provided the opportunity for all to have a voice and contribute to the initial and ongoing vision. Sites that used this shared or team approach initially continued to do so as simulation was further integrated into the curriculum.

Delegative leadership primarily involved unilateral decision-making by nursing administrators at the onset of the initiative. Simulation was presented to simulation leaders and nursing faculty members as an expectation by these leaders. Leaders who used a delegative style did not include much if any input from the simulation leader or faculty members into the overall development of a vision. However, once the expectations of the nursing administrators were made clear, the simulation leaders were given power, permission, and domain over how to incorporate simulation. One example of this was stated by a simulation leader:

> *Our Dean would tell us . . . simulation is a priority. Here are my expectations, we need to do this to enhance our curriculum and the way that we get there is totally up to you but here are my expectations (018).*

Nursing administrators who used both participatory and delegative leadership styles were able to encourage both simulation leaders and nursing faculty members to work together which resulted in a higher level of uptake than institutions where the participants reported that a laissez-faire leadership style was employed. These sites had difficulty because they did not or could not establish or convey a plan for simulation or a direction to follow. One faculty member highlighted this by stating that "the director at the time said basically . . . if you think there is a place for (simulation) to be integrated, find a place" (027).

The second strategy articulated by participants that served to maintain the direction of integrating simulation into the curriculum was the development of the simulation leader's role. In most high uptake sites, simulation leaders were given a new title, power, and autonomy with their new role. This helped nursing programs to navigate the uncharted path of integrating simulation since many simulation leaders invested considerable personal time and effort to develop expertise in this area. To do this, many simulation leaders worked toward creating a new work identity and aligning simulation with their career and educational goals. This was noted by a simulation leader who stated:

> *As far as the simulation piece, it just seemed to be a fit . . . it fell in line with what my organization needed but it also fell into line because I could focus my Masters on (simulation) in nursing education (021).*

While there was substantial personal sacrifice noted, in some cases this resulted in professional achievements such as advancing from part-time to full-time employment status. Gaining expertise provided simulation leaders a means of managing challenges which arose during the integration of simulation such as resistance or indifference among faculty members or troubleshooting equipment problems. The development of the simulation leader's role served to facilitate and direct the path of simulation into the curriculum.

3.5. Networking. Networking involves creating or seeking out a support system comprised of individuals or groups who have the same or similar interests and objectives [17, 18]. Participants in this study described networking as the creation of relationships by both the nursing administrator and simulation leader who served to move simulation forward in the nursing curriculum. These connections occurred within the institution, among different professions, outside of the institution, and across the nursing profession. Both nursing administrators and simulation leaders created support systems to gain information and share resources related to simulation. Nursing administrators primarily used networking as a means of collaborating and securing necessary or additional resources, whereas simulation leaders used it for the purpose of learning and gaining expertise.

Within the individual institutions, some nursing leaders connected with other departments representing different disciplines that included physical or occupational therapy, medicine, pharmacology, and emergency response. This strategy allowed the programs to share resources such as lab space, equipment, and, at times, personnel, which provided the potential for institutional cost-savings. Networking with colleagues from other professions within the same organization who have experience or expertise with simulation enabled simulation leaders to learn about the equipment and gain expertise in managing and organizing a lab. Additionally, this networking provided the opportunity for faculty members and simulation leaders from multiple programs to work together, conduct research, and plan and implement simulations. In some instances, these connections also led to the development of interprofessional simulations that met the needs of students in different programs.

Networking also occurred with local health care agencies such as hospitals and community health care organizations. In some cases, the nursing program would reach out to the health care agency to inform them of the educational approaches offered to nursing students through simulation. Other institutions presented simulation to local health care agencies as a means of generating potential revenue by having agencies rent out the facilities and equipment for staff training purposes. Other programs initiated these partnerships as a way to enhance interprofessional education. One administrator summed this up stating: "I felt that (simulation) was an interprofessional initiative for the whole region, that simulation would be a way to bring everybody together and raise the profile of this school" (005).

Simulation leaders also connected with other nursing professionals. These connections typically developed through simulation conferences. At the onset of this initiative, most networking was done outside the province, in the United States, since there were few nursing experts in Ontario with whom to consult. These interactions provided an opportunity to learn about nursing-specific content and for simulation leaders to develop their own expertise. Institutions that were able to support simulation leaders' attendance at conferences and thus gain expertise had an easier time integrating simulation into the curriculum.

Networking with the purpose of securing resources that benefited more than one program within the same institution and connecting with health professionals in the community both served to move simulation forward to become a faculty-wide or community affiliated initiative rather than just a nursing-specific initiative. Networking was a key strategy used by nursing leaders during the preliminary phases of the simulation initiative, but it must continue in order to advance simulation in nursing education. It needs to be actively pursued by both nursing administrators and simulation leaders.

4. Discussion

The tandem leadership between the nursing administrator and the simulation leader is similar to the definition of shared leadership that exists in the literature. Shared leadership is considered a dynamic interaction between people that focuses on achieving specific group or organizational goals [19]. While this type of leadership is discussed within the broader field of education [20], there is no discussion of how it has been applied to simulation. This is a significant finding from this study that adds to the literature on simulation. To date, much of the literature about the uptake of simulation into nursing curricula has focused on the attitudes and beliefs of faculty members [21] and the aspects that nursing faculty consider when making decisions about whether to incorporate simulation [22]. This study, on the other hand, suggests that faculty attitudes and beliefs about simulation as a teaching strategy may not be the only consideration which can facilitate or impede the adoption and incorporation of simulation. The shared leadership between the nursing administrator and the simulation leader who utilize negotiating, navigating, and networking strategies to manage change contributed significantly in the adoption and incorporation of simulation into nursing programs. Sites that had leaders working in tandem to share the workload and the responsibilities experienced a high level of uptake of simulation compared to sites that did not have these nursing leaders. Effective shared leadership involved utilization of negotiating, navigating, and networking strategies to manage change.

The role of simulation leader proved to be crucial in the process of adopting and incorporating simulation into nursing programs. The findings from this study provide insights into the complexity and diversity of this role by highlighting the multiple responsibilities and extensive workload expectations. What was discovered during this study is that the development of the role of the simulation leader was driven by the needs, requirements, and feasibility of each individual institution. This was highlighted by the lack of consistency related to workload, level of responsibility, and title. As a result, the role may become indistinguishable from the institution because it is so specifically based on the needs and resources within that organization. This can potentially lead to ambiguity about the role of simulation leaders as it relates to the broader context of the nursing culture. This is an issue for future consideration as the role of the simulation leaders becomes embedded into the organizational structure of nursing programs.

5. Strengths and Limitations

The strengths of this study included the triangulation of data sources and theoretical sampling. Triangulation of data sources was achieved by including participants who held different roles in the same institution, thus offering varied perspectives [23]. Theoretical sampling was achieved by returning to participants to clarify concepts and add further details in order to refine the emerging theoretical categories [14, 24]. This strategy was used "until no new properties emerge[d]" [14, page 96].

A limitation of this study was that the chair, dean, or the director roles within the nursing programs were grouped together under the umbrella of nursing administrator. The roles were not differentiated with respect to specific responsibilities or the permanence of the position. Inclusion of these aspects may have elicited additional findings related to the shared leadership among the nursing leaders.

6. Conclusion

Nursing leaders, specifically nursing administrators and simulation leaders who represented high uptake sites, worked in tandem and utilized negotiating, navigating, and networking strategies to impact the uptake of simulation into nursing curricula. Nursing leaders who employed these strategies were able to secure necessary resources, collaborate with key stakeholders, gain information, create a vision, and forge a course of action through uncharted territory. Insights regarding the development of the role of the simulation leader were shared and concerns about the future of this role as it relates to the broader context of the nursing profession were raised. Additionally, this study offered strategies that may be useful when planning and executing the adoption and incorporation of an innovation, specifically simulation, and offered practical approaches that may be helpful to nurse leaders when embarking upon an organizational change.

Conflict of Interests

The authors declare that they have no conflict of interests regarding the publication of this paper.

Authors' Contribution

All authors meet at least one of the following criteria: substantial contributions to conception and design or acquisition of data, analysis, and interpretation of data; drafting of the paper or revising it critically for important intellectual content. All have agreed on the final version [25].

References

[1] R. P. Cant and S. J. Cooper, "Simulation-based learning in nurse education: systematic review," *Journal of Advanced Nursing*, vol. 66, no. 1, pp. 3–15, 2010.

[2] W. M. Nehring and F. R. Lashley, "Current use and opinions regarding human patient simulators in nursing education: an international survey," *Nursing Education Perspectives*, vol. 25, no. 5, pp. 244–248, 2004.

[3] H. B. Yuan, B. A. Williams, J. B. Fang, and Q. H. Ye, "A systematic review of selected evidence on improving knowledge and skills through high-fidelity simulation," *Nurse Education Today*, vol. 32, no. 3, pp. 294–298, 2012.

[4] Nursing Secretariat, "Embracing our past, strengthening our future," in *Proceedings of the 10th Anniversary Commemorative Journal*, p. 9, Ministry of Health and Long Term Care. Government of Ontario, 2004.

[5] S. Decker, S. Sportsman, L. Puetz, and L. Billings, "The evolution of simulation and its contribution to competency," *Journal of Continuing Education in Nursing*, vol. 39, no. 2, pp. 74–80, 2008.

[6] D. M. Gaba, "The future vision of simulation in health care," *Quality and Safety in Health Care*, vol. 13, no. 1, pp. i2–i10, 2004.

[7] K. Taplay, S. M. Jack, P. Baxter, K. Eva, and L. Martin, "Organizational culture shapes the adoption and incorporation of simulation into nursing curricula: a grounded theory study," *Nursing Research and Practice*. In press.

[8] S. J. Zaccaro and Z. N. J. Horn, "Leadership theory and practice: fostering an effective symbiosis," *The Leadership Quarterly*, vol. 14, no. 6, pp. 769–806, 2003.

[9] A. Bamford-Wade and C. Moss, "Transformational leadership and shared governance: an action study," *The Journal of Nursing Management*, vol. 18, no. 7, pp. 815–821, 2010.

[10] E. H. Schein, *Organizational Culture and Leadership*, Jossey-Bass, San Francisco, Calif, USA, 4th edition, 2010.

[11] P. K. Young, C. Pearsall, K. A. Stiles, and S. Horton-Deutsch, "Becoming a nursing faculty leader," *Nursing Education Perspectives*, vol. 32, no. 4, pp. 222–228, 2011.

[12] S. Horton-Deutsch, P. K. Young, and K. A. Nelson, "Becoming a nurse faculty leader: facing challenges through reflecting, persevering and relating in new ways," *The Journal of Nursing Management*, vol. 18, no. 4, pp. 487–493, 2010.

[13] C. Pearsall, K. T. Pardue, S. Horton-Deutsch et al., "Becoming a nurse faculty leader: doing your homework to minimize risk taking," *Journal of Professional Nursing*, vol. 30, no. 1, pp. 26–33, 2014.

[14] K. Charmaz, *Constructing Grounded Theory a Practical Guide through Qualitative Analysis*, Sage, London, UK, 2006.

[15] I. Dey, *Grounding Grounded Theory: Guidelines for Grounded Theory Inquiry*, Academic Press, San Diego, Calif, usa, 1999.

[16] QSR International Pty Ltd, *Nvivo Version 9*, 2012, http://www.qsrinternational.com/products_nvivo.aspx.

[17] Merriam Webster dictionary online, 2013, http://www.merriam-webster.com/dictionary/teamorgoal.

[18] Oxford dictionary online, 2013, http://www.oxforddictionaries.com/definition/english/team.

[19] B. J. Avolio, F. O. Walumbwa, and T. J. Weber, "Leadership: current theories, research, and future directions," *Annual Review of Psychology*, vol. 60, pp. 421–449, 2009.

[20] A. Konu and E. Viitanen, "Shared leadership in Finnish social and health care," *Leadership in Health Services*, vol. 21, no. 1, pp. 28–40, 2008.

[21] N. Akhtar-Danesh, P. Baxter, R. K. Valaitis, W. Stanyon, and S. Sproul, "Nurse faculty perceptions of simulation use in nursing education," *Western Journal of Nursing Research*, vol. 31, no. 3, pp. 312–329, 2009.

[22] C. J. King, S. Moseley, B. Hindenlang, and P. Kuritz, "Limited use of the human patient simulator by nurse faculty: an intervention program designed to increase use," *International Journal of Nursing Education Scholarship*, vol. 5, pp. 1–17, 2008.

[23] L. Krefting, "Rigor in qualitative research: assessment of trustworthiness," *The American Journal of Occupational Therapy*, vol. 45, no. 1, pp. 214–222, 1990.

[24] M. Q. Patton, *Qualitative Evaluation and Research Methods*, Sage, Newbury Park, Calif, USA, 1990.

[25] International Committee of Medical Journal Editors (ICMJE), "Uniform requirements for 1 manuscripts submitted to biomedical journals: ethical considerations in the conduct and reporting of research: authorship and contributorship," 2013, http://www.icmje.org/recommendations/browse/roles-and-responsibilities/defining-the-role-of-authors-and-contributors.html.

5

An Analysis of Canadian Psychiatric Mental Health Nursing through the Junctures of History, Gender, Nursing Education, and Quality of Work Life in Ontario, Manitoba, Alberta, and Saskatchewan

Mary Smith[1] and Nazilla Khanlou[2]

[1] *Queen's University, Kingston, ON, Canada K7L 3N6*
[2] *School of Nursing, Faculty of Health, York University, 4700 Keele Street, Toronto, ON, Canada M3J 1P3*

Correspondence should be addressed to Mary Smith; mary.smith@queensu.ca

Academic Editors: N. M. C. Alexandre and R. Northway

A society that values mental health and helps people live enjoyable and meaningful lives is a clear aspiration echoed throughout our Canadian health care system. The Mental Health Commission of Canada has put forth a framework for a mental health strategy with goals that reflect the virtue of optimal mental health for all Canadians (Mental Health Commission Canada, 2009). Canadian nurses, the largest group of health care workers, have a vital role in achieving these goals. In Canada, two-thirds of those who experience mental health problems do not receive mental health services (Statistics Canada, 2003). Through a gendered, critical, and sociological perspective the goal of this paper is to further understand how the past has shaped the present state of psychiatric mental health nursing (PMHN). This integrative literature review offers a depiction of Canadian PMHN in light of the intersections of history, gender, education, and quality of nursing work life. Fourteen articles were selected, which provide a partial reflection of contemporary Canadian PMHN. Findings include the association between gender and professional status, inconsistencies in psychiatric nursing education, and the limitations for Canadian nurse practitioners to advance the role of the psychiatric mental health nurse practitioner.

1. Introduction

The account of the way Canadian psychiatric mental health nursing (PMHN) has emerged into its current state can provide an insightful perspective that fosters a better understanding of its present challenges and opportunities. This review paper examines the development of Canadian PMHN in Ontario and the western provinces since the beginning of the 20th century. Canada consists of 3 territories and 10 provinces. With a population of approximately 34,880,500, Canada had the highest growth rate of the G8 countries in the 2011/2012 period [1].

In Canada, registered nurses (RNs), registered psychiatric nurses (RPNs), licensed practical nurses (LPNs), and nurse practitioners are employed in the area of psychiatric or mental health care. RPNs are a regulated separate profession in the provinces of Manitoba, Saskatchewan, Alberta, and British Columbia (For the purposes of this paper RPN refers to registered psychiatric nurses that are only legislated in the four western provinces. In Ontario, registered practical nurses, also abbreviated to RPN, provide care in all settings and are not solely specific to or trained in the area of psychiatric mental health. When RPN is used in this paper, the reference is to registered psychiatric nurses.)

Statistics on the various types of nursing professions employed in psychiatric or mental health care can reflect pertinent conditions in relation to the Canadian mental health system. For instance, in 2010, 5.1% of all RNs in Canada were working in the mental health care sector, a slight decrease from 2007 where 5.2 were employed in this same area [2]. In Ontario alone, between 1993 and 2003, there has been a 29.4% drop in the number of nurses working in the psychiatric sector [3]. The number of RPNs increased by 3.8% since 2007 but the RPN workforce remained at 1.5%. The proportion of full time RPNs in psychiatric nursing decreased from 67.8% in 2007 to 62.2% in 2011. The RPN profession also has the highest percentage of males, 22%, of all the Canadian nursing professions [2]. According to the Canadian Nurses Association, nurse practitioners (NPs) account for 0.9% of the entire number of RNs [4]. Of the 2,486 NPs employed in Canada, 1,482 or 60% work in Ontario. The percentage of NPs working in psychiatric mental health in 2010 was 1.4% [4].

The statistics concerning the employment of nurses in the mental health care sector are meaningful when considered in light of the statistics concerning how many people in Canada suffer from mental health problems. The Canadian Community Health Survey by Statistics Canada was completed in 2003 and is scheduled again in 2013. This will enable further comparisons of how Canada fairs in terms of prevalence of mental health disorders and the mental health services available [5]. In 2003, it revealed that two-thirds of those who experience mental health problems do not receive mental health services [6]. Furthermore, persons living with mental illness may have difficulty competing for limited health care due to high rates of poverty and disability [7]. In 2012, the Institute for Clinical Evaluative Sciences and Public Health Ontario released the report "*Opening eyes, opening minds: the Ontario burden of mental illness and addictions report*" [8]. This report measures the extent of mental illnesses in Ontario in comparison with the prevalence of other medical conditions. Addictions and mental illnesses represent an enlarging burden. The need for improved accessibility of mental health services is emphasized [8]. The size of the PMHN workforce and the accessibility of services may impact mental health care for Canadians.

Historically, the deinstitutionalization trend that began in the 1960s resulted in many persons with mental illness being released into the community where a serious lack of mental health services prevailed [9]. This led to a significant portion of individuals with mental illness to become imprisoned in jails or detention centers with limited access to mental health care. Additionally, a revolving door phenomenon occurred where previously institutionalized individuals were readmitted into acute psychiatric care settings [9].

To further understand the Canadian context for PMHN, it is useful to be familiar with developments concerning mental health care in Canada. There are recent major initiatives underway in Canada with regards to mental health reform. In 2005, a national review of the Canadian mental health system took place as outlined in the Kirby report [10]. In 2006, the Standing Senate Committee on Social Affairs, Science and Technology completed the final report entitled "*Out of the shadows at last—transforming mental health, mental illness and addiction services in Canada*" [11]. As the mental health care system was considered to be fragmented, the final report made recommendations for the reformation of mental health care. The assembly of a Mental Health Commission to enable a national strategy for mental health care was emphasized by Michael Kirby, the chairman of the Standing Senate Committee on Social Affairs. Funding for the commission came in 2007, and in 2009, the Mental Health Commission of Canada released the framework "*Towards recovery and well-being: a framework for a mental health strategy for Canada*" [12]. Seven goals are set in this framework that represent how a transformed system will appear. The goals depict that everyone should have the opportunity for optimum mental health and well-being [12]. The Mental Health Commission has recognized that there is a lack of opportunities for Canadians with mental health disorders to achieve optimum mental health. This calls for key stakeholders, that is, groups interested in responding to people with mental health concerns, to address ways to further the provision of mental health care. Nurses are the largest group of healthcare providers, and nurses who provide mental health care are important stakeholders in meeting the mental health care needs of Canadians.

In 2012, the Mental Health Commission of Canada released the blueprint "*Changing directions, changing lives: the mental health strategy for Canada*" [13]. Six strategic directions are given in this report including the provision of mental health services and treatments accessible to the people who need them. Reference to the vital role nurses have in conjunction with the team of health care providers to fully achieve the strategic directions is not explicit in the 2012 report. Community health nurses are instrumental in providing mental health care in the community. In addition, NPs are becoming increasingly more common in providing primary health care within Canada. Their role in the assessment, diagnosis, and treatment of mental health disorders may be extremely useful to further the strategic direction concerning enhanced accessibility to treatment. Collectively, nurses and nurse practitioners have a critical role in the strategic direction as identified by the Mental Health Commission of Canada. A national strategy is needed, and mental health care providers will need to be included in this strategy according to the Kirby report [10]. Nurses who form the largest group of health care workers in Canada may need to be strong stakeholders in the strategic direction for mental health care in Canada. The commission has yet to clearly voice how health care and nurses will be reorganized to support accessible services and treatments.

Kirby [14] indicates the pivotal position that mental health care providers have and also addresses concerns regarding the stress levels and mental health of health care professionals themselves. Indeed this leads to concerns regarding the quality of nursing work life for PMHN and how this specialty is responding to the demands of the mental health care system. The analysis of the history of Canadian PMHN can enable a better understanding of why PMHN is the way it is today. With this understanding, opportunities for further PMHN development, education, and future research may surface.

Given the need for increased accessibility to mental health care and treatment, it is helpful to further explore how nursing will move to foster improved mental health care. At this time, there is a shortage of research studies that look at how the current nursing workforce specifically addresses improved accessibility to mental health care. Career pathways to become NPs that specifically work in mental health are lacking, where NPs may diagnosis and treat mental

TABLE 1: Studies using a gendered, critical and sociological perspective relevant to PMHN.

Author and date	Purpose	Design/methodology/approach	Province	Sample size	Findings
Wall (2010) [20]	To critique nursing research on nursing practice environments using a critical sociological perspective To propose a paradigm for future research	Review of research on nursing practice environments Sociological concepts are linked to variables in the nursing literature	Refers to nursing in general within the Canadian context	NA	Nurses' job satisfaction can be linked to gender knowledge, professionalization, and organization not just management concerns
McGibbon et al. (2010) [21]	To reformulate the nature of nursing stress with regards to context	Interviews, participant observation, and focus groups with pediatric ICU nurses Theoretical perspective uses Smith's critical sociological frame of institutional ethnography	Study occurs within the province of Ontario	23 nurses	Six main forms of stress—emotional distress, constancy of presence, burden of responsibility, negotiating hierarchical power, engaging in bodily caring, and being mothers, daughters, aunts, and sisters

health conditions. As an NP working in mental health care, the options for pursing advanced mental health nursing education in Canada are limited. PMHN education varies across Canada and unlike the United States there is no legislated psychiatric mental health nurse practitioner (PMHNP) role. Also RPNs may wish to become advanced practice nurses or PMHNPs that are able to diagnose or prescribe psychotropic medications. A regulated PMHMP's role may further the accessibility of mental health care in Canada. There are opportunities for nurses to achieve a master's degree in mental health in Manitoba; however, there are no programs in Canada that specifically yield PMHNPs that may diagnose or prescribe medications particular to mental health care. The educational programs for nurses also vary in each province in terms of content and the prerequisites. With the variety of different educational approaches to PMHN in Canada, the career path to advance nursing practice in PMHN is complicated. An RPN in the western provinces has had different preparation than an RN working in mental health care in Ontario. How these diverse PMHN educational approaches have come to be and their implications for Canadian PMHN can provide useful insights to inform future directions to PMHN in Canada.

2. Materials and Methods

2.1. Review Aims and Research Question. The purpose of this inquiry is to understand the current state of mental health nursing in Canada through the intersections of history, gender, nursing education, and quality of work life as evidenced by the existing research and literature. The research question that guided it was as follows: what does the research reveal about contemporary Canadian PMHN in terms of the junctures of history, gender, education, and quality of PMHN work life?

An integrative methodology was determined to be most suitable for this review due to the scarcity of data on the organization and efficacy of Canadian PMHN. Rigor was maintained through evaluating primary sources for methodological quality. The integrative review includes the stages of problem identification, literature search, data evaluation, data analysis, and presentation.

2.2. Integrative Review. Whittemore and Knafl [15] explain that the integrative review is particularly suited to inquiries with limited existing empirical research. Historical events in PMHN are relevant to how this field has come to be. Yet few research studies exist on Canadian PMHN, and the studies are in the form of social historical analyses that reflect on the events of the past. Moreover, there is a paucity of data pertaining to Canadian NPs specific to mental health care and NP mental health education. Sociological, critical, and social historical analyses, reports, and surveys on Canadian nursing and Canadian mental health care offered insight into the field of Canadian PMHN that furthered this inquiry (see Tables 1, 2, and 3). In the integrative review, according to Whittemore and Knafl [15], diverse methodologies may be incorporated to further a comprehensive grasp of issues suited to the complexities of health care. Both quantitative and qualitative research may contribute to the perspective concerning a phenomenon. The culmination, analysis, and evaluation of diverse data and research regarding PMHN enabled a perspective that may begin to further understanding mental health care in Canada in light of the lacking research solely pertaining to Canadian PMHN or PMHNPs.

2.3. Theoretical Perspective. A sociological perspective allows for a critical assessment of common assumptions and fosters recognition of opportunities and constraints that shape our circumstances, the interplay between societal forces and personal lives, and of human diversity [16]. In addition, the concept of gender stratification is comprehensively analyzed within sociology and is applicable to the topic of this paper. Gender stratification concerns the imbalanced division of privilege and power between females and males [17]. A sociological perspective is appropriate for this inquiry as

Table 2: History, gender, and educational implications for Canadian psychiatric mental health nursing.

Author and date	Purpose	Design/methodology/approach	Province	Sample size	Findings
Tipliski (2004) [23]	How Canadian psychiatric nursing developed into two entirely different models?	Historical analysis—case studies in the provinces of Ontario, Manitoba, and Saskatchewan	Ontario, Manitoba, and Saskatchewan	Not applicable (NA)	PMHN development can be understood through psychiatry's authority in the context of the gender limitations traditionally imposed upon women and nurse leaders Ontario nurse leaders took control of psychiatric nursing, whereas in Manitoba and Saskatchewan they did not
Dooley (2004) [24]	Historical account of Manitoba's distinct mental health nursing	Labour history—historical analysis—oral testimony of Manitoba's nursing graduates from the 1930s	Manitoba	NA	Manitoba—distinct class of PMHN giving rise to the regional differences where psychiatric nursing education is not integrated into general nursing education
Hicks (2008) [25]	Examination of factors that lead Manitoba to adopt the western style of PMHN and RPN class	Genealogical analysis from archives, interviews, and secondary sources	Manitoba	NA	RPN in Manitoba is a political, contingent development that will evolve
Hicks (2011) [27]	Historical account of professionalization of Manitoba's RPNs	Historical analysis from archives and secondary sources	Manitoba	NA	RPN profession in Manitoba arose to fill inadequately staffed mental hospitals then developed into a specialized workforce
Boschma et al. (2005) [9]	How gender shaped training, work opportunities, and professional identity of PMHN?	Social history method of analysis—interviews with questionnaires of PMH nurses who practiced between 1939–1990	Alberta	34 women, 9 men	Alberta's PMHN professional identity shaped by gendered care ethic
Boschma (2012) [26]	Exploration of how psychiatric nurses understand and create their role in Alberta	Historical analysis, case study, and oral history interviews	Alberta	NA	Alberta's present community mental health service is evolved and transformed from the prior institutional practice

nurses are employed within gendered hierarchal structures that interact and are influenced by the larger political context.

Feminist theories, emerging from a sociological perspective, address patriarchy, power structures, and gender inequality. They are concerned with the societal organization and interactions that maintain male authority and female subordination [18]. A feminist perspective enables the depiction of the social structures leading to the devaluation of women. Social order then becomes the problem rather than women themselves [18]. The intent in this work is not to devalue women or nurses but, rather, to illuminate the social structures that have persevered throughout history and have influenced PMHN education and quality of work life. The sociological perspective applied here encompasses feminist concepts.

A sociological perspective also bridges history and how things are today. Wright [19] calls this way of thinking the sociological imagination that grasps the connection between history and the way we are and the way we are becoming. The history of PMHN seen through a sociological perspective can promote an understanding of its current state.

2.4. Search Strategies. The primary literature search involved databases, the internet, and published online journals. The databases included CINAHL, PsycINFO, Evidence-Based Mental Health, Cochrane, PubMed, and ProQuest. Published online journals were accessed through Blackwell Synergy and Sage. Primary search results were then analyzed to search their references for secondary sources of interest. The databases were accessed through the York University Library, Toronto, Ontario and Queens University Library, Kingston,

TABLE 3: Canadian mental health psychiatric quality of nurses work life.

Author and date	Purpose	Design/methodology/approach	Province	Sample size	Findings
Robinson et al. (2003) [33]	To examine prevalence, distribution, correlates, and predicators of vicarious trauma and burnout among registered psychiatric nurses (RPNs) in Manitoba	Survey contained the Maslach Burnout inventory, the Traumatic Stress Institute Belief Scale (TSIBS), and a section on PTSD	Manitoba	295 surveys returned, response rate of 29%	RPNs experiencing high levels of emotional exhaustion and higher levels of personal accomplishment. No significant difference on the TSIBS
Ryan-Nicholls (2004) [34]	To address impact of health reform on RPN practice	Focus groups	Manitoba	33	Increase in independence. Insufficient preparation for new roles, current, and future shortage of RPNs
Statistics Canada (2006) Findings from the 2005 National Survey of the Work and Health of Nurses [31]	To assess work and health of Canadian nurses	Survey	All provinces	19000 nurses including RNs, licensed practical nurses (LPNs), and RPNs	Mental and physical health problems of nurses linked to work stress, low autonomy, shift work, poor physician-nurse relationships, low support, and lack of respect
Health Canada (2002): *"Our health, our future: creating quality workplaces for Canadian nurses, final report of the Canadian Nursing Advisory Committee"* [29]	To improve quality of nursing work life	6 researches & information projects	All provinces		(i) Paucity of data on licensed practical nurses and RPNs (ii) 51 recommendations (3 categories): (1) implement conditions to resolve work load, overtime, and absenteeism and decrease nonnursing tasks; (2) create professional practice environment in leadership, education, and prevention of violence and abuse; (3) monitor workplaces and health of nurses, accreditation, and research and disseminate information to keep nurses informed
Maslove and Fooks (2004) [30]	To learn what actions to implement recommendation by the Canadian Nursing Advisory Committee (CNAC) made in the 2002 *"Our health, our future: creating quality workplaces for Canadian nurses"* report	Scan of web sites, letter to stakeholders to learn what had been done, interviews with key informants, and presentation with 14 representatives from nursing stakeholders in Ottawa	All provinces	94 stakeholders, 14 key informants	Increased number of education seats for RNs, LPNs, and RPNs, workload measurement systems, increased number of full time positions, nurse mentors, and flexible scheduling—progress not uniform but concentrate in acute care rather than community; responsibility to carry out recommendations is unclear, need for CNACs, leadership position, funding, survey, accreditation, research to identify problems
Health Canada (2007): *"The working conditions of nurses: confronting the challenges"* [32]	To examine research on the state of Canada's nurses and implication for a larger health care system	Bulletin	All provinces	NA	Workplace and workforce issues require collaboration and government involvement

Ontario. Texts were borrowed through the assistance of the librarian at Waypoint Centre for Mental Health Care, Penetanguishene, Ontario.

Through combinations of keywords, topics searched for included psychiatric nurses in Canada, Canadian psychiatric nursing history, Canadian psychiatric nursing education, Canadian mental health nursing, Canadian psychiatric mental health nursing, Canadian nurses and gender, quality of life for Canadian psychiatric mental health nurses, stress experienced by psychiatric nurses in Canada, registered psychiatric nurses in Canada, work stress of nurses working in mental health, literature review on psychiatric mental health nursing in Canada, sociological perspective of psychiatric nursing, psychiatric mental health nurse practitioner, mental health nurse practitioner education, and sociology of nursing stress.

The searches included English language reports, studies, reviews, editorials, and narratives and was limited to Canadian sources and Canadian PMHN. The intent was to better understand the Canadian context of PMHN. International comparisons were beyond the scope of this undertaking. With regards to the unique Canadian historical influences shaping PMHN, 14 studies were selected as relevant. There was a lack of studies that focused solely on the Canadian PMHN experience as many reports included RPNs and RNs. RNs in the provinces east of Manitoba do not have a separate psychiatric regulation, as do the western provinces. No studies were found on the education in Canada for NPs in mental health. As a result data often combines all nurses. This made it difficult to discern the unique state of Canadian PMHN from that of all Canadian nurses.

3. Results

The results from the literature review are divided into three sections. The first section reviews the literature from 2 sources that include a critical sociological perspective. The next section considers the interrelation of history, gender, and the development of education for Canadian PMHN through the review of 6 social, historical, and analytical studies. The final section focuses on the quality of Canadian mental health psychiatric nurses work life from 6 survey reports.

3.1. Studies with a Sociological Perspective Relevant to PMHN. Wall [20] utilized a sociological outlook, as described in Section 2.3, to critique nursing practice settings and nursing research. The experiences of nurses can be further understood through a lens that encompasses professionalization and organizational influences. In addition, gender is ingrained in all of nursing where a patriarchal culture manifests. According to Wall [20], the control of medicine over nursing is evident in nursing's utilization of quantitative approaches in research that is consistent with the history of medicine. Health care, being a largely institutionalized entity, has its own way of socializing nursing and continues to place medicine at the apex of health care despite health care reformation. Conversely, Wall [20] does not comment on the socialization or culture of medicine with regards to gender, as medicine being once an overwhelmingly male profession has increased the number of female practitioners. Furthermore, the discussion by Wall [20] discusses nursing in general and does not specify particular sectors of nursing such as NPs. Nevertheless, a critical sociological paradigm may help to further understand issues in nursing and PMHN related to knowledge, gender, professionalization, and organizations [20].

McGibbon et al. [21] utilized Smith's [22] sociological frame of institutional ethnography to reconsider the stress in nursing through interviews, focus groups, and observation of pediatric intensive care nurses [21, 22]. Results suggest that stress is framed within the social structure of organizations that may have hierarchical and power-based relations. Articulating patient matters may be challenging in organizations with hierarchical systems. This may contribute to the level of stress nurses experience. Studies concerning nursing stress or vicarious trauma often neglect how gender influences the life of nurses. Theories that are utilized in nursing research may avoid gender analysis. Without a gendered analysis, occupational stress may not be illuminated or solutions may not be identified. Nursing may further benefit by utilizing a gender perspective in research to potentially unveil social patterns that may influence teamwork and collaboration. Gender, race, and class are aspects of nurses' identities but may not be within the range of the theory utilized for the research. This may lead to research that may neglect identification of concerns for nurses [21]. The critical gendered and sociological perspectives as depicted by Wall [20] and McGibbon et al. [21] provided the lens in how PMHN is perceived in relation to the following results.

3.2. Intersections of History, Gender, and Education for Canadian PMHN. Tipliski [23] contributes to the understanding of Canadian PMHN history in the study entitled "*Parting at the crossroads: the emergence of education for psychiatric nursing in three Canadian provinces,*" *1909–1955.* Gendered roles may have permitted psychiatry to maintain control of psychiatric nursing education in the western provinces. Unlike Ontario, where nurses were able to assume control over PMHN, thereby allowing PMHN incorporation into general nursing education, the provinces of Manitoba and Saskatchewan permitted psychiatry to prevent the merging of PMHN with general nursing. From here, as Tipliski explains, two different models for Canadian PMHN education developed leading to the class of the RPN that only exists in the western provinces [23]. This may have fostered a partition in the PMHN nursing force in Canada, as the RPN designation presents a separate regulation of nurses that is nonexistent east of Manitoba.

Tipliski [23] describes how the nursing leaders of Saskatchewan and Manitoba failed to assert control over nursing education. In 1955, the Canadian Nurses Association (CNA) recognized how the separate training that was occurring in the western provinces was not conducive to the efforts to professionalized nursing for all of Canada. Unfortunately, a progressive movement by the nursing leaders of that time to bring psychiatric nursing under the umbrella of general nursing in the 1950s dissolved. This left the western provinces with a split nursing educational approach where psychiatric nurse training remained separate from general nursing education and in the hands of psychiatrists [23]. Although psychiatric nursing is no longer controlled by the psychiatrists in the western provinces, separate training for RPNs remains. From this perspective, it can be appreciated how female nursing leaders in Ontario influenced historical developments to integrate psychiatric nursing education, which was consistent with earlier efforts made by CNA to converge the psychiatric nursing education with general nursing in the western provinces. Ontario nurse leaders were able to gain control over their own nursing education and practice and were aided by the government. Tipliski [23] explains how the Ontario male medical superintendents attempted to keep mental nursing separate from general nursing thus hindering the professionalization of nursing. The contributions from Nettie Fidler in 1933, a nurse graduate from the Toronto General Hospital, together with a report by Professor George Weir that recommended the merging of general with mental nursing, stimulated the progression by the Registered Nurses Association of Ontario (RNAO) to advocate for closure of the separate schools providing only mental health training [23]. It is possible that this account may overlook some of the other possibilities accounting for how PMHN developed in diverse ways, yet Tipliski [23] provides a description of the history of PMHN that may help to explain how gender dynamics influenced the development of PMHN in Canada. Despite the variation between educational approaches that resulted in the RPN designation for the provinces east of Ontario, there is a lack of evidence revealing how PMHN care varies given the differing education preparations.

Of interest is Tipliski's [23] reference to how gender may have been a factor in the development of the RPN designation of the western provinces. This relates to the feminist concepts of patriarchy. Brown [18] defines patriarchy as a social system that holds several assumptions. One assumption portrays women as being assigned a social function. In nursing, as Tipliski [23] depicts nurses were assumed to be fitting to provide care due to their female gender with their inherent ability to nurture. The view of female nurses as nurturers may have been a patriarchal belief held by the male medical superintendents. Another patriarchal assumption is that women are thought of as weaker and less strong. Tipliski [23] also considers the patriarchal context of PMHN, where the nurse leaders of the western provinces may have struggled against the authority of the medical profession. On the other hand, Tipliski [23] does not speak of the power issues between general nursing and medicine or the professionalization the regulated psychiatric nurses of the western provinces experienced.

Dooley [24] argues that the separate class of psychiatric nurses in Manitoba developed their own unique craft that is specialized for the mentally ill population. In this study, the account from Manitoba mental health nurses of the 1930s supports the view that the development of their nursing profession was the outcome of their cooperation with physicians. Female mental health nurses in Manitoba considered themselves skilled and at a higher level than the male attendants. The female nurses were often in supervisory positions directing the personal care given by the male attendants. This contrasts with Tipliski's [23] view on the separate division of psychiatric nursing being related to paternalistic structures and in which female mental nurses could not overcome male physicians and psychiatrist's domination that sought control and power. Yet the Manitoba mental health nurses that would become RPNs asserted their distinct class, and this has enabled the continuation of the separate training for mental health nursing that continues to manifest inside the western provinces. Evidence to suggest that the separate divisions of psychiatric nursing education in Canada that have any effect on the quality of mental health care has not been substantiated in research.

One must also acknowledge the circumstances that influenced Canadian women as nursing leaders in the past. For instance, Dooley [24] describes the social context of the interwar years where women were looking for ways to support themselves, and mental health nursing provided a way to live that would provide regular meals and housing for mental health nurses. From this description, it is possible that PMHN also developed in diverse ways in Canada as a result of social and economic circumstances in addition to gender influences, that have yet to be fully explored.

Hicks [25] provides further details concerning Manitoba's adoption of the RPN model. Through a genealogical analysis, the study considers historical circumstances that led to the RPN model. Gender stands out as a main influence in this movement where the male leaders of the psychiatric nursing associations of the adjacent western provinces were influential in drawing Manitoba to call for the distinct nursing class. The male nurses of the RPN psychiatric nursing associations in the western provinces developed a collegial relationship with the male attendants of Manitoba who sought RPN status. This presents an interesting insight with regards to gender, in that the men were able to increase their strength and power through the joining with the male psychiatric nurses of Manitoba. This also diverges form Tipliski's view where the psychiatric nurses were submissive to medical authority in relation to the female gender. In addition, the separate psychiatric RPN distinction was favored by the male medical superintendents as there was a lack of interest by the general nurses to work in psychiatry [25], which may have also furthered the movement towards the RPN class. Hicks [25] considers the large number of male attendants and the significance of gender in the creation of the RPN designation. Male attendants provided custodial care and sought to provide nursing care that would elevate the status of the male attendants. Unlike Dooley [24] and Tipliski [23] who focus on the female gender of nursing, Hicks [25] depicts the collegiality and support of male RPN leaders of the western provinces. The Canadian Council of Psychiatric Nursing provided support to the Manitoba attendants who sought RPN status [25]. The RPN emergence may be seen as a way for the male gender to enter into nursing in a time where nursing was culturally enshrined as a female role and the attendants of psychiatric institution sought status and class through the RPN profession. In this way, Hick's study demonstrates how male gender has influenced the history of Canadian PMHN [25].

Boschma et al. [9] examined nurses' stories that further the understanding of the development of PMHN in Alberta. RN status was recognized as being desirable for PMHN and could be achieved by mental health nurses by taking an extra 18 months of training in a general hospital after completing 2 years in a psychiatric hospital. Women were sought as nurses by the governing psychiatrists for their caring and compassionate nature. The male attendants were excluded from nursing because of their gender and became increasingly resentful. The male attendants sought recognition and professional status. Like Saskatchewan, the separate status from RNs was lobbied for by the male attendants and in 1963 registration was given to psychiatric nurses [9]. In this sense, the development of the separate RPN status stems from the gender division that favoured RN status to females leaving male mental health attendants to seek professional status by becoming RPNs. Similar to Hicks [25], Boschma et al. [9] also indicate the influence of male attendants. This differs from the view held by Tipliski [23] that mainly denotes the oppression of largely female nurses by the medical superintendents. Likewise, the account by Hicks [25] and Boschma et al. [9] also varies from the perspective by Dooley [24]. Dooley [24] explains that the female psychiatric nurses saw the RPN category as separate and offering more to the mental health care of patients than the general nurse education could offer. Despite the development of the RPN class, mental health care in Alberta continued to suffer and the need for further education continued pressure to achieve RN status [9].

Professionalization through the regulation of RPNs is described further by the interweaving of data from Boschma's case study of community mental health in Alberta [26] and Hick's historical review of psychiatric nursing in Manitoba [27]. Boschma [26] explains that Alberta graduates from the mental hospitals that started in the 1930s met with resistance from the general nursing organizations leading to the formation of the separate professional organization for RPNs. Hicks [27], consistent with Tipliski [23], indicates that the Alberta Association of Registered Nurses (AARN) had opposed the plan by superintendent Charles Baragar to establish a program to train psychiatric nurses. The AARN recommended that general nurses may complete a postgraduate psychiatric course or combine with general nursing students during a third year of training. They also suggested the hiring of general nurses who were unemployed. Baragar, however, was able to succeed in his intentions through his appeal to the minister of health, and the program was implemented. This program included a total of 4 years of instruction at the mental hospital with 2 of these years occurring at the general hospital. Male attendants were restricted from attending and had to complete a three-year psychiatric program. The male attendants went on to successfully lobby for the Alberta psychiatric professional nursing association [27]. Hicks [27] explains that the association's activities during that period may have been more union type activities rather than professional. In the 1950s, the movement to form the psychiatric nursing association was developing in Manitoba. The Canadian Nurses Association recommended combining the RN and psychiatric training programs in disapproval of the two models emerging for psychiatric nursing in Canada. Despite efforts to organize this endeavour, Canadian Nurses Association's (CNA) plans were never realized [27]. Boschma [26] and Hicks [27] further explicate that beyond the development of the RPN profession to meet the poor staffing of the mental health facilities, the profession of psychiatric nursing in the western provinces grew to deliver a much needed service that provides specialized mental health nursing differing from what general nursing could supply. The RPN profession may advance mental health nursing knowledge and care through the experiences gained from this profession's unique historical development.

3.3. Quality of Canadian Mental Health Psychiatric Nurses Work Life. In 2001, the Canadian Nursing Advisory Committee (CNAC) formed as a result of the recommendations by the Advisory Committee on Health Human Resources (ACHHR). The ACHHR's first recommendation of the *Nursing Strategy for Canada* [28] was to create the CNAC. The CNAC included nursing representatives from the three nursing professions of RNs, RPNs, and LPNs. The CNAC's main goal concerned the quality of nursing work life and the identification of provincial and territorial strategies to enhance nursing work life. With the shrinking workforce this was deemed a high priority. The CNAC's recommendations concern all nursing workplaces including settings that provide PMHN.

The CNAC commissioned 6 projects which looked at strategies to improve workplaces, costs related to absenteeism and overtime, workload issues, satisfaction of nurses in the workplace, workplace respect, and autonomy and health care organizational structures [29]. As a result, 51 recommendations were made to the ACHHR. The recommendations can be summarized into three categories. The first category concerns management issues and resources. There is a need to reduce nursing's pace and intensity, increase full time work, decrease sick time and overtime, and enable full scope of practice. The second recommendation speaks to professional work settings that foster a thriving and dedicated workforce. Respect for nurses is key to this recommendation, as well as education at the master and doctoral levels. Education for nurses should be accessible in remote and rural areas. Violence and abuse in the workplace must be addressed. In the third recommendation, monitoring of the health of nurses and workplaces and disseminating information to keep nurse abreast of initiatives and education are considered. Accreditation, awards to promote quality of nursing work life, continued research on the nursing workforce, implementation of regional nursing committee recommendations, national nursing retention, and recruitment campaigns with a heightened emphasis for diverse and aboriginal groups are a few activities mentioned within this recommendation [29].

The recommendations strive to rectify the main issues that concern the shortage of nurses, the lack of educational opportunities, the limited scope of nursing practice, and the unfavourable working conditions, which are also applicable to the RPNs and RNs who provide PMHN. However, the CNAC recommendations lack consideration of gender and its intersection with professionalization and workplace culture that culminate in the core of issues, including patriarchal culture- and power-based hierarchical organizations that impact nursing work lives [20, 21]. Lacking also from the CNAC recommendations is reference to PMHN being a stakeholder in mental health. As a stakeholder, PMHN needs to organize as a united front, so that its voice is heard. This may be challenging as more powerful stakeholders, like medicine, have traditionally dominated health care [20, 21].

Maslove and Fooks [30] conducted a study to determine the degree of implementation of the 51 CNAC recommendations made in 2002 as requested by the Office of Nursing Policy at Health Canada. Policies of the stakeholder organizations were assessed to determine their impact on facilitating the implementation of the recommendations. Their methodology included scanning of websites, sending letters to 94 stakeholders to determine their progress, and interviewing 14 informants to identify barriers and supports. The 94 stakeholders included employer organizations, the federal government, provincial/territorial governments, unions, professional associations/regulators, educators, research community, and national organizations. There was a 50% response rate from stakeholders. Findings were then shared with nursing stakeholders at a roundtable to enable feedback [30].

The recommendation to increase the number of education seats occurred in a uniform manner. However, other recommendations occurred in some areas but not all, and there was difficulty in determining what had occurred nationwide. Implementation of the recommendations including workload measurement systems, increased full time positions, analyzing sick time, increasing nurse mentors, and flexible scheduling were not consistently taking place throughout Canada. Key informants favoured regulation at the provincial versus the national level. The lack of stable funding was depicted as a barrier to implementation of the recommendation to develop secure jobs. The varying professional associations and regulatory colleges that exist in each province may complicate assigning recommendations [30]. Respondents addressed lack of interest from government regarding nursing issues. Accountability is seen as critical to implementation of the recommendations made by the CNAC. Determining what organizations should be responsible for is a priority concern, and employers need support to enable improvements that will impact nursing quality of work life [30]. Organizations may require government funding in order to implement the recommendations that will enhance nursing work environments.

Together, the CNAC's recommendations [29] and the study by Maslove and Fooks [30] include data from RPNs and general nurses who also provide psychiatric care in the provinces east of Manitoba. Issues pertaining to violence and abuse were seen as priority issues [30]. Poor working conditions may negatively impact quality care, and the lack of action and accountability by organizational and provincial territorial leaders and their support to employers [30] may adversely impact the mental health of both nurses and the Canadian population, which they serve.

Findings from the 2005 National Survey of the Work and Health of Nurses (NSWHN) [31] examined the health of Canadian regulated nurses as related to their work environment. The data as presented here was collected between 2005 and 2006. Nineteen thousand nurses inclusive of RNs, RPNs, and LPNs were surveyed with a response rate of 80%. More than one-quarter reported being physically assaulted. Of note is that 44% of males reported assault compared to 28% of female nurses. The reasons for this finding are not elaborated upon in the 2005 NSWHN. It is not known if this points to male nurses being more likely to be assaulted or more likely to report assault. Forty-four percent of nurses reported emotional abuse. High physical demands were reported by 75% of LPNs, 60% of RNs, and 45% of RPNs. Gender difference was not specified for physical demands, that is, if male or female nurses reported higher physical demands. The mental health of nurses was adversely associated with evening shifts and employment in long-term care facilities. Lack of respect and low support from coworkers and superiors were linked with poorer mental health. In addition, the mental health of nurses was also affected by elevated job strain, low autonomy and control, and poor physician relations. One in ten nurses reported having depression and needing to take time off in relation to their mental health. The finding of depression in nurses is compared with the overall employed population that utilized data from the Workplace and Employee Survey, Labour Force Survey, and the Community Health Survey [31]; however, comparisons with specific groups or professions are not explicit. Of all nurses, including both male and female, 9% experienced depression. The experience of depression by sex was not included for nurses but for all; employed the 4% of men and 7% of women experienced depression. Also at the time of this study in 2005, one-fifth reported their mental health difficulties interfering with their jobs. Quality of care was negatively affected by inadequate staffing. Thirty-eight percent of nurses felt that staffing was inadequate. Improvements in quality care were related to improved management and more staffing [31]. The findings of this survey may further illuminate the working conditions for nurses and the implications for their mental and physical health.

The Health Policy Research Bulletin (HPRB) is published usually twice yearly by Health Canada with the purpose of reinforcing the evidence that supports decision making in health policy. In 2007, the HPRB's issue, titled "*The working conditions of nurses: confronting the challenge*" [32], focused on the Canadian nurses' working conditions and implications for the country's health care system. Between 1997 and 2005 overtime by RPNs, LPNs, and RNS increased in all areas where nurses work by 58%. In light of the high overtime rates, it is questionable if the current level of full-time nursing positions in mental health care in Canada is sufficient to adequately care for those with mental illness. All areas in nursing face similar pressures concerning increased overtime and a need for more full time work; however, mental health settings entail frequent interactions with challenging and difficult behaviours. This may intensify the stress on nurses working in mental health care where there is shortage of full-time nurses.

Robinson et al. [33] conducted a study with a cross-sectional design. A survey of 1015 RPNs in Manitoba was conducted to determine the predictors, prevalence, correlates, and distribution of vicarious trauma and burnout. The survey included the Maslach Burnout Inventory, the Traumatic Stress Institute Belief Scale, and a section on post-traumatic stress disorder (PTSD) symptoms. Seventy-nine percent of the respondents were female, and 20.2% were male. Emotional exhaustion was the highest in RPNs working in community services and acute care hospitals. Constant interruptions, burdensome responsibility, increased trauma work, depersonalization, and elevated vicarious trauma scores were linked with higher emotional exhaustion levels. With regards to vicarious trauma, 21% had persistent thoughts in relation to client trauma, and 30% experienced a heightened level of arousal. Client trauma is the exposure to a stressful experience that overwhelms a person's coping mechanism. Fifty-five percent of those involved in client trauma met one criteria of PTSD, and 48% responded that symptoms were troublesome to some degree. Lack of peer support and skills to deal with trauma could be rectified by increased education and team building. The RPNs in this study also reported a high level of personal accomplishment, which is associated with low burnout [33]. Personal accomplishment includes the perception that clients are improving and the RPNs have the skills necessary to help individuals with mental health disorders. The study is significant in that it mirrors the results of the studies in the preceding discussion concerning nursing quality of work life. Stress is evident in nurses working in mental health care and impacts the mental health of the caregivers. On the other hand, personal accomplishment was high amongst the RPNs, and this may decrease burnout. How this impacts client care requires further study.

Ryan-Nicholls [34] studied the repercussions of health reform in RPNs. Seven focus groups with RPNs from a diversity of health care settings took place in Manitoba over a nine-month period. The themes that emerged consisted of changes from institutional care to the community, variations in professional position, primary and secondary care and prevention, lack of provincial communication, and consistency amongst policies. Deinstitutionalization was considered to have largely impacted the practice setting of RPNs. This change led to an extension of their roles in many different settings including emergency departments, treatment centers, and acute psychiatry. RPN professional status has required a move to more autonomous roles within the primary care setting where professional competence is emphasized. Emphasis on health promotion and prevention is in contrast to the traditional approaches that focused on treating illnesses in institutionalized settings. Study participants described lack of consistency with mental health standards, protocols, and policies in the region. This was not conducive to the provision of mental health services [34].

In the same study, the RPNs became more familiar with the growing emphasis client-centered care and the need for mental health consumers to be involved in the decision making process. The transition from the traditional institutionalized care where decisions were made for the clients had left some RPNs feeling unprepared and concerned that the client may not choose what is best for them. The importance of engaging the family has become more apparent and this contrasts to the way care was provided in the past where family involvement was limited in the institutional setting [34]. The education of RPNs and RNs is essential to meet the changing approaches to caring for those with mental illness and the growing recognition of the impact of social determinants of health on the health and well-being of diverse populations. There is scant research that clearly indicates how the diverse educational preparation of nurses working in psychiatric care impacts the quality of care for persons with mental health disorders. Given the burden of mental illness in Canada there is need for more research that analyzes the psychiatric educational preparation of nurses in relation to accessibility to mental health care and therapeutic and treatment outcomes. Client-centered care requires advocacy and involvement with family and community beyond the confines of institutional care and this may require increased education specific to the changing dynamics of mental health care within the community setting.

According to Ryan-Nicholls [34], the shortage of RPNs is a concern of the existing RPNs. Previously, it was believed that deinstitutionalization would perhaps leave RPNs without jobs. Now, there are not enough RPNs to fill the vacant positions. In addition, participants in the focus groups discussed concern about the 2-year diploma program changing into the 4-year baccalaureate degree for RPNs, graduating only 15 students per year as compared to 60 students per year from the diploma program [34]. Therefore, the issues for RPNs parallel to the issues of the broader nursing workforce, where the shift to higher education has impacted the size of the nursing workforce, but at the same time the nursing graduates of today have increased knowledge to meet the current challenges of health care.

4. Discussion

The diversity between the organization of PMHN and education between the western provinces and the rest of Canada has connections with events of the past and intersects with gender, professionalization, and the predominating organizational culture. The historical analyses of nursing may foster additional inquiries that may benefit nursing knowledge through learning from past approaches and gaining new perspectives.

Overall PMHN in Canada is challenged to further itself to meet the lack of accessible mental health services. There is evidence that nurses are stressed, and there is a need to enhance a coordinated national approach for advanced degrees in PMHN. The lack of a uniform approach to PMHN education in Canada has consequences for the further development of PMHN and may generate barriers to further PMHN to meet the growing mental health care challenges. The implementation of standards by the Canadian Federation of Mental Health Nursing is brought to the discussion here in order to explain how standards are an important way to address the diverse forms of PMHN education. The standards foster an overarching educational approach for PMHN that enables quality PMHN practice. In 2006, the third edition of the Canadian *standards for psychiatric-mental health nursing* was released in an effort to prompt nurses to adopt the standards into daily practice and further nursing reflection on their work [35]. The latest standards were developed after consultation with Canadian consumers of mental health across Canada. Beal et al. [36] acknowledge that systemic issues, that is, labeling, stigma, caregiver, and treatment role, affect PMHN but emphasize the need for nurses to know their clientele to foster therapeutic relationships. Systemic factors including workforce size, workload, violence in the workplace, nursing scope of practice, and accessibility to PMHN may have important implications for PMHN and their daily practice. PMHN education strives to produce nurses whose practice meets or exceedes the standards [36]. However, systemic factors must be addressed to foster PMHN's delivery of high quality care that are consistent with the *standards for psychiatric-mental health nursing*. Furthermore, as an influential and strong stakeholder that can affect change in mental health care, PMHN may benefit from a uniform educational process throughout Canada.

Also of concern is the mental health of nurses who experience high stress. As nurses are mostly women and nurses form the largest group of health care providers, the ramifications for the health and productivity of the Canadian society are especially disconcerting if the majority of nurses are experiencing reduced quality of work life. As Wall [20] and McGibbon et al. [21] point out, a sociological paradigm enables the discussion of sensitive issues including the gendered impact over nursing and the need for research from a perspective that views critically the influence of gender on quality of nursing work life. The labour divisions in organizations where nurses practice are entrenched in hierarchal power struggles that undermine nursing knowledge and autonomy and contribute to poor quality of work life and stress.

4.1. Limitations of Review. There were limitations encountered in this review. Although several studies were found in relation to the history of PMHN for the western provinces and Ontario, no studies were located that convey the full PMHN history of eastern Canada. While there were government documents concerning the quality of work life for all nurses, it was difficult to abstract information specific to PMHN from these documents. For instance, although the NSWHN found a high incidence of depression amongst nurses, the percentage of nurses in PMHN experiencing depression was not given. It is acknowledged that the whole puzzle of what PMHN is like in Canada is not complete. Furthermore, as NPs are becoming more established within the Canadian health care system there is a need for increased research that reveals NP mental health care initiatives and activities. At present, there is a lack of research pertaining to Canadian NPs employed in mental health and their quality of work life. Despite this, the findings reported here depict important points regarding the issues that concern all of PMHN and how they impact the provision of mental health care for Canadians.

4.2. Implications for Nursing Practice. While NPs have made significant progress in achieving prescriptive authority in the area of primary care, minimal movement has occurred regarding the feasibility of NPs specializing in mental health. In Canada, there are no educational programs or legislated provisions for NPs who wish to specialize as a psychiatric NP or who already have extensive experience providing mental health care [37]. The existing situation for NPs practicing within mental health care settings is hampered by the absence of recognition for the psychiatric mental health nurse practitioner (PMHNP) in Canada. Prescriptive authority can only be obtained in Ontario through registration in the extended class in the designated specialties, NP paediatrics, NP-Primary Health Care and NP-Adult. The educational programs that prepare NPs for these specialties focus on the medical and physiological aspects of the specialties with limited content on mental health [37]. In 2011, open prescribing became possible for Ontario NPs. The Nursing Act, 1991, no longer stipulates the prescribing of only listed medications by NPs [38]. With the exception of medications under the Controlled Drugs and Substances Act, NPs are now able to prescribe medications commonly used in mental health care. This allows NPs to further their care for clients needing mental health care; however, it may also point to the need for comprehensive mental health training for NPs. It beckons further exploration if the existing mental health nursing programs offered throughout Canada could enable the development of PMHNP programs that would enable RNs or RPNs and NPs to obtain the competencies of the PMHNP. Communities with insufficient mental health care resources may be better served by nurses with an expanded scope of practice with specialized mental health education. In addition, although there have been changes to legislation, specifically regulation 965 of the Public Hospitals Act, that gives admitting and discharging privileges to NPs; changes to the mental health act have not been made and regulated forms enabling admission to a hospital for psychiatric assessment cannot be completed by Canadian NPs [37]. When the NP is the person's main care provider, it would seem prudent that the NP should be involved in decisions concerning psychiatric admission and discharge.

The variability of PMHN in Canada presents both challenges and opportunities to the advancement of PMHN education. Given the challenge for increased accessibility to mental health care services and treatments, the development of already existing nursing programs in Canada could bond by striving to achieve the same psychiatric educational nursing standards. To further mental health care it may be possible for all nursing programs to uphold the same standards for psychiatric nursing education. The CNA motioned a resolution in 2005 to include RPNs as it was recognized that a separate national level for RPNs would hinder professional nursing practice and the power for Canadian nurses to advocate for change [39]. Amending the division between RPN and RNs and to enable certification and eligibility of CNA membership for both groups may strengthen the Canadian PMHN workforce. Gallop [40] considers how the education system in Canada lacks prospects for nurses working in mental health to obtain advanced degrees in PMHN, although, as previously mentioned, there is new potential for RPNs and nurses to obtain master degrees specializing in mental health nursing west of Ontario. As mental health care is no longer confined to institutional settings and mental health training is pertinent to all areas of health care, the necessity for advanced mental health education is relevant to all health care settings where nurses practice. Nursing needs to facilitate advanced education in mental health so that people within the primary care setting also benefit from the knowledge and expertise of nurses who have additional mental health education. Bridging programs or additional educational opportunities for psychiatric nurses wishing to broaden their knowledge specifically to prescribe psychiatric treatments or medications may be helpful. Partnerships between provincial nursing bodies to foster national standards for PMHN education and bridging programs to a PMHNP program if developed may represent new opportunities for all Canadian nurses. The report entitled "*Canadian nursing education in Canada statistics,*" *2009-2010* [41], conducted by the Canadian Nurses Association (CNA) and the Canadian Association of Schools of Nursing (CASN), reveals an increase of 64.3% from 2009 to 2010 for graduates for doctoral programs [41]. In 2010, 47.6% of NPs had a master's, and 0.8% of NP had a doctorate degree [4]. More nurses and NPs are acquiring advanced degrees. With this trend for advanced education, it is likely that mental health education for all nurses and nursing research pertaining to mental health and PMHN will flourish. Advanced PMHN education offers possibilities to further mental health care for Canadians.

5. Conclusion

PMHN in Canada must take action to meet the goals as set out by the Mental Health Commission of Canada. National standards for psychiatric nursing education for all Canadian nursing education programs may positively impact mental health care. Advanced education for PMHN including the development of a Canadian PMHNP program may further the accessibility of psychiatric treatments. Psychiatric mental health education for all nurses will complement primary health care and the provision of mental health care in general hospitals and community settings. Efforts to unite and form partnerships with the varying groups providing PMHN at a national level may empower PMHN as a powerful stakeholder in mental health care reform. Also, the mental health of nurses in light of their quality of work life is a red flag for all leaders in the Canadian health care system. There is a need to understand the circumstances of nurses with regards to occupational stress and barriers to advanced education in mental health nursing. Although the full picture of what Canadian mental health nursing looks like today cannot be fully realized by this synthesis, important issues facing PMHN have been identified through the analysis of history and application of a critical and gendered sociological lens. Another chapter on the evolution of Canadian PMHN has yet to be written; hopefully, it will entail how PMHN works together with all stakeholders equally to provide the best care possible.

References

[1] Statistics Canada, "Canada's population estimates: age and sex," 2012, http://www.statcan.gc.ca/daily-quotidien/120927/dq120927b-eng.pdf.

[2] Canadian Institute for Health Information, "Regulated Nurses: Canadian Trends, 2006 to 2010," 2012, https://secure.cihi.ca/free_products/Regulated_Nurses_EN.pdf.

[3] M. Alameddine, A. Laporte, A. Baumann et al., "Where are nurses working? Employment patterns by sub-sector in Ontario, Canada," *Healthcare Policy*, vol. 1, no. 3, pp. 65–86, 2006.

[4] Canadian Nurses Association, "2010 Workforce Profile of Nurse Practitioners in Canada," 2012, http://www2.cna-aiic.ca/CNA/documents/pdf/publications/2010_NP_Profiles_e.pdf.

[5] Statistics Canada, "Canadian Community Health Survey—Mental Health (CCHS)," 2012, http://www23.statcan.gc.ca/imdb/p2SV.pl?Function=getSurvey&SDDS=5015&lang=en&db=imdb&adm=8&dis=2.

[6] Statistics Canada, "Canadian Community Health Survey: Mental Health and Well Being," 2003, http://www.statcan.gc.ca/daily-quotidien/030903/dq030903a-eng.htm.

[7] Health Canada, "Sharing the Learning. The Health Transition Fund. Ottawa: Health Canada," 2002, http://www.hc-sc.gc.ca/hcs-sss/alt_formats/hpb-dgps/pdf/pubs/2002-htf-fass-prim/2002-htf-fass-prim-eng.pdf.

[8] S. Ratnsingham, J. Cairney, J. Rehm, H. Manson, and P. A. Kurdyak, "Opening eyes, opening minds: the ontario burden of mental illness and addictions report," An ICES/PHO Report, Institute for Clinical Evaluative Sciences and Public Health Ontario, Toronto, Canada, 2012, http://www.oahpp.ca/resources/documents/reports/opening-eyes-mental-health/PHO-ICES%20Opening%20Eyes%20Opening%20Minds%20Report%20-%20Oct%202012%20final.pdf.

[9] G. Boschma, O. Yonge, and L. Mychajlunow, "Gender and professional identity in psychiatric nursing practice in Alberta, Canada, 1930–75," *Nursing Inquiry*, vol. 12, no. 4, pp. 243–255, 2005.

[10] M. J. Kirby, "Mental health reform for Canada in the 21st century: getting there from here," *Canadian Public Policy: Analyse de Politique*, vol. 31, sl, pp. 5–12, 2005.

[11] The Standing Senate Committee on Social Affairs, Science and Technology, "Out of the shadows at last: transforming mental health, mental illness and addiction services in Canada," 2006, www.parl.gc.ca/39/1/parlbus/commbus/senate/com-e/soci-e/rep-e/rep02may06-e.htm.

[12] Mental Health Commission Canada, "Toward recovery and well being: a framework for a mental health strategy for Canada," 2009, http://www.mentalhealthcommission.ca/SiteCollectionDocuments/boarddocs/15507_MHCC_EN_final.pdf.

[13] Mental Health Commission of Canada, "Changing directions, changing lives: the mental health strategy for Canada," 2012, http://strategy.mentalhealthcommission.ca/pdf/strategy-images-en.pdf.

[14] M. Kirby, "Mental health in Canada: out of the shadows forever," *Canadian Medical Association Journal*, vol. 178, no. 10, pp. 1320–1322, 2008.

[15] R. Whittemore and K. Knafl, "The integrative review: updated methodology," *Journal of Advanced Nursing*, vol. 52, no. 5, pp. 546–553, 2005.

[16] J. J. Macionis and L. M. Gerber, *Sociology*, Pearson Education Canada, Toronto, Canada, 5th edition, 2005.

[17] R. J. Brym, *New Society: Sociology for the 21st Century*, Harcourt Canada, Toronto, Ontario., 2001.

[18] L. S. Brown, "Feminist therapy," in *Handbook of Psychological Change: Psychotherapy Process and Practice for the 21st Century*, C. R. Snyder and R. E. Ingram, Eds., pp. 358–380, Wiley, New York, NY, USA, 2000.

[19] M. C. Wright, *The Sociological Imagination*, Oxford University Press, New York, NY, USA, 1959.

[20] S. Wall, "Critical perspectives in the study of nursing work," *Journal of Health, Organisation and Management*, vol. 24, no. 2, pp. 145–166, 2010.

[21] E. McGibbon, E. Peter, and R. Gallop, "An institutional ethnography of nurses' stress," *Qualitative Health Research*, vol. 20, no. 10, pp. 1353–1378, 2010.

[22] D. Smith, *The Everyday World as Problematic: A Feminist Sociology*, University of Toronto Press., Toronto, Canada, 1987.

[23] V. M. Tipliski, "Parting at the crossroads: the emergence of education for psychiatric nursing in three Canadian provinces, 1909–1955," *Canadian Bulletin of Medical History*, vol. 21, no. 2, pp. 253–279, 2004.

[24] C. Dooley, "'They gave their care, but we gave loving care': defining and defending the boundaries of skill and craft in the nursing service of a Manitoba mental hospital during the great depression," *Canadian Bulletin of Medical History*, vol. 21, no. 2, pp. 229–251, 2004.

[25] S. C. Hicks, *From Barnyards to Besides to Books and Beyond: The Evolution and Professionalization of Registered Psychiatric Nursing in Manitoba, 1955–1989*, University of ManitobaCanada, 2008.

[26] G. Boschma, "Community mental health nursing in Alberta, Canada: an oral history," *Nursing History Review*, vol. 20, pp. 103–135, 2012.

[27] B. Hicks, "Gender, politics, and regionalism: factors in the evolution of registered psychiatric nursing in Manitoba, 1920–1960," *Nursing History Review*, vol. 19, pp. 103–126, 2011.

[28] Advisory Committee on Health Human Resources, *The Nursing Strategy for Canada*, Health Canada, Ottawa, Canada, 2000.

[29] Health Canada, "Our Health, Our Future: Creating Quality Workplaces for Canadian Nurse, Final Report of the Canadian Nursing Advisory Committee, Advisory Committee on Health Human Resources," 2002, http://www.hc-sc.gc.ca/hcs-sss/alt_formats/hpb-dgps/pdf/pubs/2002-cnac-cccsi-final/2002-cnac-cccsi-final-eng.pdf.

[30] L. Maslove and C. Fooks, "Our Health, Our Future: Creating Qualtiy Workplaces for Canadian Nurses: A Progress Report on Implementing the Final Report of Canadian Nursing Advisory Committee," Canadian Policy Research Networks, 2004, http://www.cprn.org/documents/30762_en.pdf.

[31] Statistics Canada, Special Surveys Division, "Findings from the 2005 National Survey of the Work and Health of Nurses," 2006, http://www.statcan.gc.ca/daily-quotidien/061211/dq061211b-eng.htm.

[32] Health Canada, "The working conditions of nurses: Confronting the Challenges," 2007, http://www.hc-sc.gc.ca/sr-sr/alt_formats/hpb-dgps/pdf/pubs/hpr-rps/bull/2007-nurses-infirmieres/2007-nurses-infirmieres-eng.pdf.

[33] J. R. Robinson, K. Clements, and C. Land, "Workplace stress among psychiatric nurses: prevalence, distribution, correlates, & predictors," *Journal of Psychosocial Nursing and Mental Health Services*, vol. 41, no. 4, pp. 32–41, 2003.

[34] K. D. Ryan-Nicholls, "Impact of health reform on registered psychiatric nursing practice," *Journal of Psychiatric and Mental Health Nursing*, vol. 11, no. 6, pp. 644–653, 2004.

[35] Canadian Federation of Mental Health Nurses, "The Canadian Standards for Psychiatric-Mental Health Nursing (3rd ed.)," 2006, http://cfmhn.ca/sites/cfmhn.ca/files/CFMHN%20standards%201.pdf.

[36] G. Beal, A. Chan, S. Chapman et al., "Consumer input into standards revision: changing practice," *Journal of Psychiatric and Mental Health Nursing*, vol. 14, no. 1, pp. 13–20, 2007.

[37] C. Forchuk and R. Kohr, "Prescriptive authority for nurses: the Canadian perspective," *Perspectives in Psychiatric Care*, vol. 45, no. 1, pp. 3–8, 2009.

[38] College of Nurses of Ontario, "NP Diagnostic and Prescriptive Authority," 2012.

[39] Canadian Nurses Association, "Resolution 2. Inclusion of Psychiatric Nurses," 2005, http://www.cna-nurses.ca/CNA/about/meetings/resolutions_2005/resolutions_02_e.aspx.

[40] R. Gallop, "Advanced practice psychiatric nursing in Canada," International society of psychiatric nurses [ISPN], 2007, http://www.ispn-psych.org/html/what_canada.html.

[41] Canadian Nurses Association (CNA) and the Canadian Association of Schools of Nursing (CASN), "Nursing Education in Canada Statistics, 2009-2010," 2012, http://www2.cna-aiic.ca/CNA/documents/pdf/publications/Education_Statistics_Report_2009_2010_e.pdf.

6

Study on Situational Influences Perceived in Nursing Discipline on Health Promotion: A Qualitative Study

Meimanat Hosseini,[1] Tahereh Ashk Torab,[2] Mohammad Hossein Taghdisi,[3] and Safar Ali Esmaeili Vardanjani[4]

[1] *Department of Community Health Nursing, Faculty of Nursing and Midwifery, Shahid Beheshti University of Medical Sciences, International Branch of Shahid Beheshti University of Medical Sciences, Tehran, Iran*
[2] *Department of Medical-Surgical, Faculty of Nursing and Midwifery, Shahid Beheshti University of Medical Sciences, Tehran, Iran*
[3] *Department of Health Promotion, Faculty of Tehran University of Medical Sciences, Tehran, Iran*
[4] *Shahrekord University of Medical Science, Shahrekord, Iran*

Correspondence should be addressed to Tahereh Ashk Torab; t_ashktorab@sbmu.ac.ir

Academic Editors: A. Green and B. Roberts

Introduction and Objectives. Nurses, as behavioral models, play a key role in health promotion, and their attitudes towards health promotion highly influence their health and performance. The aim of this study is to explore nursing students' perception of studies in nursing discipline as a situational influence on health promotion. *Materials and Methods.* This study was conducted using directed content analysis, by means of 20 deep semistructured interviews with nursing students. The participants were selected on purposive sampling. Data was analyzed by the qualitative content analysis method. All interviews were recorded, transcribed, and reviewed, and all codes were extracted and summarized. The codes were subcategorized on the basis of centralization and were categorized after review of subcategories, and finally, a theme was determined. *Findings.* The theme of nursing discipline's situational influence on nursing students' health promotion was revealed. This theme consisted of "choosing the field," "unfavorable environmental factors," "negative impacts of studies in nursing discipline on health," "positive effects of studies in nursing discipline on health", "needs," "attractiveness (aesthetics)," and "coping with negative situational influences in nursing discipline." *Conclusion.* The perception of studies in nursing discipline as a health-promoting behavior is under influence of social environment. Considering the importance of the students' positive perception of the existing situation, it is essential to pay attention to their attitudes and perceptions so that they can provide better services to patients.

1. Introduction

The increased rate of health care costs and the concerns about inefficiency of patient care has led to greater support of health promotion concept and its propagation among health care personnel, particularly nurses [1].

Health promotion is a process which enables people to control their health [2]. Health-promoting behavior is an important concept in nursing [3] and should be considered as a healthy nursing or interactive method which promotes health [4].

Nurses are the biggest group to render services to patients [5] and take a significant role in public health promotion [6]. According to statistics published by Nursing Organization, nurses constitute 50% of the entire 600,000 personnel in Iran's health system [7]. Nurses, as behavioral models and professional caretakers, play a key role in health promotion, and their beliefs on the importance of health promotion are part of their work [8].

Pender states that cognitive variables such as situational influences along with particular behavioral variables can help determine health-promoting behaviors of people [9]. Situational influences directly [10] and indirectly affect the behaviors and the commitment to action planning [11]. These influences embrace health-promoting behaviors, conceptions of possible choices, need characteristics and aesthetic aspects of the environment [12]. Situational influences, such as choices, may increase or decrease commitment to or participation in health-promoting behaviors [13]. Since behavior is dependent on the surrounding environment, it may be affected by situational factors [14], and this influences a person's behavior [15].

The results of studies have revealed that nursing students' view of occupational situation is highly personal. These students often think there is a relation between the status of a profession and judgments regarding the value of a job, and their attitude towards nursing is under influence of several factors such as negative attitude of parents and unreal images of nurses shown in TV [16].

In order to attract more people to nursing profession, a positive image of nursing needs to be developed by the public society and nursing education center. It should also be mentioned that experiences and concerns of nursing students are a permanent theme of professional pressure [17].

The considerable point is that according to studies, the conception of nursing affects the student's decision to enter, continue or discontinue nursing profession [18]. Unsupported by their families or their faculties, students have frequently made decision to continue or discontinue their studies in spite of their desires. A research on, 1,000 American students revealed that students believe that nursing includes a physical challenge and the respect for nursing profession is of a low level. On the other hand, another study has revealed that students have selected nursing discipline owing to good job opportunity, job safety, salary, and interest. Furthermore, friends, families, relatives, media, and society have been noted as contributing factors in choosing nursing discipline [17].

Nursing students should be able to do activity in cultural context of nursing profession easily and confidently. The students who feel accepted in this context experience less anxiety. On the other hand, immoral and inaccurate activities are connected with being not accepted in cultural groundwork [19].

In a broad library search, researchers found no research on the relation between study of nursing discipline as a situational factor and health-promoting behavior, neither in Iran nor in other countries. However, the shortage of nursing forces all over the world, including Iran, has been considered to be a serious challenge [20], the cause of which might be the effect of nurses' perception of nursing discipline on their health-promoting behaviors. On the other hand, it is not known what effect the perception of studies in nursing discipline has on students' health-promoting behaviors. Therefore, this research was conducted to explore nursing students' perception of studies in nursing discipline as a situational influence on health promotion.

2. Materials and Methods

Nursing research, like nursing itself, deals with different and complicated phenomena [21]. The present study is part of a broader research which was performed by qualitative method with a content analysis approach. Qualitative content analysis is a story-like data content analysis in order to determine prominent themes and patterns among themes [22]. The phenomenon under study in this research is study of nursing discipline as a situational influence. 20 nursing students from nursing faculties of medical universities of the city of Tehran participated in individual semistructured interviews. The participants were chosen by purposive sampling method from June up to November 2012 until data saturation. After choosing the participants, interviews were performed in leisure times at classes or rooms allocated by managers of the faculties or work office of researcher or open area of the faculties, however the participants wished. In researches performed in natural environment, the main responsibility of the researcher is to obtain consent of the participants in a conscious way [22]. In line with this objective, after obtainment of verbal consent from participants and completion of letter of informed consent by them, deep semi-structured interviews consisting of four questions were performed based on the guidance of the interview's questions. Deep interview helps the researcher to make a mental interpretation from the stories told by participants and to assess the facts as they clarify the phenomenon under study. During the dialogue between interviewer and interviewee, meaningful and relevant subjects are produced [23]. Data was collected using deep, semi-structured interviews and making field notes. All interviews were recorded on an MP3 player. The interview's questions were based on health-promoting behaviors and delineation of nursing students' perception of their academic field as a situational influence on their health-promoting behavior. Minimum and maximum times of individual interviews were 19 : 30 and 71 : 25, respectively. To prevent data collection bias, all interviews were performed by one researcher. Among moral points of this research were compliance with the principle of secrecy and confidentiality of the participants' names and information in all steps, making them confident about protection of their secrets and the right of withdrawal in any part of the research.

In this research, data was analyzed by directed content analysis method, in which primary encoding is started with a theory or relevant research findings [24]. The aim of directed content analysis is to validate or develop a conceptual framework or theory. The existing theory or research can help concentration on the research question. By using the existing theory or research, the researchers start with determined concepts and variables as primary coding classifications. Then, operational definitions of each category class are determined by using the theory [25]. Since Pender's model was the basis of this research on health-promoting behaviors, the researchers used directed content analysis, and categories were determined on the basis of Pender's Health Promotion Model [26].

Based on this, one of the researchers first performed an interview and made field notes and then studied them line by line accurately, underlining key words and sentences and coding each. After coding was completed, the interview was restudied to see if any possible code is found. Next, the codes were merged and summarized, and similar codes were classified. This way the primary classifications of the data were obtained. Then, the researcher tried to perform the same process for the categorizations as well. Finally, the subcategories were located in categories on the basis of common characteristics and dimensions.

The rigor of qualitative research is shown through the researcher's attention to discovered information and its confirmation. The aim of accuracy in qualitative studies is to show the authenticity of participants' experiences. Credibility, dependability, confirmability and transferability are terms which constitute practical methods for supporting rigor of a research [27]. In this study, credibility of the data was achieved by long-term investigation of the research subject by researcher, allocation of sufficient time to gather data, interview, observation of the examinees during the sessions, data control by participants and review of extracted codes. To achieve dependability of the data, the researchers used the validity of research findings. To achieve confirmability of the data, audit trial was used. For this purpose, a detailed report of the process leading to conclusion has been presented, whereby enabling the pursuit of research process and actions taken by researchers. To achieve transferability of the data, data were accurately investigated by external supervisors.

3. Findings

Twenty nursing students from nursing faculties of medical universities of the city of Tehran participated in individual semi-structured interviews. The participants were 6 male and 14 female nursing students who were studying in the 1st to 8th semesters of Bachelor's Degree course of studies. Four of the participants were married and sixteen were single. Six of them were working as nurse, one was working in a profession other than nursing and thirteen were unemployed. Five participants were living in dormitory, fourteen were living with their families, and one was living with friends.

Data analysis indicated that the main theme of nursing's situational influence on health promotion included 227 meaning units, 35 subcategories, and 7 categories as follows: "choosing the field," "unfavorable environmental factors," "negative impacts of studies in nursing discipline on health," "positive effects of studies in nursing discipline on health," "needs," "attractiveness of nursing discipline" and "coping with negative situational influences in nursing discipline."

Studying in university had been perceived as a situational influence on health promotion, in such a manner that one of the participants said that

> *"Because of my age the only important thing is studying. Any other thing doesn't matter ... educational future is important ... that is why I say success in the most important aspect of life still makes me feel healthier." (Participant No. 10)*

The students said that they have used the subjects learnt in nursing discipline for their health promotion. Almost all participants in this research believed that studying in nursing discipline is a factor contributing to their health promotion. In this respect, a student said that

> *"Well, the field we are studying is very effective in health promotion. It has helped me think more profoundly about the things which I used to skip very easily." (Participant No. 7)*

The use of subjects to diagnose disease and identify probable diseases by observing the patients hospitalized in hospital ward was mentioned as the health-promoting behavior.

> *"Well, personally I try to review things learnt in the class by checking them in myself... anyway as we go to the wards and see the patients, it makes us think and see what problems we have and what problems we don't have." (Participant No. 2)*

The significant role of nursing education was a considerable aspect in paying attention to oneself and to family members and everyday activities in line with health promotion, which the participants believed in:

> *"Well, the most important thing is the education I was given in all fields. Since I am married and have baby, I have to be more careful than others, in all my works ... and the training I can give to my child, about what he should do." (Participant No. 8)*

3.1. Choosing Nursing Discipline. The conception of having a good occupational future and the feeling of safety owing to good financial situation were among the reasons for choosing nursing discipline, so that good job opportunity of this discipline had overcome the lack of interest in that:

> *"You can be relaxed when you think no matter if you don't like nursing; there will be job for that ... anyway you will have a job. I think one of the reasons; actually the main reason that I chose it was its good job opportunity". (Participant No. 13)*

Furthermore, there was a belief of having better situation in terms of health-promoting behaviors in the case of studying a better discipline:

> *"If I hadn't come to university and hadn't had academic studies, I would certainly have had worse behavior. If I had studied a better discipline, my behavior would certainly have been even better and I would've had better mental conditions and better self-confidence." (Participant No. 1)*

3.2. Unfavorable Environmental Factors. The low status of nursing in public society had been perceived as a factor contributing to reduction of health level. The effect of lack of respect and value in public society was considered to be connected with field comparison:

> *"When you go somewhere else like hospital or the public society, you see people treat nursing as a very ordinary job, not a job that is serving them, so they don't respect it." (Participant No. 1)*

Negative comments of medical personnel and the colleagues in regards to nursing were another issue that the participants considered as a negative impact on their health promotion. They believed that the biggest occupational damage is inflicted by their colleagues:

"In hospital you see that both physicians and nurses have this opinion. I mean the nurses themselves inflict the biggest damage to this job. When you see such behavior you become very upset that even your colleagues don't respect you." (Participant No. 1)

The negative attitude of the community, family, and relatives influenced the value of nursing discipline as stated by the students, the effect of which was shown by reduction of interest in nursing:

"At first, I was very interested in nursing. But later when I saw the attitude of others, I started to dislike it. Now I don't like nursing at all. I mean the thing for which I made so much effort is now valueless for me." (Participant No. 10)

3.3. The Negative Impacts of Studies in Nursing Discipline on Health. The students pointed to negative impacts of studies in nursing discipline, particularly in internship courses. These negative impacts were worse in internship courses in which they dealt with mental problems of patients:

"Internship courses which deal with mental problems have a very bad psychological effect on nurses." (Participant No. 6)

To see patients' pain and sorrow in clinical environments was mentioned as a factor influencing the students. This impact was conveyed to students through the feeling of sympathy and altruism:

"Our work in hospital includes such sad experiences. For example, someone who had an accident came from another city to hospital in Tehran. He ordered one of his relatives in his city to buy platinum and bring for him in Tehran. But his relative was killed in his way to Tehran in an accident and his money was wasted as well. The poor guy experienced another disaster in addition to his accident. By seeing that, a feeling of sadness comes to your heart instinctively and unconsciously, because he is a human being like you." (Participant No. 5)

The negative impacts of work in hospital were more severe in an internship course because, in addition to negative impacts of seeing patients and their problems on the students, it caused a feeling of depression and aimlessness:

"The practical course we are passing has depressed us. In addition, we don't know exactly how we should pass this year." (Participant No. 3)

Physical tiredness caused by intensive academic programs was another negative influence resulting from studies in nursing discipline, as the result of which the students could not do their daily affairs:

"For example, during the course of this semester, when we came from university we were too tried. Sleeping was the only thing we could do. Well, no time remained for us to think about something or do something funny or think about our nutrition to see what our body needs." (Participant No. 14)

The students who had emigrated from other cities to Tehran to study nursing expressed another problem as well. They said that limitations of living in dormitory and missing their family members influenced their health:

"Living in dormitory has some limitations. Unconsciously, when a person is in some public place like dormitory, some works are limited automatically." (Participant No. 5)

The negative impact of living in dormitory had been conceived as a shocking change which had made the participants unable to do any activity and had influenced all their life planning:

"When I was in dormitory, I had free time but I didn't know who to do. I could neither do exercise nor study my lessons. At least in the first semester I was in such conditions. I was really in shock." (Participant No. 13)

3.4. The Positive Effects of Studies in Nursing Discipline. The perception of being different from ordinary people of the society and having more knowledge was among positive effects of studies in nursing discipline. By way of better care of oneself, nursing discipline could have positive effect on health:

"Well, I differ from other people. I have more knowledge on medical treatment. You imagine someone like my mother who has studied another field of study. Well, she has no much knowledge like me. She cannot take care of herself." (Participant No. 2)

Performing examinations, familiarity with health standards, and preventive activities were among the positive things in nursing discipline. Awareness about health standards and activities resulted in compliance with health requirements:

"I think the minimum difference between us and other people who don't have this information are that we know what things are good or bad for health; for example, we know what things cause problem for heart, kidney, etc. At least we know the standards, so we can comply with them." (Participant No. 6)

The ability to diagnose diseases by help of academic studies in nursing discipline was another point which had positive effect on health promotion:

> *"As a person who has studied nursing, I can easily diagnose diseases." (Participant No. 2)*

The arrival to nursing profession was a factor which increased the responsibility of the participants to both themselves and their family members. They felt that since they have chosen nursing discipline they will try more to promote their health level. The source of this effort was the insight in health-promoting behaviors:

> *"Since I have studied nursing discipline and entered this profession, I am responsible towards my family as well as myself... before I entered this discipline I didn't have so much knowledge. But when I studied nursing I gained the knowledge I needed. When you become familiar with a series of diseases, you know what to do to prevent them. Well, such diseases may exist in my family as well." (Participant No. 18)*

The arrival to nursing discipline had caused the students to become curios about their own health. Enthusiasm for more studies and screening tests stimulated them to have periodical tests and identify probable diseases:

> *"On the other hand, as I had become a nurse, I liked to study more and know about things. So I worked on my own screening system. For this purpose I went and had myself tested once every 3-4 months." (Participant No. 12)*

3.5. Needs. The need to have a healthier body in nursing discipline was one of considerable conceptions among the students, which made them observe health-promoting behaviors including nutrition and exercise:

> *"Well, I used to eat fast foods so much. But when I started exercise, I stopped eating fast foods for a couple of years. Another reason was our field of study, namely nursing." (Participant No. 4)*

Giving priority to health in order to be able to take care of patients better was another need conceived by the participants:

> *"The first priority is our own health and the second is other's health. When you are not healthy you won't be able to help others." (Participant No. 19)*

Among needed actions in the faculty to promote students' health was to design a system in hospitals to separate work area of physicians from that of nurses and protect the dignity of nurses. Independency of nursing faculties was mentioned as a need:

> *"If a system is designed in hospitals to separate work area of physicians from nurses, so that nurses are not ordered by physicians too much, it would be very better. They should respect each other. The main head of the students who go to hospital should be the faculties, not hospital or head nurse." (Participant No. 19)*

Furthermore, the participants believed that it is necessary to protect themselves against the risks of the work environment as far as possible. In this matter, how to make body contact with a patient was expressed by students:

> *"Considering the job we have, it is mentally hard. We have such challenges as how to contact with patients in work environment, how to protect ourselves against probable risks as far as possible." (Participant No. 6)*

3.6. Attractiveness of Nursing Discipline (Aesthetics). One of the things done by students was to compare the status of nursing discipline with other fields such as medicine. In this case, the participants had a feeling of humility and humbleness:

> *"Well, when you see in the society that your status and dignity in lower than somebody else, say a student of medicine or a general practitioner, you feel they are more important than you and an unconscious sense of humility appears in you." (Participant No. 1)*

The participants compared the problems of their own discipline with students of other fields. This problem was more severe in their internship course:

> *"A nine-day internship course which is 1 credit has only one permitted absence. Imagine that someone has cold and needs a two-day absence in the middle of the week. It results in deletion of that credit. These are problems that I think students of other fields don't have." (Participant No. 6)*

The participants believed that the subjects they had studied are only about the patient. They felt that their mental and physical needs had been disregarded and that they had been sacrificed for patients and health team personnel:

> *"Whatever we study is about patient. There should be some lessons about our own health as well. They should teach us a little about our health and how to comply with health standards. This way we can learn our own mental health not the patient's mental health. We always have to be sacrificed for patients and medical team." (Participant No. 6)*

One of the participants who had immigrated to Tehran to study nursing pointed out to conditions of dormitory and compared it with his own home. He expressed that while living in dormitory had enhanced his tolerance, at the same time, it had restricted him to much extent:

> *"My problem is being away from my family. Despite it is enhancing my tolerance; it prevents me from being what I like to be." (Participant No. 5)*

3.7. Coping with Negative Influences in Nursing. Among the ways of coping with negative influences in the field of nursing are to try to establish more friendships, communicate with family, do funny things have entertainment with friends, and be happy in resting times in internship courses. Moreover, to have no mental and emotional problems was among considerable things that they pointed to in connection with coping and preventing the problems:

> *"We try to enhance our friendship. For example, we try to have fun in rest times or go out with each other to mentally refresh a little. We also try to contact our family members. I think that is the only solution. This way the students can overcome their mental or emotional problems. If a person is emotionally weak, she gets into trouble." (Participant No. 6)*

In connection with negative impact of nursing on physical problems resulting from tiredness and fatigue, the participants mentioned they consume drugs to alleviate pain as one of the methods:

> *"When I went home at night after C.C.U internship, I applied salicylate to sleep. I couldn't sleep without that." (Participant No. 6)*

The participants who lived in dormitory expressed gradual adaptation to bad conditions of dormitory as a strategy to cope with negative impacts. They hoped to adapt more to dormitory in the next semesters:

> *"There was beetle in the room and the food was bad. In the second semester I am starting to adapt. There are still many things I cannot accept. But I hope it gets better until third or fourth semester." (Participant No. 13)*

Also, good interperson relation in dormitory was expressed as a strategy of coping with probable problems of living with other students:

> *"In dormitory we should protect our rights and behave in such a manner to neither oppress others or to be oppressed. We should respect the rights of others and at the same time we should not let others to order us frequently and consider us a weak person, otherwise we will suffer for the following four years." (Participant No. 16)*

Cooperation in compliance with environmental health standards in dormitory was another strategy of coping with environmental issues of dormitory. The students did so as they were aware of the effects of such cooperation:

> *"Despite the dormitory have some servants who clean the dormitory every day, the students themselves also clean the dormitory, even the toilets, in cooperation with each other. We all cooperate with each other and try to maintain the dormitory in the best manner." (Participant No. 5)*

The research findings are shown in Figure 1.

4. Discussion and Conclusion

The most common influence on the nurses' concentration on health promotion is their personal attitudes [6]. Students have a wide range of perceptions about nursing [17]. In this research, the participants believed that studies in nursing discipline can be a situational factor contributing to their health promotion lifestyle. They expressed that they have used the subjects learnt in nursing discipline to promote their health and their family members' health. In this respect, studies have indicated that nursing comprehensive programs have had positive effects on nursing students, such as considerable improvement of health responsibility and increase of physical, personal, and professional practice use. These changes last for one to seven years [28].

The students enumerated the lack of personal interest, lack of respect for nursing, and negative attitude of the public towards nursing as unfavorable environmental factors. They believed that the biggest damage is inflicted on them by their own colleagues. Negative attitude to nursing and lack of respect for nursing in the society were considered to be connected with field comparison. In this respect, the findings of a research conducted by Kemppainen et al. indicated that cultural aspects of the organization in which nurses' work contributes to their health-promoting activities. This cultural context may be supportive or disappointing [6]. In a study with qualitative approach by content analysis method, it was indicated that the problems of communication with students are one of the important factors contributing to reduction of their interest in nursing discipline. According to the data obtained by analyzing handwritings, all nursing students pointed to cultural-social issues as one of the important factors contributing to reduction of their interest in nursing. This main theme embraced a wide range of factors contributing to reduction of motivation, among which were low dignity and improper conception of the society [29]. The findings have indicated that, in contemporary history, negative image and low dignity of nursing have been among the causes of nurse shortage in Muslim and Arab societies. These negative images of nursing are being continued, and nursing is being considered as a job that requires no skill, has low income, is womanish, and is less important than other healthcare jobs [30].

In the present study, nursing discipline has been selected mostly due to its good job opportunity. In other words, the feeling of financial safety was the reason for choosing this field. In this connection, 68 interviews have been made about Saudi Arabian nurses' conception of nursing as a job. The findings indicated that despite negative conceptions of gender in nursing, the conception of good job opportunity of this field was increasing [30].

In this research, nursing's negative impacts on the students' health were mostly mental problems and feeling of tiredness, in such a way that intensiveness of the courses had made them unable to have good nutrition, meet their physical and mental needs and have sufficient entertainment and rest. In this matter, the studies performed on nurses have indicated several themes that evaluate health promotion in nurses as weak. Among the things expressed are insufficient sleep,

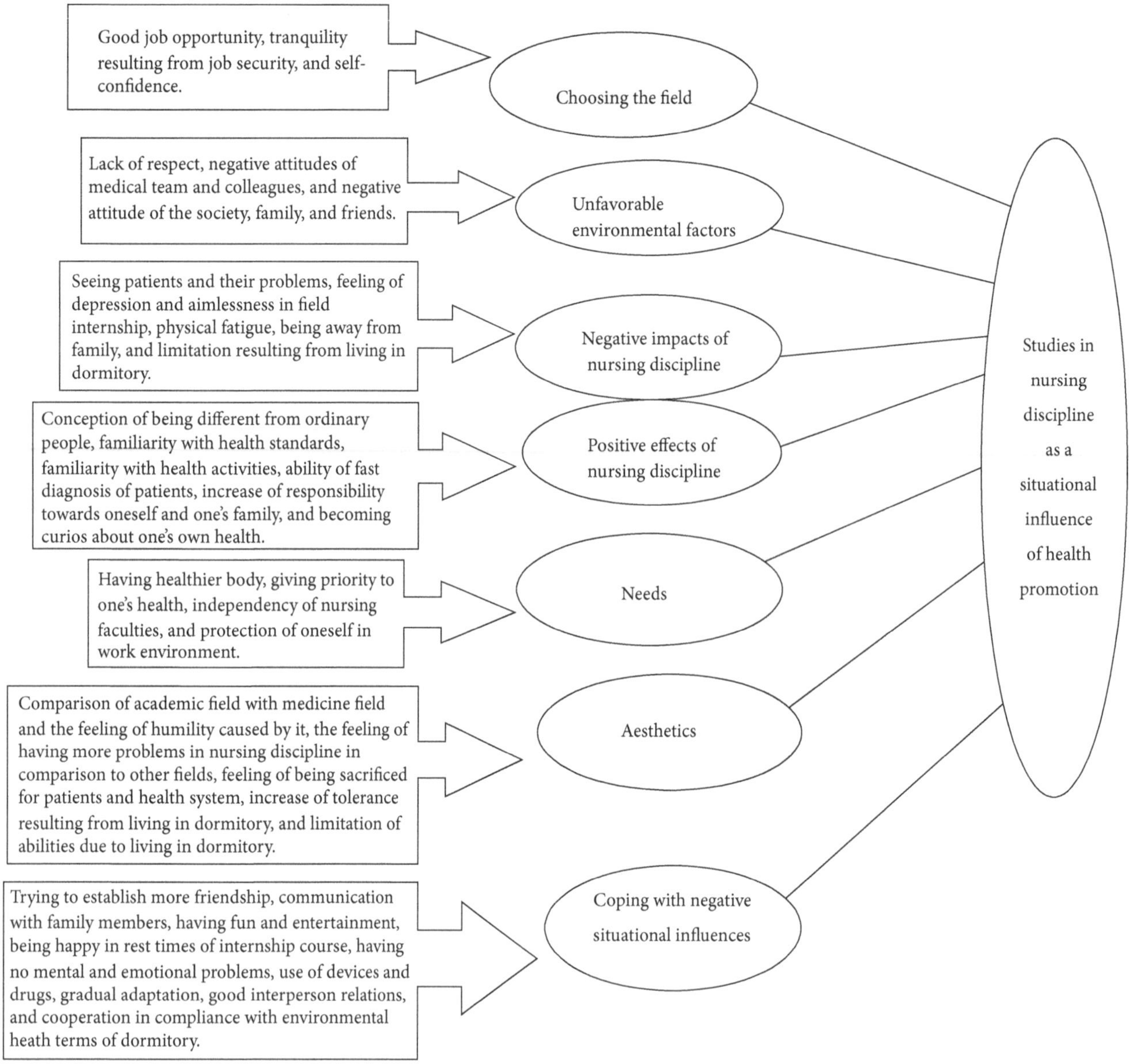

FIGURE 1: Theme, categories, and subcategories of situational influences perceived in nursing discipline.

smoking and improper nutrition in surgery room nurses, the need to improve health activities in special care units nurses, improper nutrition and exercise in American-African nurses, and the need to concentrate on nutrition, exercise, and stress management [28].

Among the positive effects of studies in nursing discipline enumerated by the participants were having more knowledge than the public community, ability of early diagnosis of their diseases, awareness about health standards and better care of oneself. Studies have indicated that passing nursing discipline subjects which concentrate on health promotion has undeniable effects on the increase of students' level of knowledge. A research made by Hong et al. showed that there is a positive meaningful relation between health promoting lifestyle and courses and subjects of health-promotion passed in nursing discipline [31].

The students expressed the need to have a healthier body in nursing discipline in order to take better care of patients, which resulted in improvement of health-promoting behaviors such as nutrition and exercise. In order to advocate healthy life style and to be an effective model, nurses are expected to pay more attention to their own health [1].

The participants also expressed that nursing faculties should be independent. According to the previous studies, nursing can be studied as a mummified job in which old and stereotyped values have highly remained. The main motivation to become a nurse is the desire for independency, flexibility, and altruism. In order to enhance nursing profession, professors and clinical supervisors should consider nursing students' attitudes as an important point of education and develop them in different environments [32].

Among the issues expressed by the participants was comparison of nursing's status with other fields of study. They compared the problems of their field with the problems faced by students of other fields and estimated their health to be in a lower level. Furthermore, the students who lived in dormitory had conceived the dormitory's environment as unpleasant. Two studies have indicated that stressful environments result in unhealthy solutions such as smoking and improper nutrition, which in turn causes harmful behaviors having negative impact on patients' health and reduction of efficiency of the nurses as health promoters [33]. According to findings of a research on the attitudes of others towards nurses' health-promoting behaviors, the participants felt that their efforts had been understood positively by patients. However, some of the participants believed that their work environment is unsupportive [34].

In the present research, the participants believed that the subjects they have learnt are merely about patients. They felt that they had been sacrificed for patients and medical team. In this respect, McElligott et al. believed that nurses often use holistic approaches to consult patients on health promotion. However, studies have denoted that there are weak health-promoting behaviors in the nurses themselves [28].

Among the strategies of coping with negative influences in nursing discipline are establishment of more friendships, communication with family members, having fun and entertainment with friends and family, and being happy in rest times of internship courses. In this respect, the results of studies have indicated that excessive occupational needs, fear of errors, unsafe work environment and weak communications are among health promotion obstacles for nurses. The inclusion of welfare programs in work place will have a positive effect on health promotion and results in improvement of health, enhancement of creativity, satisfaction, and reduction of health care costs [28].

5. Limitations and Recommendations

Since the present research studied a limited number of students, its generalization to other conditions and situations must be performed with caution. It is recommended that some research be made on the perceived situations of nursing in broader dimensions and in other educational levels of nursing discipline.

Conflict of Interests

The authors declare that they have no conflict of interests.

Acknowledgments

This study is a part of a thesis and research project approved by Shahid Beheshti University of Medical Sciences. The authors would like to thank the International Branch of Shahid Beheshti University of Medical Sciences for its financial support and all the participants who sincerely expressed their feeling and views of nursing's situational influences on their health promotion and enabled researchers to carry out this study.

References

[1] L. Haddad, D. Kane, D. Rajacich, S. Cameron, and R. Al-Ma'aitah, "A comparison of health practices of Canadian and Jordanian nursing students," *Public Health Nursing*, vol. 21, no. 1, pp. 85–90, 2004.

[2] B. K. Lee, S. M. Yanicki, and J. Solowoniuk, "Value of a health behavior change reflection assignment for health promotion learning," *Education for Health: Change in Learning and Practice*, vol. 24, no. 2, pp. 1–13, 2011.

[3] D. Chhim, *Comparison of health promotion lifestyles of family nurse practitioner students and non-nursing students [M.S. thesis of Science in Nursing]*, California State University, Long Beach, Calif, USA, 2009.

[4] L. Liimatainen, M. Poskiparta, A. Sjögren, T. Kettunen, and P. Karhila, "Investigating student nurses' constructions of health promotion in nursing education," *Health Education Research*, vol. 16, no. 1, pp. 33–48, 2001.

[5] J. Needleman, E. T. Kurtzman, and K. W. Kizer, "Performance measurement of nursing care: state of the science and the current consensus," *Medical Care Research and Review*, vol. 64, no. 2, pp. 10–43, 2007.

[6] V. Kemppainen, K. Tossavainen, and H. Turunen, *Nurses' Role in Health Promotion Practice: An Integrative Review*, Health Promotion International Advance Access, Health Promotion InternationalShahid Beheshti University of Medical Science, 2012, http://heapro.Oxfordjournals.org/.

[7] Medical Group News Website, "Chief of Nursing Council of Iran said if they do not hire 23 thousand nurses, community nurses do what they did in year 83," 2012, http://www.pezeshk.us/?p=24236.

[8] Y. C. Hesiao, M. Y. Chen, Y. M. Gau, L. L. Hung, S. H. Chang, and H. M. Tsai, "Short-term effects of a health promotion course for Taiwanese nursing students," *Public Health Nursing*, vol. 22, no. 1, pp. 74–81, 2005.

[9] K. A. Coey-Boerner, *The relationship between social support and health-promoting lifestyle behaviors in uninsured adults [M.S. thesis of Science in Nursing]*, Family Nurse practitioner at university of Wisconsin, Oshkosh, Wis, USA, 2010.

[10] K. K. Paraska and C. C. Clark, *Health Promotion in Nursing Practice*, Jones and Bartlett Learning, Sudbury, Mass, USA, 1st edition, 2011.

[11] A. Robotham and M. Frost, *Health Visiting: Specialist Community Public Health Nursing*, Elsevier, New York, NY, USA, 2nd edition, 2005.

[12] J. B. Butts and K. L. Rich, *Philosophies and Theories for Advanced Nursing Practice*, Jones and Bartlett Learning, Sudbury, Mass, USA, 2011.

[13] S. H. Rankin, K. D. Stallings, and F. London, *Patient Education in Health and Illness*, Lippincott Williams & Wilkins, Philadelphia, Pa, USA, 5th edition, 2005.

[14] R. D. Galloway, "Health promotion: causes, beliefs and measurements," *Clinical Medicine and Research*, vol. 1, no. 3, pp. 249–258, 2003.

[15] A. W. Finkelman and C. Kenner, *Professional Nursing Concepts: Competencies for Quality Leadership*, Jones and Bartlett Learning, Sudbury, Mass, USA, 2010.

[16] E. D. S. Cockrell, *Pre nursing student's perceptions of the nursing profession [M.S. thesis of Science]*, Graduate Faculty of the Louisiana State University and Agricultural and Mechanical College, School of Human Resource and Workforce Development, 2002.

[17] T. Eman, S. Cowman, and A. Edgar, "A triangulation study: Bahraini nursing students' perception of nursing as a career," *Journal of Nursing Education and Practice*, vol. 2, no. 3, pp. 81–92, 2012.

[18] P. Grainger and C. Bolan, "Perceptions of nursing as a career choice of students in the Baccalaureate nursing program," *Nurse Education Today*, vol. 26, no. 1, pp. 38–44, 2006.

[19] K. L. Rush, B. McCracken, and C. Talley, "Nursing students' self-perceptions as insiders in the practice culture," *Nurse Education in Practice*, vol. 9, no. 5, pp. 314–321, 2009.

[20] C. Duffield and L. O'Brien-Pallas, "The causes and consequences of nursing shortages: a helicopter view of the research," *Australian Health Review*, vol. 26, no. 1, pp. 186–193, 2003.

[21] G. LoBiondo-Wood and J. Haber, *Nursing Research: Methods and Critical Appraisal for Evidence-Based Practice*, Mosby, St. Louis, Mo, USA, 2006.

[22] D. F. Polit and C. T. Beck, *Essentials of Nursing Research. Appraising Evidence for Nursing Practice*, Wolters Kluwer Health, Lippincott Williams & Wilkins, Philadelphia, Pa, USA, 7th edition, 2010.

[23] P. Mongkhonsiri, *The mindful self: sence of self and health promotion lifestyle behaviors among Thai college women [Ph.D. thesis of Philosophy in Nursing]*, Massey University, Palmerston North , New Zealand, 2007.

[24] Y. Zhang and B. M. Wildemuth, "Qualitative analysis of content," in *Applications of Social Research Methods to Questions in Information and Library Science*, B. Wildemuth, Ed., Libraries Unlimited, Westport, Conn, USA, 2009.

[25] H. Hsieh and S. E. Shannon, "Three approaches to qualitative content analysis," *Qualitative Health Research*, vol. 15, no. 9, pp. 1277–1288, 2005.

[26] N. J. Pender, C. L. Murdaugh, and M. A. Parsons, *Health Promotion in Nursing Practice*, Pearson Education, Boston, Mass, USA, 6th edition, 2011.

[27] H. J. S. Speziale and D. R. Carpenter, *Qualitative Research in Nursing. Advancing the Humanistic Imperative*, Lippincott Williams & Wilkins, Philadelphia, Pa, USA, 3rd edition, 2003.

[28] D. McElligott, K. L. Capitulo, D. L. Morris, and E. R. Click, "The effect of a holistic program on health-promoting behaviors in hospital registered nurses," *Journal of Holistic Nursing*, vol. 28, no. 3, pp. 175–183, 2010.

[29] M. N. Kalyani, F. Sharif, M. Moattari, N. Jamshidi, and S. Karami, "Decrease in motivation of nursing students: a qualitative study," *Iranian Journal of Nursing Research*, vol. 6, no. 21, pp. 47–58, 2011.

[30] L. A. Gazzaz, *Saudi nurses' perception of nursing as an occupational choice: a qualitative interview study [Ph.D. thesis of Philosophy]*, University of Nottingham, 2009.

[31] J. F. Hong, S. Sermesri, and B. Keiwkarnka, "Health-promoting lifestyles of nursing students in Mahidol University," *Journal of Public Health and Development*, vol. 5, no. 1, pp. 27–40, 2007.

[32] E. D. Lyckhage and E. Pilhammar, "The importance of awareness of nursing students' denotative images of nursing," *Journal of Nursing Education*, vol. 47, no. 12, pp. 537–543, 2008.

[33] S. P. Davis, "Commentary: nurses as champions of health promotion," *Southern Online Journal of Nursing Research*, vol. 8, no. 3, 2011, http://www.snrs.org/.

[34] E. Rash, "Advanced practice nursing students' perceptions of health promotion," *Southern Online Journal of Nursing Research*, vol. 8, no. 3, 2008, http://www.resourcenter.net/images/snrs/files/sojnr_articles2/vol08num03art03.html.

7

Prevention, Rehabilitation, and Mitigation Strategies of Cognitive Deficits in Aging with HIV: Implications for Practice and Research

David E. Vance

School of Nursing, University of Alabama at Birmingham, Birmingham, AL 35222, USA

Correspondence should be addressed to David E. Vance; devance@uab.edu

Academic Editors: P. Di Giulio, S. McClement, and R. Northway

Highly active antiretroviral therapy has given the chance to those living with HIV to keep on living, allowing them the opportunity to age and perhaps age successfully. Yet, there are severe challenges to successful aging with HIV, one of which is cognitive deficits. Nearly half of those with HIV experience cognitive deficits that can interfere with everyday functioning, medical decision making, and quality of life. Given that cognitive deficits develop with more frequency and intensity with increasing age, concerns mount that as people age with HIV, they may experience more severe cognitive deficits. These concerns become especially germane given that by 2015, 50% of those with HIV will be 50 and older, and this older cohort of adults is expected to grow. As such, this paper focuses on the etiologies of such cognitive deficits within the context of cognitive reserve and neuroplasticity. From this, evidence-based and hypothetical prevention (i.e., cognitive prescriptions), rehabilitation (i.e., speed of processing training), and mitigation (i.e., spaced retrieval method) strategies are reviewed. Implications for nursing practice and research are posited.

1. Introduction

Highly active antiretroviral therapy (HAART) helps treat and prevent the spread of HIV [1–4] but also provides the opportunity for people to age with this disease [5]. This is welcome news to the 33 million people worldwide who are living with this disease [6]. Still, this population represents an enormous strain on the healthcare system of many countries grappling with this disease. For example, in South Africa approximately 17.8% of those between 18 and 49 are infected with HIV [6, 7], which means they must make difficult decisions in allocating resources and rationing healthcare [8–10]. All of this is occurring within the larger context of worldwide aging. The fastest growing age group on the planet is those 60 and older which constitutes 700 million people, and this cohort will swell to 2 billion by 2050 [11].

In part due to the unprecedented and historical event of global aging [12] along with HAART increasing the lifespan of those infected with HIV, the number of older adults with HIV is increasing ([5]; Figure 1). In the United States, it is projected that by 2015, half of those with HIV will be 50 and older [13, 14]. Although many are aging with this disease, later-life infections also occur. Those 50 and older account for 15% of all new diagnoses [15]. All of this ushers in new concerns such as how to promote quality of life and facilitate successful aging with HIV.

According to P. B. Baltes and M. M. Baltes [16], successful aging requires competencies in eight areas: length of life, biological health, cognitive efficiency, mental health, social competence, productivity, personal control, and life satisfaction. If one possesses a sufficient amount of these competencies, one is considered to be aging successfully. However, some of these competencies may be more important in promoting successful aging than others. In particular, cognitive efficiency or cognitive health, just like physical health, is often taken for granted until it is compromised. It can be argued that optimal cognitive functioning is needed to help promote biological health (i.e., remembering to take medication [17]), mental health (i.e., being able to exert enough cognitive energy to consciously switch attention from dwelling on negative thoughts to positive thoughts [18]), social competence (i.e., attending to details in conversation

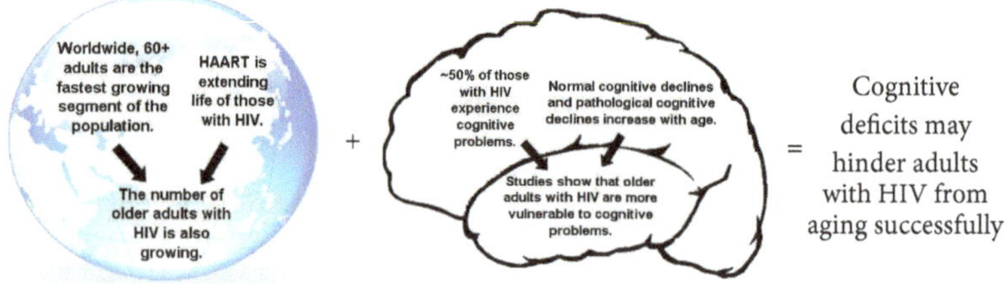

FIGURE 1: Older adults with HIV will be more at risk for cognitive deficits.

[19]), personal control (i.e., decision making such as in finances [20, 21]), and life satisfaction (i.e., remembering and reflecting on personal events and deriving meaning [22–24]). Based on this argument, optimal cognitive functioning is one of the most important competencies needed to help adults with HIV age successfully.

Unfortunately, HIV not only affects the immune system, but it also produces neurological sequelae often resulting in cognitive deficits [25, 26]. In a cross-sectional study, Heaton and colleagues [27] administered a neuropsychological battery to 1,555 adults with HIV (M_{age} = 43.2; SD = 8.5) from six sites across the United States. In this sample, 52% of patients exhibited observed cognitive deficits; specifically, 33% exhibited asymptomatic neurocognitive deficits, 12% exhibited mild neurocognitive disorder, 5% exhibited confounded neurocognitive deficits, and 2% exhibited HIV-related dementia. In fact, studies have shown that even after 1 year of being diagnosed with HIV, changes in brain chemistry and metabolism are evident which correspond to poorer cognitive performance [28–30].

Given that increasing age is associated with more cognitive complaints, cognitive deficits, and the risk for pathological cognitive aging (i.e., Alzheimer's disease, vascular dementia, and Lewy body dementia) [31–33], concerns mount that as people age with HIV, they may become more vulnerable for developing such cognitive deficits and dementia (Figure 1; [34–38]). As highlighted in Figure 1, this risk is further increased since HIV produces systemic inflammation and neuroinflammation which may accelerate normal aging and brain aging, respectively [39–42]. In a recent study, Vance et al. [43] administered a comprehensive neuropsychological and everyday functioning battery to four groups of participants: (1) 47 younger adults with HIV (<50), (2) 31 older adults with HIV (50+), (3) 43 younger adults without HIV (<50), and (4) 41 older adults without HIV (50+). These researchers found that as a group, the older adults with HIV performed the worst on all 9 measures; furthermore, significant main effects for both age and HIV were found in a variety of cognitive domains including executive functioning and reasoning, speed of processing, memory, and fine psychomotor ability.

Similarly, in a sample of 59 adults with and 55 adults without HIV, Baldewicz and colleagues [44] administered a neuropsychological battery every 6 months to them for over 8 years. Over time, those with HIV exhibited significant declines in speed of processing and fine motor speed compared to their HIV-negative counterparts. Also, those who progressed to AIDS (a CD4+ lymphocyte count less than 200 cells/mm^3) experienced the worst declines in cognitive functioning. Likewise, in a sample of 182 adults with HIV, Valcour and colleagues [45] found that older adults with HIV were nearly three times more likely to develop HIV-associated dementia than younger adults with HIV. This and other studies reinforce the prevalence of such a cognitive vulnerability phenotype in older adults with HIV [17, 36, 46–52].

Thus, the purpose of this paper is to provide an overview on the cognitive sequelae observed in adults with HIV, especially as they age and are more vulnerable to such cognitive deficits. In doing so, the known and possible mechanisms of such cognitive deficits are examined within the context of cognitive reserve. Next, within this context, prevention, rehabilitation, and mitigation strategies are examined; this paper includes both known evidence-based strategies as well as potential strategies that might be effective in augmenting cognition in this population. Finally, general directions and implications for nursing practice and research are posited.

2. Cognitive Reserve and Neuroplasticity

The brain's ability to efficiently process information by using existing and alternative neural networks in lieu of damage or disease-related insults (e.g., transient ischemic attack) is referred to as cognitive reserve [53–57]. In its most simplistic form, cognitive reserve refers to the complexity, efficiency, and strength of the neural connections in the brain; it is from these intricate connections in which neurons communicate to each other and convey information that cognition emerges. The more intricate and efficient these connections, the faster neural communication is transmitted and the more complex the thoughts that can emerge from such communication. However, this complexity also produces a protective effect. For example, if some of the neural connections are severed due to disuse, traumatic brain injury, or disease-related insults, information can be rerouted through alternative neural pathways so that neural information can still be communicated and cognition can continue to function. This simplistic explanation can be seen in Figure 2. In the left panel, a neural system that is operating at peak efficiency is represented. Information from neuron A at level 1 is able to transmit neural information through many pathways down to level 3 where it needs to go; however, as indicated by the dark bold lines, there may be a preferred path that is used more consistently which reflects over learning (i.e., routine). This

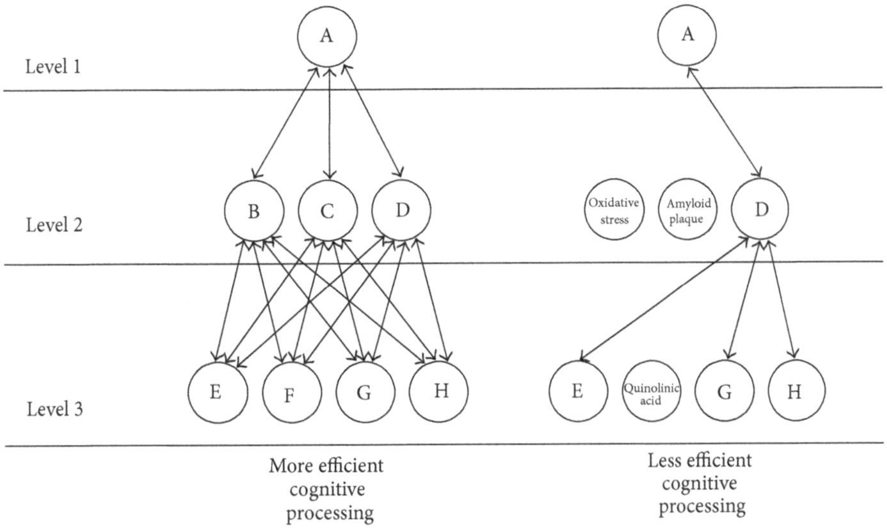

FIGURE 2: Neural communication and cognitive reserve. Circles represent neurons and arrows represent neural pathways.

routine path reflects a strong neural pathway. In contrast, in the right panel of Figure 2, the neural system is not operating at peak efficiency. Neurons B, C, and F are compromised by oxidative stress, amyloid plaques, and quinolinic acid, respectively. Because neurons B, C, and F are not functional due to damage or neural death, the number of paths leading from level 1 to level 3 is dramatically reduced. So this neural system will be more vulnerable to cognitive disruption because there are generally less efficient pathways available in communicating neural information. Furthermore, cognitive efficiency would decrease more as the existing neurons are compromised. Thus, the greater one's cognitive reserve (i.e., number and strength of connections between neurons), the more one is able to withstand neurological insults and maintain cognitive efficiency.

Many factors affect cognitive reserve such as health status, stress and negative emotion, substance use, genetics, and environment [53, 58–61]; however, the underlying process that increases or decreases cognitive reserve is positive neuroplasticity and negative neuroplasticity, respectively [62]. Positive neuroplasticity refers to the nervous system's ability to increase the number and strength of connections between neurons in response to novel stimuli. Likewise, negative neuroplasticity refers to the nervous system's ability to decrease the number and strength of connections (i.e., atrophy) between neurons in response to lack of novel stimuli. This process of cognitive reserve and cognition is well documented in animal studies that use the enriched environmental paradigm and human studies involving taxi drivers, older adults, and those with dementia.

The enriched environmental paradigm used with rats [63, 64] and dogs [65] epitomizes these concepts. For example, genetically similar rats (i.e., from the same colony) are randomly placed to live in one of three conditions: impoverished, standard, or enriched environments. In the impoverish environment, rats are placed one to a cage, so these rats have no other rats with which to socialize and interact. In the standard environment, rats are placed three to a cage, so these rats have other rats with which to socialize and interact. In the enriched environment, several rats are placed to a cage that contains toys for them to explore, so these rats have other rats with which to socialize and interact and have toys with which to explore and interact. Otherwise, the rats receive identical food, water, and other care. After exposure to these environments for a set period of time (i.e., several weeks to several months depending on the study), researchers placed these rats in mazes to test their memory and spatial abilities. Rats placed in the impoverished environment performed statistically worse on maze tasks than those rats placed in the standard environment; likewise, rats placed in the standard environment performed statistically worse on maze tasks than those rats placed in the enriched environment [56, 63]. These findings suggest that being placed in an impoverished environment leads to worse cognitive functioning (i.e., maze performance); this is indicative of negative neuroplasticity. Similarly, these findings suggest that being placed in an enriched environment leads to better cognitive functioning (i.e., maze performance); this is indicative of positive neuroplasticity [61]. Further analyses confirm that changes in brain chemistry and brain morphology correspond to cognitive functioning (i.e., maze performance) in rats. Specifically, more dendritic connections between neurons and higher levels of brain neurotrophic factor were observed in the brains of rats in the enriched environment compared to rats in the standard and impoverished environments; likewise, this same pattern of findings was found in the brains of rats in the standard environment compared to rats in the impoverished environment [66–69].

Just as rats were exposed to novel and complex stimuli in the enriched environmental paradigm, humans are also exposed to various levels of novel environmental stimuli that can also produce neuroplastic changes that either increase or decrease cognitive reserve. A seminal study investigating this phenomenon in humans is the London Taxi Driver Study

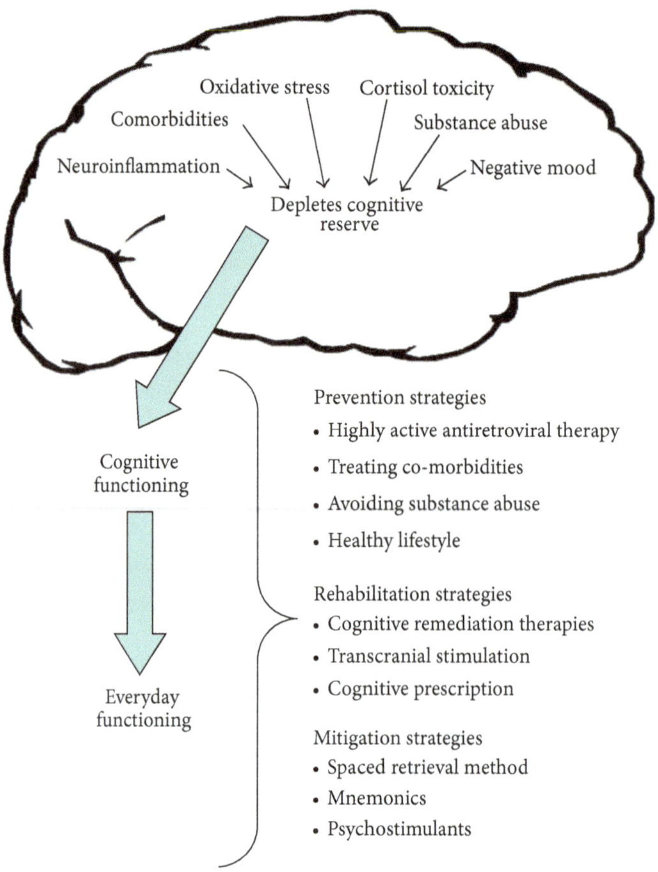

FIGURE 3: The effects of HIV on brain function and preventive, rehabilitative, and mitigation strategies.

[70, 71]. In this naturalistic study, researchers examined two groups of people (i.e., London taxi drivers and London bus drivers) who underwent two different training conditions for their jobs. In order for London taxi drivers to earn their license, they had to engage in a 2 to 4 year training program whereby they had to familiarize themselves with London's 25,000 streets and learn how to navigate through them, as well as recall many points of interest along the way. This intense training program represents an enriched environment. The London bus drivers did not participate in such an intense training program in order to qualify for their license. In addition, bus drivers were assigned a route that changed little. This lack of training represents a standard or impoverished condition. MRIs of the brains of these taxi drivers were compared to brains of London bus drivers; this revealed significantly larger midposterior hippocampi (brain structures necessary for encoding and consolidating memory) in taxi drivers than bus drivers. Interestingly, the more years of being a taxi driver was associated with larger hippocampi; however, such an association was not found for this group of bus drivers. Thus, this study shows that exposure to novel and challenging stimuli may actually change brain morphology in humans.

These principles of neuroplasticity and cognitive reserve have also been demonstrated in a seminal study focusing on older adults. Boyke et al. [72] administered a brain MRI (i.e., Time 1) to 69 community-dwelling older adults (M_{age} = 60; 50–67) and then attempted to teach them how to juggle in a 3-ball cascade pattern. Approximately 3 months later, after 25 of these participants learned how to successfully juggle for at least 1 minute, brain MRIs (i.e., Time 2) were administered again. Then approximately 3 months later, brain MRIs (i.e., Time 3) of these participants were administered after they stopped juggling. These researchers observed that the nucleus accumbens and hippocampi increased in size from Time 1 to Time 2 as people learned to juggle; this reflects positive neuroplasticity and a change in brain morphology indicative of increased cognitive reserve. Likewise, it was observed that these same brain structures decreased in size from Time 2 to Time 3 as people stopped juggling; this reflects negative neuroplasticity and a change in brain morphology indicative of decreased cognitive reserve.

These studies demonstrate that exposure to stimulating and enriching activities promotes positive neuroplasticity and may increase cognitive reserve. Meanwhile, these studies also provide evidence that being exposed to nonstimulating and nonenriching activities promotes negative neuroplasticity and may decrease cognitive reserve. In fact, many studies are investigating how these principles of neuroplasticity and cognitive reserve may be used to protect against age-related cognitive impairment and dementia [24, 54, 73, 74]. For example, Roe and colleagues [75] investigated whether educational attainment, an indicator of being exposed to stimulating activities that may increase cognitive reserve, is related to the delay in the onset of cognitive symptoms of Alzheimer's-related dementia in a sample of 37 adults with and 161 adults without this disease. Using radiotracers and positron emission tomography to measure the amount of fibrillar beta-amyloid (i.e., amyloid plaques) as an indicator of disease severity, these researchers observed that even in the presence of high levels of fibrillar beta-amyloid which impedes neural communication (Figure 1), those with high levels of education (and essentially more cognitive reserve) performed better cognitively. Thus, this study suggests that even when amyloid plaques may reduce the number of connections between neurons, remaining neural connections, which reflect cognitive reserve, allow information to be rerouted to other neurons which supports continued cognitive functioning. This rerouting process of cognitive reserve is observed in other systems in the body. For example, in occlusive coronary heart disease where blood vessels are blocked, coronary collateral arteries circumvent such blockage by providing an alternative route for circulation, which reduces the risk of myocardial ischemia [76]. By having such alternative and redundant function, such bodily systems, whether they are nervous or circulatory, can continue in lieu of diseases and insults. Such information becomes quite germane considering the variety of insults that can compromise cognitive reserve in those aging with HIV [77].

3. Mechanisms of Cognitive Deficits

As highlighted in Figure 3, several mechanisms endemic to HIV and normal aging can be damaging to the brain, deplete cognitive reserve, and diminish cognitive functioning. Although by no means exhaustive, some of the most widely recognized mechanisms are neuroinflammation; comorbidities; oxidative stress; and cortisol toxicity, negative affect, and substance abuse.

3.1. Neuroinflammation. Inflammation is an immune response to pathogens, disease, injury, and oxidative stress and is a fundamental component in the healing process. Although normally a good biological process, prolonged inflammation causes tissue damage and can result in neurodegeneration and impair neurogenesis [78]. Unfortunately, even when HIV is controlled through HAART, the body still responds to the virus by producing cytokines (i.e., molecules that increase or decrease immune response) that modulate the immune system, thus creating inflammation in the body and neuroinflammation in the brain. In fact, the accelerated aging observed in HIV is often attributed to this inflammation; for this reason, HIV is considered a "slow burner" inflammation disease as well as an immunodeficiency disease [79].

The link between neuroinflammation and cognitive functioning has been well established [78, 80–82].

For example, in a large sample of older adults, Yaffe and colleagues [83] examined the association between cognitive functioning as measured by the Modified Mini-Mental State Examination and inflammation as measured by serum levels of inflammatory molecules (i.e., IL-6, TNF-α, and CRP) at baseline and over 2 years. These researchers found that those with the highest tertile of CRP and IL-6 at baseline and 2 years later performed significantly poorer on this cognitive test at baseline and 2 years compared to those in the lowest tertile for these inflammatory markers. In fact, those in the highest tertile had a 24% increased risk of cognitive decline over 2 years.

Similarly, this neuroinflammation observed in HIV has been attributed to many of the cognitive deficits that are observed in this population [84]. To exemplify this, Thompson and colleagues [85] compared MRI brain scans of 26 adults with HIV treated with HAART to 15 adults without HIV. These researchers found that even in these medically stable adults with HIV, thinning was observed in the prefrontal parietal cortices compared to the control group. Such cortical thinning is attributed to the inflammation and neuroinflammation that is occurring with this disease. Thus, addressing neuroinflammation may be an area ripe for cognitive intervention.

3.2. Comorbidities. That which affects the body also affects the brain. Given this basic principle, it is not surprising that comorbidities such as heart disease, liver disease such as hepatitis C, and renal disease also affect neurological and cognitive functioning [86]. For example, untreated hypertension leads to small-vessel cerebrovascular disease that creates white matter lesions; these small lesions are basically damaged neural tissue [87, 88]. Using MRIs, de Leeuw and colleagues [87] found that in a sample of 1,077 community-dwelling older adults (M_{age} = 51; 60–90 years) the duration of hypertension corresponded to more periventricular and subcortical white matter lesions. In addition, these researchers found that those adults with untreated hypertension experienced more of such lesions in both of these brain areas.

In another example, Bruehl and colleagues [89] compared the cognitive functioning of 41 adults with type 2 diabetes to 47 adults without type 2 diabetes matched on age, gender, and education. These researchers found that those with type 2 diabetes performed more poorly on cognitive tests compared to those without type 2 diabetes. In fact, MRI scans revealed that those with type 2 diabetes also had decreased volume in their prefrontal cortex (the brain region needed for executive functioning and reasoning) and hippocampi (the brain structures needed for memory). Further analysis revealed that the decreased volume of the prefrontal cortex was statistically correlated to poorer glycemic control. This study and several others [90, 91] revealed a similar association between comorbidities and cognitive functioning [86]. Such comorbidity and cognitive deficits are of concern given that HAART can create or exacerbate such comorbidities and that such comorbidities (e.g., heart disease and hypercholesterolemia) are highly prevalent in older adults with HIV [49, 92–94].

3.3. Oxidative Stress. Oxygen is needed by the body to perform a host of functions, yet oxygen itself is a corrosive element and damages tissues. In particular, reactive oxygen species, sometimes referred to as free radicals, interact with tissues and produce a variety of cellular and molecular changes that cause inflammation [95]. To counteract the detrimental effects of such reactive oxygen species, the body utilizes an intricate system of antioxidant mechanisms whereby such effects are minimized or rendered inert. Sadly, such antioxidant mechanisms become less efficient with increased age. As such, these reactive oxygen species damage tissues; this is frequently referred to as oxidative stress [96]. In particular, reactive oxygen species can damage mitochondria (i.e., the energy producing organelle in cells) which subsequently impair cell function. But reactive oxygen species can also progressively damage DNA over time. Since DNA is used to generate cells and tissue, this accumulated damage results in less efficient tissues being produced resulting in poor systemic functioning. In fact, the effects of oxidative stress on mitochondria and DNA are one of the prevailing theories on the causes of aging [52, 95].

The brain, being composed of neural tissue, is also negatively affected by oxidative stress. This effect has been observed in well-controlled rat and human studies. Singh and colleagues [97] compared rats that received food enriched with folic acid, an antioxidant, over an 8-week period to same age rats that received standard food. These researchers found that those rats that received folic acid performed better than their counterparts on maze, active avoidance, and passive avoidance tests which served as indicators of cognitive functioning. Upon further examination, lipid perioxidant, a proxy of aging, was significantly lower in the brains of the folic acid fed rats. This and other studies suggest that foods rich in antioxidants can be neuroprotective and support cognitive reserve [98, 99].

In humans, this protective relationship has also been observed. In a sample of 1,389 older adults (60–70 years), Akbaraly and colleagues [100] examined plasma selenium (an antioxidant) levels and cognitive functioning over 9 years. Using a series of linear and logistic models, these researchers found that a decline in selenium was associated with a decline in cognitive functioning. With the abundance of evidence supporting antioxidant supplementation on brain health and cognition, such supplementation could provide some protection against age-related neurodegenerative diseases [101–104].

3.4. Cortisol Toxicity, Negative Affect, and Substance Abuse. HIV is a stigmatizing disease that can produce an intense emotional reaction for those infected [105]. Unfortunately, one's emotional state, specifically experiencing severe negative affect or mood, can obviously impact cognition in at least three ways: (1) it increases cortisol levels, (2) it competes for existing cognitive resources, and (3) it can result in poor coping techniques (i.e., substance abuse). First, a negative emotional state is associated with increased cytokines (an inflammatory molecule) and stress hormones like cortisol that over time can cause inflammation which can impair or damage neural tissue [106]. In particular, stress, anxiety, and depression can lead to a response of the hypothalamic-pituitary-adrenal axis whereby glucocorticoids (i.e., cortisol) are secreted [107]. Although cortisol is needed by the body to suppress the immune system, increase energy production, and help metabolize proteins, fats, and carbohydrates during periods of stress [108], prolonged exposure can damage the brain, in particular hippocampal neurons [109, 110]. In a cross-sectional study of 967 older adults (50–70 years), Lee and colleagues [111] found that higher levels of salivary cortisol levels were predictive of poorer cognitive functioning across multiple domains (i.e., speed of processing, verbal memory, visual memory, learning, and executive functioning). In a longitudinal study of 538 older adults (70–79 years), Karlamangla and colleagues [112] found that higher levels of urinary cortisol levels at baseline were predictive of poorer cognitive functioning seven years later. Furthermore, this association was still observed after taking into consideration age, gender, education, blood pressure, smoking, and cardiovascular disease. Thus, such dysregulation of the hypothalamic-pituitary-adrenal axis and subsequent long-term exposure of cortisol may slowly deplete cognitive reserve and increase the risk of developing cognitive deficits.

Second, ruminating over such negative affect can compete for cognitive resources that otherwise could normally be allocated to other tasks [18]. For example, it is difficult to concentrate on and switch attention to a complex accounting problem (e.g., balancing one's checkbook) when one is also dwelling on a severe emotional problem that is consuming one's mental resources. In fact, many studies clearly demonstrate that depression, stress, and anxiety are associated with poorer cognitive functioning [86]. Using the analogy of a computer virus, negative affect can slow down speed of processing which can detrimentally impact cognitive functioning. Sadly, as a group, older adults with HIV do experience considerable negative affect and generally have a fragile social network to help cope with such aversive emotional states [113]. For example, in a sample of 914 older adults with HIV, Grov and colleagues [114] observed that 63% of their sample experienced clinically significant levels of depressive symptomatology. Similarly, Kalichman et al. [115] found in a sample of 113 middle-aged and older men with HIV that 27% thought about taking their life within the past week; clearly, such suicidal ideation can consume normal rational thought processes. Ostensibly, negative affect is present in this clinical population and it may be severe enough to interfere with cognitive functioning.

Third, poor coping skills with such negative affect can also lead to poorer cognitive function such as through engagement with alcohol and substance use [116–118]. Current and past alcohol and substance abuse can produce obvious neurological problems that negatively impact cognitive functioning [119, 120]. In particular, glial cells, which support neuronal functioning and aid in forming connections between neurons, are compromised by many substances; this leaves neurons more vulnerable to oxidative stress and cortisol toxicity [53, 121]. Alcohol and substance abuse has also been shown to reduce hippocampi size and cognitive functioning in adolescence; because of this reduced growth and diminished cognitive reserve, such adolescents may be more vulnerable to developing cognitive deficits in later life [122]. In a sample of 98 adults with HIV, Fazeli and colleagues

[123] found that self-reported alcohol and substance use was predictive of poorer cognitive functioning. This and other studies support these general findings [47, 77].

4. Prevention Strategies

Implementing strategies of protecting cognition is not often considered until one observes such loss in a friend or family member. Yet, prevention strategies to avoid cognitive loss are obviously preferred rather than relying on rehabilitation and mitigation strategies that may be only moderately effective. Although by no means exhaustive, a few of the more salient strategies of preventing cognitive deficits in adults aging with HIV are receiving HAART, treating comorbidities, treating depression and anxiety, avoiding substance abuse, and engaging in a healthy lifestyle [38].

4.1. HAART. Treating HIV with HAART so that the virus does not compromise the immune system and thus prevent opportunistic infections, which can also impact brain health, is the most obvious strategy for preventing cognitive deficits in this population [124]. In 59 adults with HIV who were either HAART-naïve or about to change their HAART regimen due to treatment failure (i.e., the medication was no longer suppressing viral replication), Parsons et al. [125] assessed the cognitive functioning of these participants at baseline (before taking HAART) and six months later (after taking HAART). These researchers found that those participants who achieved successful viral suppression also experienced improvements in their cognitive functioning compared to those who did not achieve successful viral suppression.

Despite HAART's ability to protect and improve cognitive functioning in adults with HIV [126, 127], four caveats must be considered when using these medications. First, the HAART medications are not equally effective in crossing the blood brain barrier; in other words, some medications are more efficient at entering the brain and hindering the detrimental effects of HIV than others [128]. For example, within one of the class of HAART medications known as nucleoside reverse transcriptase inhibitors, the medications tenofovir, zalcitabine, and didanosine do not cross the blood brain barrier well while zidovudine and abacavir do so very well. Therefore, prescribing HAART medications to address cognitive deficits must take this penetration of the blood brain barrier into consideration. (For more information, Letendre and colleagues [128] provide a schema for which HAART medications have lower, intermediate, and high blood brain barrier penetration.)

Second, a high adherence rate (i.e., 95%) to HAART is needed to achieve viral suppression and avoid drug resistance and viral mutation [129, 130]. Unfortunately, poor medication adherence can lead to cognitive problems [17]; likewise, cognitive problems can lead to poor medication adherence [131–133]. For these reasons, effective strategies are needed to remember to take one's medications consistently. (For an example of such medication adherence strategies, see the spaced retrieval method in the Mitigation Strategies section of this paper.)

Third, some of the HAART medications can be neurotoxic. For example, efavirenz, a nonnucleoside reverse transcriptase inhibitor, increases the risk of developing cognitive deficits [134]. Although the exact mechanism of these neurotoxic effects is unknown [126], it has been suggested that nonnucleoside reverse transcriptase inhibitors in particular may adversely affect brain metabolism and damage neuronal mitochondria [30, 126, 135].

Finally, HAART creates metabolic syndromes that can either cause or exacerbate comorbidities such as hypercholesterolemia, hypertension, heart disease, and diabetes [94]. These comorbidities have been shown to negatively impact brain health and cognitive functioning [86]. In addition, such comorbidities can produce extra stress on other bodily systems by increasing inflammation and oxidative stress which also impairs neurons [78].

4.2. Treating Comorbidities. As mentioned, the presence of comorbidities exacts a burden on the brain resulting in less cognitive reserve and more cognitive deficits. As such, preventing such comorbidities through healthier lifestyles and treating such comorbidities through medication to restore physiological homeostasis represent a practical strategy for maintaining or improving cognitive functioning. Treating comorbidities with the appropriate medication has been shown in several studies to exert cognitive benefits [86]. For example, in a sample of 18,999 older women (70–81 years), Logroscino et al. [136] examined the effects of different type 2 diabetes treatments on cognitive functioning over a two-year period. These researchers found that those women with type 2 diabetes treated with oral hypoglycaemic agents performed at the same level cognitively to women without type 2 diabetes at baseline and two years later; however, women with type 2 diabetes treated with insulin performed poorer cognitively in comparison. Meanwhile, those women with type 2 diabetes not being treated cognitively performed the worst in general at baseline and two years later.

Similarly, although it is well established that hypertension and heart disease can negatively impact cognitive functioning [137–139], treating such conditions medically can mitigate their affect. Viamonte and colleagues [140] examined the cognitive functioning of 315 community-dwelling older adults without heart disease to 185, 41 and 56 community-dwelling older adults treated for hypertension, heart disease, or a combination of both, respectively. These researchers found that there were no cognitive differences between these groups; this and other studies [141, 142] support the idea that medically treating such comorbidities as hypertension can yield cognitive benefits or protect against the development of cognitive deficits. Thus, with the average number of comorbidities for adults with HIV in their 50s and +60s being 4.40 and 4.52, respectively [94], addressing such comorbidities is an obvious way to support cognitive reserve and cognitive functioning.

4.3. Treating Depression and Anxiety. The prevalence of depression and anxiety across each decade of life for adults with HIV hovers around 40% and 20%, respectively [94]. As already mentioned (see Cortisol, Negative Affect, and Substance Abuse section), there is a strong (and possible causal) connection between negative mood and cognition in this clinical population [143]. In fact, in a sample of 107 adults with HIV, Thames and colleagues [144] found that those who experienced elevated levels of depression reported more cognitive problems. Thus, treating psychiatric comorbidities may also be important for protecting and improving cognitive functioning [145]; in fact, several studies show this. Claypoole and colleagues [146] found that in a sample of 78 adults with HIV suffering from depression and treated with antidepressants for 12 weeks reported significantly fewer cognitive problems and improved on objective measures of cognitive functioning. Given the strong connection between negative mood and cognitive functioning via the hypothalamic-pituitary-adrenal axis [107], treating psychiatric comorbidities such as depression and anxiety should be considered as a potential treatment of cognitive deficits in this clinical population.

4.4. Avoiding Substance Abuse. Substance abuse has been shown in several studies to negatively impact cognitive functioning in normal adults and adults with HIV [123, 147, 148]. Yet, some studies do not support these findings; surprisingly, these findings are mixed [149, 150]. For example, in a sample of 399 adults with HIV categorized into three groups of substance users (134 with no substance use, 131 with nonsyndromic substance use, and 134 with syndromic substance use matched on CD4 nadir, depressive symptomatology, and literacy level), Byrd and colleagues [151] found out the same prevalence of cognitive deficits across these groups, regardless of substance use engagement. In fact, those with a history of cocaine or marijuana use actually had higher levels of verbal fluency. In making sense of these findings, it is important to note that substance use is a complex behavior. For example, some adults who abuse substances may have more cognitive reserve and can withstand such neurological insults than others; thus, cognitive deficits may not always manifest in lieu of substance abuse, and this could explain some of the mixed findings. Another likely explanation of these mixed findings is that many adults who once engaged in substance abuse may have experienced cognitive recovery once abstinent or reduced the level of substance use. For instance, Iudicello and colleagues [152] followed 83 methamphetamine users over a 1-year period and found that those who were able to abstain performed similarly to a healthy matched control while those who continued using did not show cognitive improvement. Other studies also confirm cognitive recovery after abstinence or reduction of use for alcohol, marijuana, and other substances [153–155]. Finally, it has been shown that the recency of substance abuse may be the strongest predictor of experiencing cognitive deficits [156, 157]. Given this evidence, it becomes more certain that not only avoidance of substance abuse is recommended, but reducing or abstaining can improve cognitive functioning.

4.5. Healthy Lifestyle. Related to avoidance of substance abuse, a healthy lifestyle can produce positive outcomes to one's quality of life, to the body, and to the brain. The impact of physical exercise, mental exercise, healthy social interactions and social support, good nutrition, and good sleep on brain health and cognition cannot be emphasized enough [49, 158–160]. In fact, some of these healthy lifestyle factors can also reduce inflammation and oxidative stress that can be damaging to the brain [49, 53]. For example, in several studies, foods rich in polyphenols and antioxidants, which can reduce such oxidative stress and inflammation, have been found to be associated with better cognitive functioning in older adults [161–163]. In fact, green tea, which is rich in polyphenols, has been found to reduce astrogliosis in HIV-1 tat-transgenic mice [164]. Thus, similar cognitively beneficial effects for diet as well as other healthy lifestyle factors may also be observed in adults with HIV.

5. Rehabilitation Strategies

Cognitive deficits that may occur when aging with HIV may be mild or moderate enough such that rehabilitation strategies may be effective in restoring cognitive functioning to near previous levels. But it is also important to note that cognitive deficits may emerge because of transitory conditions (e.g., poor sleep hygiene, negative mood, and thiamine deficiency) that may be addressed by just some simple changes in lifestyle [38]; for that reason, cognitive prescriptions are listed as a potential rehabilitation strategy. Although by no means exhaustive, two other rehabilitation strategies presented (i.e., cognitive remediation therapy and transcranial stimulation) represent novel ways of bolstering positive neuroplasticity and cognitive reserve.

5.1. Cognitive Prescriptions. Given the advantages that a healthy lifestyle exerts on cognitive health, Vance and colleagues [165] have incorporated such advantages into a holistic, individualized behavioral program, called cognitive prescriptions, that may be used to support cognitive reserve and cognitive functioning. In this regard, it may be considered as both a preventative and rehabilitation strategy. Cognitive prescriptions target several lifestyle areas known to affect cognitive functioning; these include intellectual exercise, physical exercise, social engagement, mood support, sleep hygiene, good nutrition, and substance use. In its most basic form, the nurse clinician uses motivational interviewing techniques [166] and dialogues with the patient to determine what goals he or she wishes to pursue in each lifestyle area; from this, specific behavioral goals are developed with clear objective steps for reaching such goals utilizing standard behavioral therapy techniques [167]. Such goals are represented in a highly visual way and displayed in a prominent place (i.e., refrigerator and bathroom mirror) to encourage compliance and facilitate tracking of outcomes. In addition, if certain goals are achieved or need to be altered, the program can easily accommodate the change of old goals for new goals.

For example, if the patient enjoyed painting years ago but has gotten out of the habit but is still interested in doing so, the goal may be to paint one hour a week or paint one 5 × 5 inch painting a week (whatever the patient thinks is appropriate); it is important to make the goals very specific and concrete. This is a goal that may serve in either the intellectual exercise area or, if it is relaxing to the patient, the mood support area. In another example, the patient may be experiencing bouts of insomnia which can obviously impact cognitive functioning [168]. Thus, a goal may be to (1) go for a 30-minute walk every evening and (2) take a warm bath before going to bed to relax. Again, motivational interviewing techniques are used to determine that these are intrinsically appealing activities for the patient. As before, these goals may serve simultaneously in the physical exercise area, the mood support area, and the sleep hygiene area. The advantages of cognitive prescriptions are that they represent a concrete way of supporting positive neuroplasticity and cognitive health [24, 55, 56] while simultaneously addressing other areas to promote overall health and quality of life.

5.2. Cognitive Remediation Therapy. Cognitive remediation therapy represents a collection of various strategies with the expressed purpose to either improve a particular cognitive ability such as memory, executive functioning and reasoning, and psychomotor ability or improve overall cognition. It consists of specially designed cognitive exercises that can also be delivered through several venues such as pencil-and-paper, videotape/DVDs, computer programs (i.e., gaming technology), and class-type workshops [169, 170]. For example, in a sample of 159 community-dwelling normal older adults (65–92), Vance and colleagues [171] randomized these participants into two groups—the internet training (control) condition and the speed of processing training (experimental) condition. Those in the internet training condition engaged in approximately ten hours of exercises designed to improve their skills in learning how to use the worldwide web; however, these exercises were only designed to increase factual knowledge of the internet and not to improve any fluid cognitive abilities. Those in the speed of processing training condition engaged in approximately ten hours of computer exercises designed to improve their visual speed of processing and visual attention as measured by a computer test called the Useful Field of View (UFOV) test. These speed of processing exercises administered in a game-type format required these participants to identify quickly presented objects (i.e., between 17 and 500 milliseconds) in the center of the screen and locate a peripheral object on the screen. Using a double-staircase method in the program, when participants answered incorrectly, the presentation speed was automatically reduced for the next trial, but when participants answered correctly, the presentation speed was automatically increased for the next trial. Thus, this training program forced participants to use their visual speed of processing abilities at their maximum level, and thereby pushed their threshold ability to improve. It was found that those who engaged in the speed of processing training condition improved on measures of visual speed of processing and attention (i.e., UFOV and Starry Night) compared to those in the internet training condition. In addition, the treatment effects were observed even two years after training ceased.

This study is particularly germane to adults with HIV. Marcotte and colleagues [172] found that in a sample of 68 adults with HIV that half experienced cognitive deficits in visual speed of processing as measured by UFOV. This finding is of particular concern given that deficits observed on UFOV tend to increase with age and are found to be associated with poor driving outcomes [170, 173]. Thus, compromised driving skills, as well as other everyday functions that also depend on this cognitive ability, may be a concern as adults continue to age with HIV.

Fortunately, cognitive remediation therapy has been used, similar to the previous study protocol [171], to improve speed of processing in middle-aged and older adults with HIV (M_{age} = 51.55; range 40.7–70.6). In this pre-post two-group experimental design study, Vance et al. [174] randomized these 46 adults into either a speed of processing training condition (n = 22) or to a no-contact control condition (n = 24). Like the previous study, those in the speed of processing training condition received approximately 10 hours of training over a 4-to-6-week period. Compared to the control condition, those assigned to the speed of processing condition significantly improved on UFOV as well as the Timed Instrumental Activities of Daily Living test, a measure of speeded everyday functioning such as looking up phone numbers and identifying items on a shelf of food. Although more work must be done in determining if these findings are consistent with a larger HIV-positive sample and whether the training will improve functioning in other areas such as medication adherence or driving behavior, cognitive remediation therapy represents a viable and noninvasive approach for rehabilitating cognitive abilities in those experiencing cognitive deficits.

However, a caveat about using such cognitive remediation therapies is warranted. Not all cognitive remediation training programs commercially available are the same. Some are designed to improve general cognition while others target particular cognitive abilities such as memory. In selecting such a cognitive remediation therapy, one must be mindful of the research and evidence supporting their use and effectiveness given that some have been tested more thoroughly than others [170, 175].

5.3. Transcranial Stimulation. Transcranial stimulation is a strategy in which either magnetic currents or electrical currents are applied to the scalp over certain brain regions with the goal of enhancing cognitive functioning or in some cases inhibiting certain maladaptive behaviors such as addictions or depression [176–178]. In this paper, focusing more on transcranial direct current stimulation (tDCS), because of relatively cheaper cost and easier access and use than transcranial magnetic stimulation, administration of this particular strategy has been shown to improve cognitive functioning in several studies [179–183]. For example, Lindenberg and colleagues [184] examined brain activity patterns during a motor activity in 20 stroke patients with hemiparesis (i.e., weakness on one side of the body) before and after occupational/physical therapy with half randomized to receive five concurrent sessions with tDCS and the other half randomized to receive five concurrent sham sessions (i.e., without tDCS). Occupational/physical therapy, in conjunction with tDCS, was found to increase neural activity of the ipsilesional motor cortex and resulted in improved motor function as assessed by the Upper Extremity Fugl-Meyer instrument.

Unfortunately, the exact mechanism in which tDCS increases (or in some cases decreases) such neural activity is not fully understood. It has been suggested that tDCS is able to connect remote regions of the brain which may possibly boost existing cognitive ability [179]. More specifically, Nitsche [185] hypothesized that such direct current alters the electrical current across neural membranes. Anodal stimulation (versus cathodal stimulation) in particular flows from the electrode into the scalp and into the brain, pulling the electrical currents of neurons across the surface of the cerebral cortex a few millivolts making them more prone to depolarization. Thus, when signals arrive from other neurons, they are more responsive and more likely to fire which can aid in learning and perhaps promote positive neuroplasticity. In support of this hypothesis, increased activity in the cerebral cortex has been found after utilizing tDCS.

In a recent study, Clark and colleagues [181] used a series of single-blind, randomized studies to examine the effects of tDCS on learning a complex visual task (i.e., identifying concealed objects) in 96 healthy adults. Participants played a virtual reality environment game called "DARWARD Ambush!" in which they had to identify where lethal objects such as bombs were concealed in the pictures based on feedback. These researchers fastened a 10 cm^2 sponge electrode over the right inferior frontal cortex near F10 (i.e., directly over the sphenoid bone). Participants received the direct current 5 minutes before starting the exercise and 30 minutes within the training. Clark and colleagues found that anodal 2.0 milliamp current resulted in significantly better learning that 0.1 milliamp exposure. Other studies have also found that anodal 2.0 milliamp exposure over F10 and F8 (i.e., left prefrontal cortex) may be effective in improving learning and that the effects on learning may last for several hours afterwards [179, 180].

Although tDCS has not been used to boost cognitive functioning in adults with HIV, it has been considered as a possible treatment for depression [186]. In a small sample of 8 adults with HIV suffering from depression, Knotkova and colleagues [187] administered tDCS anodal current over the F3 area (the region of the scalp that corresponds to the dorsolateral prefrontal cortex) and the cathodal current over the contralateral supraorbital region at 2.0 milliamps for 20 minutes for 8 to 10 sessions over consecutive days. These researchers found that depression scores significantly decreased; in fact, they also found that the Mini-Mental State Exam scores improved or remained unchanged. Perhaps because depression can compete for cognitive resources, abating depression may indirectly boost cognitive functioning [86]. Although this is a small pilot study, it does show that tDCS was well tolerated. Given that tDCS was shown to improve learning and cognition in normal adults as seen in Clark and colleagues' [181] study, perhaps this approach could be used with older adults with HIV to rehabilitate cognitive functions that may have declined.

6. Mitigation Strategies

Once cognitive deficits develop, if rehabilitation strategies are not effective in improving existing cognitive abilities, then mitigation strategies should be considered to compensate for the loss of cognitive functioning. Fortunately, the gerontological literature is replete with several cognitive tools such as spaced retrieval method and numerous mnemonics which can easily be translated to those aging with HIV. In addition, some psychopharmacological agents such as psychostimulants may be used to bolster cognitive functioning for brief periods; unfortunately, the use of such medication-related mitigation strategies is not without some potential side effects and other patient costs.

6.1. Spaced Retrieval Method. The spaced retrieval method is a formalized memory strategy used to help people retain a discrete unit of information or fact such as a telephone number or an address [188]. The key to this strategy is to recall the information over progressively longer periods of time until it is finally consolidated into one's long-term memory (Figure 4). For example, the fact to be remembered is presented and then repeated back immediately, then after 30 seconds, 1 minute, 2 minutes, 4 minutes, 8 minutes, and finally 16 minutes. In this stair step recall procedure, if the fact cannot be recalled at any time, then the fact to be remembered is presented again to the person and then it is to be recalled after the previous time point in which the person successfully recalled the fact. This back and forth process continues until the information can be successfully recalled after 16 minutes; once the fact can be recalled after 16 minutes without cues, the information is fully consolidated into one's long-term memory.

Spaced retrieval method has been used in many clinical populations with memory problems including those with aphasia, traumatic brain injury, and early stage dementia [189, 190]. Neundorfer and colleagues [191] used a combination of spaced retrieval method and external mnemonics (i.e., notes and lists) to help 10 older adults with HIV (M_{age} = 50; 50–60) who had executive functioning and memory problems to perform two everyday tasks (e.g., remembering to take medications on time and remembering to attend clinic appointments). These researchers delivered this intervention in eight 30-minute sessions over 4 weeks. In general, the combination of spaced retrieval method and external memory aids was found to be effective in helping those participants compensate for their cognitive problems and successfully complete their everyday tasks. Since this strategy is simple to use and does not require any special equipment, it represents a viable tool for those older adults with HIV experiencing cognitive deficits that interfere with everyday functioning.

6.2. Mnemonics. As just mentioned, spaced retrieval method is a very specific mnemonic that has been shown to be helpful in compensating for cognitive deficits. However, several other mnemonic strategies may also be helpful for older adults with HIV including method of loci, chunking, and external memory aids. All of these strategies are easy to use and do not require any special equipment.

Method of loci is a mnemonic for remembering sequential information by visualizing the information to be remembered with landmarks of a familiar path or items within one's home or a regular routine [192]. For example, as seen in

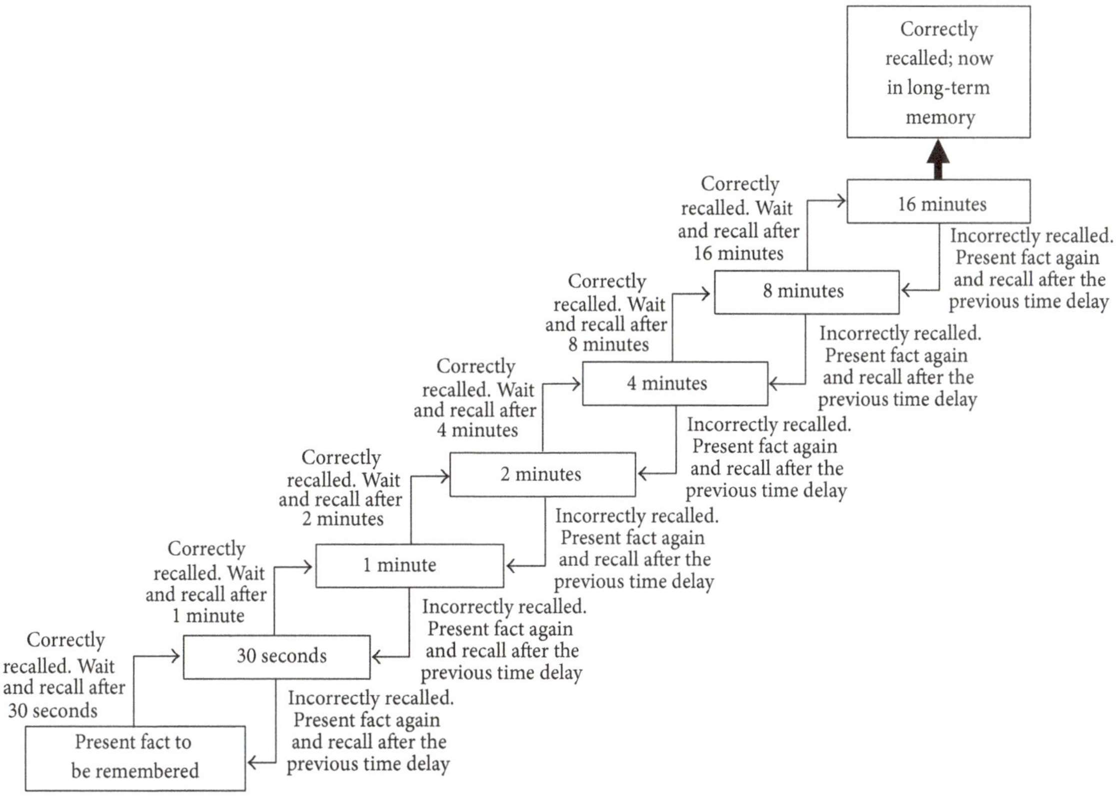

FIGURE 4: Stair step approach of the spaced retrieval method.

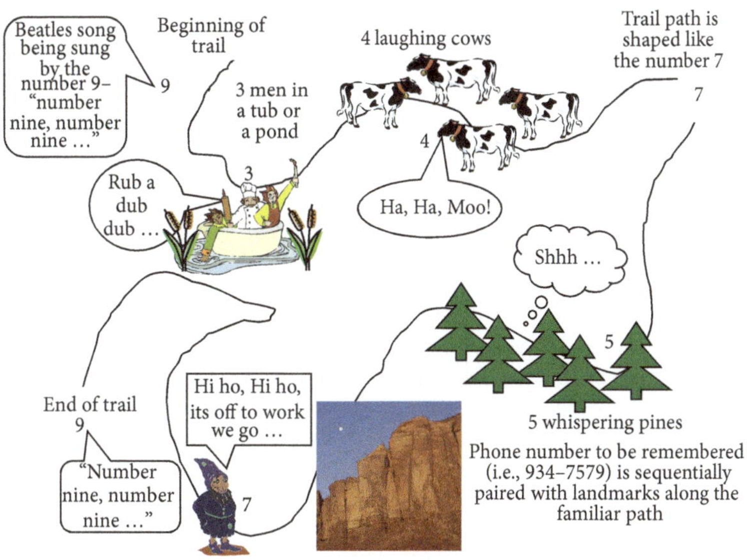
Beatles song being sung by the number 9–"number nine, number nine ..."
Beginning of trail
9
3 men in a tub or a pond
3
Rub a dub dub ...
4 laughing cows
4
Ha, Ha, Moo!
Trail path is shaped like the number 7
7
Shhh ...
5
5 whispering pines
Hi ho, Hi ho, its off to work we go ...
7
End of trail
9
"Number nine, number nine ..."
Phone number to be remembered (i.e., 934–7579) is sequentially paired with landmarks along the familiar path

FIGURE 5: Example of how to use method of loci.

Figure 5, if one needs to memorize a phone number, one may visualize the numbers along a familiar trail. So if the number is 934–7579, one can imagine that a large nine is singing the Beattle's song "Number 9" at the trail head; then along the path one can imagine 3 men in a tub in the pond nearby. Further down the path, one can imagine 4 loud laughing cows in a meadow and then image how the trail seems to curve as to make the number 7. As one continues down the path, one can imagine 5 whispering pines and then a 7 at a large outcropping of rocks and then another number 9 concluding with singing the "Number 9" song. The more novel, vivid, and detailed one makes these associations, the more likely the associations will be successfully recalled. For example, with the outcropping of rocks, one can imagine seven dwarves living in them. Likewise, method of loci could be used to assist with HIV disease management such as pairing watching the nightly news with taking one's HIV medication; that way when someone watches the evening news as part of their normal routine schedule, they can use the news program as a mnemonic to remember to take their medication on time.

Chunking is another technique one can employ to recall information [192, 193]. Using a phone number as another example, to memorize the same series of number (i.e., 934–7579), one can memorize the first three digits as a chunk and then the last four digits as a chunk and then assemble them together. In fact, this is how many actors memorize long monologues, by committing separate sections to memory in chunks and then weaving them together. Similarly, in memorizing one's medication regimens, one may memorize one medication protocol at a time and then put them together.

Finally, external memory aids can be quite effective and easy to use strategies to recall information [192]. It can be something as simple as a checklist on one's refrigerator detailing as to when to take one's medications, or it can be an app on a cell phone reminding one to attend his or her medical appointment, or it can even be a partner/friend encouraging one to check his or her blood pressure. Much of this is self-explanatory and falls within the realm of "common sense"; however, its usefulness and utility in assisting with everyday functioning for those suffering from cognitive deficits cannot be underscored enough.

6.3. Psychostimulants. Two psychostimulants have been found to improve cognitive functioning in adults with HIV: methylphenidate (Ritalin) and modafinil. Although methylphenidate has not been studied in adults with HIV in a large randomized clinical trial, several studies have found it to improve cognition in normal healthy adults [194], those with multiple sclerosis [195], and those with attention deficit disorder [196]. In a placebo-controlled, single-blind crossover study involving 16 adults with HIV, Hinkin and colleagues [197] found that methylphenidate (once daily 30 mg dose) abated cognitive slowing as measured by a computerized neuropsychological measure. Methylphenidate may improve cognitive functioning in adults with HIV in one of two ways. First, methylphenidate is a dopamine agonist [196]. Given that some adults with HIV experience lower levels of dopamine [198], methylphenidate may be an effective strategy to increase levels of dopamine in the brain and thus mitigate such cognitive deficits. Second, methylphenidate has also been shown to lower the levels of triglycerides, low density lipoprotein cholesterol, and total cholesterol [199]. Since higher cholesterol levels are associated with more cognitive deficits in adults with HIV [200] and 65.8% of older adults (60+) with HIV experience higher levels of hypercholesterolemia [94], methylphenidate represents another strategy for addressing such cognitive problems by treating this common comorbidity.

Modafinil has also been shown to improve cognitive functioning and abate fatigue in adults such as in those with attention deficit disorder [201]. In a heterogenous sample of 103 adults with HIV (51%, 40%, and 20% with a substance use history, depression diagnosis, and a hepatitis C diagnosis, resp.), McElhiney et al. [202] randomized participants to receive 4 weeks of modafinil or a placebo. These researchers found that those assigned to the modafinil condition experienced more objective global cognitive gains and fewer subjective cognitive complaints compared to those in the placebo condition. In addition, no adverse effects were observed; thus, this supports the use of modafinil as a strategy to mitigate such cognitive deficits.

Although psychostimulants such as methylphenidate and modafinil have been shown to improve cognition in adults including those with HIV, other medications such as acetylcholinesterase inhibitors, herbal and alternative supplements, omega-3 fatty acids, and hormone replacement therapy may not be as effective in mitigating such cognitive deficits. Acetylcholinesterase inhibitors are traditionally used to treat adults with Alzheimer's disease and related dementias. However, in a sample of 168 community-dwelling older adults without dementia but with memory complaints, Yesavage and colleagues [203] administered donepezil (an acetylcholinesterase inhibitor) over one year and found that it was not effective in improving cognitive functioning. This study suggests that this medication may only be effective in those with dementia, not those with cognitive deficits. Likewise, although some studies suggest that herbal and alternative supplements such as ginseng and ginkgo biloba may protect against cognitive deficits or even improve cognitive functioning, in general such strategies have not been found to be effective [204–206]. In fact, such herbal and alternative supplement may interfere with HAART, medication adherence, and medical treatment [130, 207]. Omega-3 fatty acids have also been considered as a possible avenue for enhancing cognitive functioning given that it is has been shown to be important for brain development and synaptic plasticity. Unfortunately, the findings have been mixed; clearly more research is needed in this area [208].

Finally, similar to herbal and alternative supplements, hormone replacement therapy has been touted by some as a possible strategy to prevent dementia and improve cognitive [209, 210]; unfortunately, in general both estrogen and testosterone replacement therapies have been shown to be ineffective in improving cognition in adults [211, 212]. In fact, some studies suggest that estrogen replacement therapy in women may actually increase the risk for dementia by 2-fold [213] and that testosterone replacement therapy in men may increase the risk for liver disease, heart failure, prostate cancer, hyperviscosity, and erythrocytosis [214].

7. Implications for Nursing Practice

As mentioned, 52% of those with HIV experience some degree of cognitive deficit [27]; however, this means that 48% do not and function within normal parameters. Clearly, some individuals with HIV are more resistant to such cognitive deficits. Therefore, one of the most important points of nursing practice is to monitor cognitive functioning in adults with HIV to determine who is experiencing such problems [215]. Such monitoring can occur in a number of ways.

First, nurses can administer cognitive screeners or cognitive self-report instruments to patients such as the Mini-Mental Status Exam [216], the Montreal Cognitive Assessment [217], or the Cognitive Failures Questionnaire [218]. These are simple-to-use tools and require little training in administering and interpreting results. Second, nurses can assess for cognitive changes by observing patients' behaviors such as forgetting medical appointments, word finding difficulty, and outward signs of confusions (e.g., walking in the wrong direction to leave the clinic). If patients have a caregiver, friend, or partner that accompanies the visit, questions regarding cognitive status can be directed to them about their loved ones' cognitive functioning (e.g., Have you seen any change in your friend's memory over the past three months? Does your partner get lost easily?). Finally, patients can be asked directly to report any perceived problems with memory, attention, and cognitive functioning. If patients report such problems, referrals to a psychologist or neurologist can be made. A caveat about this last approach is that patients may not be accurate about their self-appraisal of their cognitive functioning. In fact, many adults with HIV also experience metacognitive problems; in other words, they have difficulty thinking about and evaluating their own thinking [219, 220]. For example, in a sample of 46 adults with HIV, Hinkin and colleagues [221] administered a neuropsychological battery to this sample along with asking them to rate their cognitive ability. From this, nearly 1/3 (37%) overestimated their cognitive ability and nearly 1/3 (26%) underestimated their cognitive ability; meanwhile, nearly 1/3 (37%) accurately estimated their cognitive ability which matched their actual objective cognitive functioning. As such nurses must be aware that even when assessing patients' cognitive functioning, caution should be used in relying solely on self-report since it may not be accurate; thus, a combination of assessments strategies would be preferred to triangulate and validate cognitive functioning and determine the need for specific prevention, remediation, or mitigation strategies. (For a decision tree as to how to assess cognitive functioning in patients with HIV, see Vance et al. [220] for more details.)

Another important point of nursing practice in this area is to convey to patients that the health and lifestyle decisions that they make today will influence the amount of cognitive reserve they will have to weather neurological insults in later life. For those aging with HIV who are more susceptible to heart disease, hypercholesterolemia, diabetes, and other conditions known to impact cognitive functioning [86], this point cannot be emphasized enough. Thus, preventive strategies as discussed in this paper should be suggested as a way of not only protecting cognitive functioning, but may be a way to also ameliorate physical health and improve quality of life.

8. Implications for Nursing Research

Although many areas of research have already been suggested as potential research vectors to prevent, rehabilitate, and mitigate cognition in adults with HIV, several areas of research must continue to examine such strategies to help older adults with HIV age successfully; this is very important given that successful cognitive aging is needed to effectively engage in disease management (e.g., medication adherence and attending clinic visits) and everyday functioning (e.g., safe driving behavior). Lindl et al. [48] highlighted several interesting strategies that may be considered to address cognition in future research. These include nanoparticle delivery of HAART, insulin and insulin-like substances, lithium, and memantine.

As mentioned earlier, not all HAART medications are effective in crossing the blood brain barrier and delivering the medication to where it needs to be [128, 222]; this is unfortunate since the brain is considered an HIV reservoir [223]. To confront this problem, researchers are considering nanoparticle delivery of HAART so that it can cross the blood brain barrier better resulting in more bioavailability of the medication to control HIV [48, 224, 225]. If effective, this approach could potentially reduce the impact HIV has directly on the brain, not to mention that it could reduce the number of HIV reservoirs in the body.

Insulin, insulin-like growth factor-1, and neurotrophin intranasal delivery has been suggested as a way to compensate for the neural damage caused by diabetes, stroke, diabetes, Alzheimer's disease, and HIV. Small preliminary studies have been encouraging in that both short-term memory and long-term memory have been improved along with mood and odor detection [48, 226]. This is especially relevant because as adults age with HIV, they may also experience olfactory and related chemosensory declines as well [227, 228]. In a recent double-blind study of 104 adults with mild cognitive impairment or mild-to-moderate Alzheimer's disease, Craft and colleagues [229] randomized participants to receive 4 months of intranasal delivery of (1) 20 international units of insulin a day, (2) 40 international units of insulin a day, or (3) a placebo. In this intent-to-treat analysis, these researchers found those who received the 20 international units of insulin showed improved memory and those in either insulin condition had better preserved cognitive functioning compared to those in the placebo condition. Although this has not been tested in adults with HIV, this does represent a promising vector of research.

Lithium has been suggested as a possible medication to improve cognitive functioning in adults with HIV. In a small 12-week pilot study with 8 adults with HIV experiencing cognitive deficits, Letendre and colleagues [230] found that an open-label use of lithium (300 mg daily) resulted in improved cognition. Similarly, in a small 10-week pilot study with 15 adults with HIV also with cognitive deficits, Schifitto and colleague [231] did not find cognitive improvement with an open label use of lithium (300 mg twice daily); however, these researchers did find several changes in biomarkers (i.e., increased fractional anisotropy) reflective of improved brain health. Although lithium use may not be appropriate for everyone (i.e., those who are pregnant or with renal disease [196, 232, 233]), these initial findings are encouraging because the medication was well tolerated in both studies.

Memantine has also been suggested as a possible medication to improve cognitive functioning in adults with

HIV since memantine decreases glutamate excitotoxicity in both Alzheimer's disease and HIV-disease models in mice. In a pilot study with 140 adults with HIV, Schifitto and colleagues [234] found that after 16 weeks of taking memantine (10 mg daily escalated to 40 mg daily), magnetic resonance spectroscopy showed that memantine may exert protective properties for frontal white matter and the parietal cortex. Unfortunately, cognitive benefits were not observed during this 16-week period; however, additional time on memantine may be needed before benefits are observed. In a similar study involving a sample of 99 adults with HIV with cognitive deficits, Zhao and colleagues [235] randomized the participants to receive either memantine (escalated up to 40 mg daily) or a placebo. These researchers found that those in the memantine condition experienced cognitive improvement after 12 weeks compared to those in the placebo condition. Out of these 99 participants, 45 were followed over a 48-week period; unfortunately, the cognitive improvements were no longer detected but this could have been due to developed tolerance to the medication which suggests that it may be useful in only the short term. Fortunately, memantine was well tolerated in both studies and represents an area in need of more investigation.

Studies must also consider how to improve cognitive functioning to improve everyday functioning. As mentioned, Marcotte and colleague [172] observed that in comparison with those without HIV, adults with HIV experience more severe deficits in Useful Field of View—a cognitive measure of visual attention and visual speed of processing. These cognitive abilities are obviously necessary for safe driving and needed to avoid motor vehicle crashes. There is growing concern that as adults with HIV age, these cognitive abilities will atrophy and predispose them for unsafe driving [236]. Fortunately, Ball et al. [237] found that in a sample of 908 community-dwelling older adults without HIV those who received speed of processing training had a 50% reduction in at-fault motor-vehicle crashes six years after training compared to those randomized to the control group. Since this speed of processing training was shown to improve Useful Field of View in a pilot study sample ($n = 22$) of middle-aged and older adults with HIV (see Cognitive Remediation Therapy section [174]), such cognitive remediation therapy may improve driving safety in this cognitively vulnerable group; however, more research is needed on a larger sample of drivers to determine the effectiveness of such therapy on driving.

9. Conclusion

Although the process of aging along with HIV can have negative consequences on brain health through oxidative stress, neuroinflammation, and other mechanisms, this does not mean that all individuals with this disease will experience cognitive deficits. In fact, although Heaton and colleagues [27] found that 52% of adults with HIV experienced some degree of cognitive deficits, it is important to note that 48%, nearly half, do not. Clearly, there are many individuals aging with this disease who are less vulnerable to the detrimental effects aging and HIV exert on the brain. So there is room for optimism concerning successful cognitive aging with HIV; in fact, studies investigating why certain individuals age well cognitively with this disease are obviously warranted. Perhaps such fortunate individuals have greater cognitive reserve or have engaged in preventative strategies (i.e., healthy lifestyle) to avoid cognitive deficits. For those who unfortunately experience such cognitive deficits, hope is not lost either. Several rehabilitative strategies such as speed of processing training and mitigation strategies such as spaced retrieval method have been shown to be effective in this clinical population. Likewise, other strategies such as transcranial direct current stimulation has been shown to benefit older adults [238] and such approaches may be of use to those aging with HIV. Regardless, more prevention, rehabilitation, and mitigation cognitive research is needed to evaluate the effectiveness of such strategies as the number of older adults with HIV grows.

References

[1] J. V. Fernández-Montero, P. Barreiro, J. Del Romero, and V. Soriano, "Antiretroviral drugs for pre-exposure prophylaxis of HIV infection," *AIDS Review*, vol. 14, no. 1, pp. 54–61, 2012.

[2] M. W. Hull and J. Montaner, "Antiretroviral therapy: a key component of a comprehensive HIV prevention strategy," *Current HIV/AIDS Reports*, vol. 8, no. 2, pp. 85–93, 2011.

[3] C. J. McCabe, S. J. Goldie, and D. N. Fisman, "The cost-effectiveness of directly observed highly-active antiretroviral therapy in the third trimester in HIV-infected pregnant women," *PLoS ONE*, vol. 5, no. 4, Article ID e10154, 2010.

[4] E. Wood, M. J. Milloy, and J. S. Montaner, "HIV treatment as prevention among injection drug users," *Current Opinions in HIV/AIDS*, vol. 7, no. 2, pp. 151–156, 2012.

[5] D. E. Vance and F. P. Robinson, "Reconciling successful aging with HIV: a biopsychosocial overview," *Journal of HIV/AIDS and Social Services*, vol. 3, no. 1, pp. 59–78, 2004.

[6] UNAIDS, *AIDS Epidemic*, World Health Organization, Geneva, Switzerland, 2009, http://www.unaids.org/en/media/unaids/contentassets/dataimport/pub/report/2009/jc1700_epi_update_2009_en.pdf.

[7] UNAIDS, "Global report: UNAIDS Report on the Global AIDS Epidemic 2010," Joint United Nations Programme on HIV/AIDS, 2010.

[8] G. Meyer-Rath, A. Brennan, L. Long et al., "Cost and outcomes of paediatric antiretroviral treatment in South Africa," *AIDS*, vol. 27, no. 2, pp. 243–250, 2012.

[9] G. Meyer-Rath, A. Miners, A. C. Santos, E. Variava, and W. D. Venter, "Cost and resource use of patients on antiretroviral therapy in the urban and semi-urban public sectors of South Africa," *Journal of the Acquire Immunodeficiency Syndromes*, vol. 61, no. 3, pp. e25–e32, 2012.

[10] C. Ogunmefun, I. Friedman, N. Mothibe, and T. Mbatha, "A national audit of home and community-based care (HCBC) organisations in South Africa," *AIDS Care*. In press.

[11] United Nations, "Population ageing and development," 2009, http://www.un.org/esa/population/publications/ageing/ageing2009chart.pdf.

[12] C. Farrelly, "Global aging, well-ordered science, and prospection," *Rejuvenation Research*, vol. 13, no. 5, pp. 607–612, 2010.

[13] J. B. Kirk and M. B. Goetz, "Human immunodeficiency virus in an aging population, a complication of success," *Journal of the American Geriatrics Society*, vol. 57, no. 11, pp. 2129–2138, 2009.

[14] G. Smith, *Aging Hearing: HIV Over Fifty, Exploring the New Threat*, Senate Committee on Aging, Washington, DC, USA, 2006.

[15] Centers for Disease Control and Preventions, *HIV/AIDS Among Person Aged 50 and Older: CDC HIV/AIDS Facts*, US Department of Health and Human Services, Washington, DC, USA, 2008.

[16] P. B. Baltes and M. M. Baltes, "Psychological perspectives on successful aging: the model of selective optimization with compensation," in *Successful Aging: Perspectives from the Behavioral Sciences*, P. B. Baltes and M. M. Baltes, Eds., pp. 1–34, Cambridge University Press, Cambridge, UK, 1990.

[17] B. W. Becker, A. D. Thames, E. Woo, S. A. Castellon, and C. A. Hinkin, "Longitudinal change in cognitive function and medication adherence in HIV-infected adults," *AIDS and Behavior*, vol. 15, no. 8, pp. 1888–1894, 2011.

[18] D. E. Vance, J. A. Ross, L. Moneyham, K. F. Farr, and P. Fordham, "A model of cognitive decline and suicidal ideation in adults aging with HIV," *Journal of Neuroscience Nursing*, vol. 42, no. 3, pp. 150–156, 2010.

[19] L. J. Byom and L. Turkstra, "Effects of social cognitive demand on theory of mind in conversations of adults with traumatic brain injury," *International Journal of Language and Communication Disorders*, vol. 47, no. 3, pp. 310–321, 2012.

[20] E. Widera, V. Steenpass, D. Marson, and R. Sudore, "Finances in the older patient with cognitive impairment: 'He didn't want me to take over'," *Journal of the American Medical Association*, vol. 305, no. 7, pp. 698–706, 2011.

[21] A. D. Thames, V. Streiff, S. M. Patel, S. E. Panos, S. A. Castellon, and C. H. Hinkin, "The role of HIV infection, cognition, and depression in risky decision-making," *Journal of Neuropsychiatry and Clinical Neuroscience*, vol. 24, no. 3, pp. 340–348, 2012.

[22] A. R. Giovagnoli, A. M. da Silva, A. Federico, and F. Cornelio, "On the personal facets of quality of life in chronic neurological disorders," *Neurology*, vol. 21, no. 3-4, pp. 155–163, 2009.

[23] N. S. Schutte, T. Searle, S. Meade, and N. A. Dark, "The effect of meaningfulness and integrative processing in expressive writing on positive and negative and life satisfaction," *Cognition and Emotion*, vol. 26, no. 1, pp. 144–152, 2012.

[24] D. E. Vance, "Increasing cognitive reserve may promote successful cognitive aging," *Nursing*, vol. 2, pp. 27–32, 2012.

[25] M. Reger, R. Welsh, J. Razani, D. J. Martin, and K. B. Boone, "A meta-analysis of the neuropsychological sequelae of HIV infection," *Journal of the International Neuropsychological Society*, vol. 8, no. 3, pp. 410–424, 2002.

[26] N. Sacktor, R. H. Lyles, R. Skolasky et al., "HIV-associated neurologic disease incidence changes: multicenter AIDS Cohort Study, 1990–1998," *Neurology*, vol. 56, no. 2, pp. 257–260, 2001.

[27] R. K. Heaton, D. B. Clifford, Franklin et al., "HIV-associated neurocognitive disorders persist in the era of potent antiretroviral therapy (CHARTER Study)," *American Academy of Neurology*, vol. 75, pp. 2087–2096, 2010.

[28] M. R. Basso and R. A. Bornstein, "Estimated premorbid intelligence mediates neurobehavioral change in individuals infected with HIV across 12 months," *Journal of Clinical and Experimental Neuropsychology*, vol. 22, no. 2, pp. 208–218, 2000.

[29] M. R. Lentz, W. K. Kim, H. Kim et al., "Alterations in brain metabolism during the first year of HIV infection," *Journal of Neurovirology*, vol. 17, no. 3, pp. 220–229, 2011.

[30] B. C. Schweinsburg, M. J. Taylor, O. M. Alhassoon et al., "Brain mitochondrial injury in human immunodeficiency virus-seropositive (HIV+) individuals taking nucleoside reverse transcriptase inhibitors," *Journal of NeuroVirology*, vol. 11, no. 4, pp. 356–364, 2005.

[31] K. Ritchie and J. Touchon, "Mild cognitive impairment: conceptual basis and current nosological status," *The Lancet*, vol. 355, no. 9199, pp. 225–228, 2000.

[32] J. A. Schneider, Z. Arvanitakis, L. Yu, P. A. Boyle, S. E. Leugans, and D. A. Bennett, "Cognitive impairment, decline and fluctuations in older community-dwelling subjects with Lewy bodies," *Brain*, vol. 135, part 10, pp. 3005–3014, 2012.

[33] D. E. Vance, P. L. Fazeli, J. Kaur, P. Pearce, and T. McGuiness, "Neuropsychology and cognitive health in healthy older adults: a brief overview for psychiatric nurses," *Journal of Psychosocial Nursing and Mental Health Services*, vol. 50, no. 6, pp. 30–37, 2012.

[34] J. T. Becker, O. L. Lopez, M. A. Dew, and H. J. Aizenstein, "Prevalence of cognitive disorders differs as a function of age in HIV virus infection," *AIDS*, vol. 18, supplement 1, pp. S11–S18, 2004.

[35] K. P. High, V. Valcour, and R. Paul, "HIV infection and dementia in older adults," *Clinical Infectious Diseases*, vol. 42, no. 10, pp. 1449–1454, 2006.

[36] N. Sacktor, R. Skolasky, O. A. Selnes et al., "Neuropsychological test profile differences between young and old human immunodeficiency virus-positive individuals," *Journal of NeuroVirology*, vol. 13, no. 3, pp. 203–209, 2007.

[37] L. A. Wendelken and V. Valcour, "Impact of HIV and aging on neuropsychological function," *Journal of Neurovirology*, vol. 18, no. 4, pp. 256–263, 2012.

[38] D. E. Vance and T. C. Struzick, "Addressing risk factors of cognitive impairment in adults aging with HIV: a social work model," *Journal of Gerontological Social Work*, vol. 49, no. 4, pp. 51–77, 2007.

[39] P. Ancuta, A. Kamat, K. J. Kunstman et al., "Microbial translocation is associated with increased monocyte activation and dementia in AIDS patients," *PLoS ONE*, vol. 3, no. 6, Article ID e2516, 2008.

[40] T. H. Burdo, M. R. Lentz, P. Autissier et al., "Soluble CD163 made by monocyte/macrophages is a novel marker of HIV activity in early and chronic infection prior to and after antiretroviral therapy," *Journal of Infectious Diseases*, vol. 204, no. 1, pp. 154–163, 2011.

[41] T. H. Burdo, J. Lo, S. Abbara et al., "Soluble CD163, a novel marker of activated macrophages, is elevated and associated with noncalcified coronary plaque in HIV-infected patients," *Journal of Infectious Disease*, vol. 204, no. 8, pp. 1227–1236, 2011.

[42] N. Thieblemont, L. Weiss, H. M. Sadeghi, C. Estcourt, and N. Haeffner-Cavaillon, "CD14loWCD16high: a cytokine-producing monocyte subset which expands during human immunodeficiency virus infection," *European Journal of Immunology*, vol. 25, no. 12, pp. 3418–3424, 1995.

[43] D. E. Vance, P. L. Fazeli, and C. A. Gakumo, "The impact of neuropsychological performance on everyday functioning between older and younger adults with and without HIV," *Journal of the Association of Nurses in AIDS Care*. In press.

[44] T. T. Baldewicz, J. Leserman, S. G. Silva et al., "Changes in neuropsychological functioning with progression of HIV-1 infection: results of an 8-year longitudinal investigation," *AIDS and Behavior*, vol. 8, no. 3, pp. 345–355, 2004.

[45] V. Valcour, C. Shikuma, B. Shiramizu et al., "Age, apolipoprotein E4, and the risk of HIV dementia: the Hawaii Aging with HIV Cohort," *Journal of Neuroimmunology*, vol. 157, no. 1-2, pp. 197–202, 2004.

[46] M. Cherner, R. J. Ellis, D. Lazzaretto et al., "Effects of HIV-1 infection and aging on neurobehavioral functioning: preliminary findings," *AIDS*, vol. 18, supplement 1, pp. S27–S34, 2004.

[47] D. J. Hardy and D. E. Vance, "The neuropsychology of HIV/AIDS in older adults," *Neuropsychology Review*, vol. 19, no. 2, pp. 263–272, 2009.

[48] K. A. Lindl, D. R. Marks, D. L. Kolson, and K. L. Jordan-Sciutto, "HIV-associated neurocognitive disorder: pathogenesis and therapeutic opportunities," *Journal of Neuroimmune Pharmacology*, vol. 5, no. 3, pp. 294–309, 2010.

[49] L. Malaspina, S. P. Woods, D. J. Moore et al., "Successful cognitive aging in persons living with HIV infection," *Journal of NeuroVirology*, vol. 17, no. 1, pp. 110–119, 2011.

[50] E. E. Morgan, S. P. Woods, L. Delano-Wood, M. W. Bondi, and I. Grant, "Intraindividual variability in HIV infection: evidence for greater neurocognitive dispersion in older HIV seropositive adults," *Neuropsychology*, vol. 25, no. 5, pp. 645–654, 2011.

[51] V. Valcour, R. Paul, J. Nevhaus, and C. Shikuma, "The effects of age and HIV on neuropsychological performance," *Journal of the International Neuropsychological Society*, vol. 17, no. 1, pp. 190–195, 2011.

[52] V. Valcour and B. Shiramizu, "HIV-associated dementia, mitochondrial dysfunction, and oxidative stress," *Mitochondrion*, vol. 4, no. 2-3, pp. 119–129, 2004.

[53] R. D. Fields, *The other Brain: from Dementia to Schizophrenia, How New Discoveries about the Brain are Revolutionizing Medicine and Science*, Simon & Schuster, New York, NY, USA, 2009.

[54] R. Restak, *Think Smart: A Neuroscientist's Prescription for Improving Brain's Performance*, Penguin, New York, NY, USA, 2009.

[55] Y. Stern, "Cognitive reserve," *Neuropsychologia*, vol. 47, no. 10, pp. 2015–2028, 2009.

[56] D. E. Vance and M. Crowe, "A proposed model of neuroplasticity and cognitive reserve in older adults," *Activities, Adaptation and Aging*, vol. 30, no. 3, pp. 61–79, 2006.

[57] D. E. Vance and M. A. Wright, "Positive and negative neuroplasticity: implications for age, related cognitive declines," *Journal of Gerontological Nursing*, vol. 35, no. 6, pp. 11–17, 2009.

[58] C. L. Haass-Koffler and S. E. Bartlett, "Stress and addiction: contribution of the corticotropin releasing factor (CRF) system in neuroplasticity," *Frontiers in Molecular Neuroscience*, vol. 5, article 91, 2012.

[59] S. Koganemaru, K. Domen, H. Fukuyama, and T. Mima, "Negative emotion can enhance human motor cortical plasticity," *European Journal of Neuroscience*, vol. 35, pp. 1637–1645, 2012.

[60] D. E. Vance, "Implications of positive and negative neuroplasticity on cognition in HIV," *Medical Science Monitor*, vol. 16, no. 4, pp. HY3–HY5, 2010.

[61] D. E. Vance, A. J. Roberson, T. M. Mcguinness, and P. L. Fazeli, "How neuroplasticity and cognitive reserve protect cognitive functioning," *Journal of Psychosocial Nursing and Mental Health Services*, vol. 48, no. 4, pp. 23–30, 2010.

[62] D. E. Vance, J. Kaur, P. L. Fazeli et al., "Neuroplasticity and successful cognitive aging: a brief overview for nursing," *Journal of Neuroscience Nursing*, vol. 44, no. 4, pp. 218–227, 2012.

[63] M. C. Diamond, "An optimistic view of the aging brain," *Generations*, vol. 17, no. 1, pp. 31–33, 1993.

[64] S. Kobayashi, Y. Ohashi, and S. Ando, "Effects of enriched environments with different durations and starting times on learning capacity during aging in rats assessed by a refined procedure of the Hebb-Williams maze task," *Journal of Neuroscience Research*, vol. 70, no. 3, pp. 340–346, 2002.

[65] N. W. Milgram, E. Head, S. C. Zicker et al., "Learning ability in aged beagle dogs is preserved by behavioral enrichment and dietary fortification: a two-year longitudinal study," *Neurobiology of Aging*, vol. 26, no. 1, pp. 77–90, 2005.

[66] V. Paban, M. Jaffard, C. Chambon, M. Malafosse, and B. Alescio-Lautier, "Time course of behavioral changes following basal forebrain cholinergic damage in rats: environmental enrichment as a therapeutic intervention," *Neuroscience*, vol. 132, no. 1, pp. 13–32, 2005.

[67] L. Petrosini, P. De Bartolo, F. Foti et al., "On whether the environmental enrichment may provide cognitive and brain reserves," *Brain Research Reviews*, vol. 61, no. 2, pp. 221–239, 2009.

[68] S. Urakawa, H. Hida, T. Masuda, S. Misumi, T. S. Kim, and H. Nishino, "Environmental enrichment brings a beneficial effect on beam walking and enhances the migration of doublecortin-positive cells following striatal lesions in rats," *Neuroscience*, vol. 144, no. 3, pp. 920–933, 2007.

[69] H. Van Praag, G. Kempermann, and F. H. Gage, "Neural Consequences of environmental enrichment," *Nature Reviews Neuroscience*, vol. 1, no. 3, pp. 191–198, 2000.

[70] E. A. Maguire, D. G. Gadian, I. S. Johnsrude et al., "Navigation-related structural change in the hippocampi of taxi drivers," *Proceedings of the National Academy of Sciences of the United States of America*, vol. 97, no. 8, pp. 4398–4403, 2000.

[71] E. A. Maguire, K. Woollett, and H. J. Spiers, "London taxi drivers and bus drivers: a structural MRI and neuropsychological analysis," *Hippocampus*, vol. 16, no. 12, pp. 1091–1101, 2006.

[72] J. Boyke, J. Driemeyer, C. Gaser, C. Büchel, and A. May, "Training-induced brain structure changes in the elderly," *Journal of Neuroscience*, vol. 28, no. 28, pp. 7031–7035, 2008.

[73] C. Brayne, P. G. Ince, H. A. D. Keage et al., "Education, the brain and dementia: neuroprotection or compensation?" *Brain*, vol. 133, part 8, pp. 2210–2216, 2010.

[74] S. Gauthier and C. Ballard, *Management of Dementia*, Informa Healthcare USA, New York, NY, USA, 2nd edition, 2009.

[75] C. M. Roe, M. A. Mintun, G. D'Angelo, C. Xiong, E. A. Grant, and J. C. Morris, "Alzheimer disease and cognitive reserve: variation of education effect with carbon 11-labeled pittsburgh compound B uptake," *Archives of Neurology*, vol. 65, no. 11, pp. 1467–1471, 2008.

[76] C. Berry and K. P. Balachandran, "Importance of collateral circulation in coronary heasrt disease," *European Heart Journal*, vol. 28, no. 3, pp. 278–291, 2007.

[77] J. M. Foley, M. L. Ettenhofer, M. S. Kim, N. Behdin, and S. A. Castellon, "Cognitive reserve as a protective factor in older HIV-positive patients at risk of cognitive decline," *Applied Neuropsychology: Adult*, vol. 19, no. 1, pp. 16–25, 2012.

[78] A. C. Satori, D. E. Vance, L. Z. Slater, and M. Crowe, "The impact of inflammation on cognitive function in older adults: implications for healthcare practice and research," *Journal of Neuroscience Nursing*, vol. 44, no. 4, pp. 206–217, 2012.

[79] A. C. Hearps, T. A. Angelovich, A. Jaworowski, J. Mills, A. L. Landay, and S. M. Crowe, "HIV infection and aging of the innate immune system," *Sexual Health*, vol. 8, no. 4, pp. 453–464, 2011.

[80] B. T. Baune, G. Ponath, J. Golledge et al., "Association between IL-8 cytokine and cognitive performance in an elderly general population-The MEMO-Study," *Neurobiology of Aging*, vol. 29, no. 6, pp. 937–944, 2008.

[81] J. P. Godbout and R. W. Johnson, "Age and neuroinflammation: a lifetime of psychoneuroimmune consequences," *Neurologic Clinics*, vol. 24, no. 3, pp. 521–538, 2006.

[82] G. Ravaglia, P. Forti, F. Maioli et al., "The clock-drawing test in elderly Italian community dwellers: associations with sociodemographic status and risk factors for vascular cognitive impairment," *Dementia and Geriatric Cognitive Disorders*, vol. 16, no. 4, pp. 287–295, 2003.

[83] K. Yaffe, K. Lindquist, Penninx et al., "Inflammatory markers and cognition in well-functioning African-American and white elders," *Neurology*, vol. 61, no. 1, pp. 76–80, 2003.

[84] I. Kusao, B. Shiramizu, C. Y. Liang et al., "Cognitive performance related to HIV-1-infected monocytes," *Journal of Neuropsychiatry and Clinical Neuroscience*, vol. 24, no. 1, pp. 71–80, 2012.

[85] P. M. Thompson, R. A. Dutton, K. M. Hayashi et al., "Thinning of the cerebral cortex visualized in HIV/AIDS reflects CD4+ T lymphocyte decline," *Proceedings of the National Academy of Sciences of the United States of America*, vol. 102, no. 43, pp. 15647–15652, 2005.

[86] D. E. Vance, K. I. Larsen, G. Eagerton, and M. A. Wright, "Comorbidities and cognitive functioning: implications for nursing practice and research," *Journal of Neuroscience Nursing*, vol. 43, no. 4, pp. 215–224, 2011.

[87] F. E. de Leeuw, J. C. de Groot, M. Oudkerk et al., "Hypertension and cerebral white matter lesions in a prospective cohort study," *Brain*, vol. 125, no. 4, pp. 765–772, 2002.

[88] D. Liao, L. Cooper, J. Cai et al., "Presence and severity of cerebral white matter lesions and hypertension, its treatment, and its control: the ARIC study," *Stroke*, vol. 27, no. 12, pp. 2262–2270, 1996.

[89] H. Bruehl, O. T. Wolf, V. Sweat, A. Tirsi, S. Richardson, and A. Convit, "Modifiers of cognitive function and brain structure in middle-aged and elderly individuals with type 2 diabetes mellitus," *Brain Research*, vol. 1280, pp. 186–194, 2009.

[90] O. I. Okereke, J. H. Kang, N. R. Cook et al., "Type 2 diabetes mellitus and cognitive decline in two large cohorts of community-dwelling older adults," *Journal of the American Geriatrics Society*, vol. 56, no. 6, pp. 1028–1036, 2008.

[91] H. Umegaki, T. Hayashi, H. Nomura et al., "Cognitive dysfunction: an emerging concept of a new diabetic complications in the elderly," *Geriatrics and Gerontology International*, vol. 13, no. 1, pp. 28–34, 2012.

[92] G. Guaraldi, G. Orlando, S. Zona et al., "Premature age-related comorbidities among HIV-infected persons compared with the general population," *2011 Clinical Infectious Diseases*, vol. 53, pp. 1120–1126.

[93] K. K. Oursler, J. L. Goulet, S. Crystal et al., "Association of age and comorbidity with physical function in hiv-infected and uninfected patients: results from the veterans aging cohort study," *AIDS Patient Care and STDs*, vol. 25, no. 1, pp. 13–20, 2011.

[94] D. E. Vance, M. Mugavero, J. Willig, J. L. Raper, and M. S. Saag, "Aging with HIV: a cross-sectional study of comorbidity prevalence and clinical characteristics across decades of life," *The Journal of the Association of Nurses in AIDS Care*, vol. 22, no. 1, pp. 17–25, 2011.

[95] S. Hekimi, J. Lapointe, and J. Wen, "Taking a "good" look at free radicals in the aging process," *Trends in Cell Biology*, vol. 21, no. 10, pp. 569–576, 2011.

[96] S. Asha Devi, "Aging brain: prevention of oxidative stress by vitamin E and exercise," *The Scientific World Journal*, vol. 9, pp. 366–372, 2009.

[97] R. Singh, S. S. Kanwar, P. K. Sood, and B. Nehru, "Beneficial effects of folic acid on enhancement of memory and antioxidant status in aged rat brain," *Cellular and Molecular Neurobiology*, vol. 31, no. 1, pp. 83–91, 2011.

[98] J. A. Joseph, B. Shukitt-Hale, N. A. Denisova et al., "Reversals of age-related declines in neuronal signal transduction, cognitive, and motor behavioral deficits with blueberry, spinach, or strawberry dietary supplementation," *Journal of Neuroscience*, vol. 19, no. 18, pp. 8114–8121, 1999.

[99] J. A. Joseph, B. Shukitt-Hale, N. A. Denisova et al., "Long-term dietary strawberry, spinach, or vitamin E supplementation retards the onset of age-related neuronal signal-transduction and cognitive behavioral deficits," *Journal of Neuroscience*, vol. 18, no. 19, pp. 8047–8055, 1998.

[100] T. N. Akbaraly, I. Hininger-Favier, I. Carrière et al., "Plasma selenium over time and cognitive decline in the elderly," *Epidemiology*, vol. 18, no. 1, pp. 52–58, 2007.

[101] J. A. Joseph, B. Shukitt-Hale, G. Casadesus, and D. Fisher, "Oxidative stress and inflammation in brain aging: nutritional considerations," *Neurochemical Research*, vol. 30, no. 6-7, pp. 927–935, 2005.

[102] S. A. Mandel, T. Amit, O. Weinreb, and M. B. H. Youdim, "Understanding the broad-spectrum neuroprotective action profile of green tea polyphenols in aging and neurodegenerative diseases," *Journal of Alzheimer's Disease*, vol. 25, no. 2, pp. 187–208, 2011.

[103] C. B. Pocernich, M. L. B. Lange, R. Sultana, and D. A. Butterfield, "Nutritional approaches to modulate oxidative stress in Alzheime's disease," *Current Alzheimer Research*, vol. 8, no. 5, pp. 452–469, 2011.

[104] C. C. Tangney, Y. Tang, D. A. Evans, and M. C. Morris, "Biochemical indicators of vitamin B12 and folate insufficiency and cognitive decline," *Neurology*, vol. 72, no. 4, pp. 361–367, 2009.

[105] L. Z. Slater, L. Moneyham, D. E. Vance, J. L. Raper, M. Mugavero, and G. Childs, "Support, stigma, health, coping, and quality of life in older gay men with HIV," *Journal of the Association of Nurses in AIDS Care*, vol. 24, no. 1, pp. 38–49, 2013.

[106] R. M. Reynolds, "Glucocorticoid excess and the developmental origins of disease: two decades of testing the hypothesis," *Psychoneuroendocrinology*, vol. 38, no. 1, pp. 1–11, 2013.

[107] T. Jones and M. D. Moller, "Implications of hypothalamic-pituitary-adrenal axis functioning in posttraumatic stress disorder," *Journal of the American Psychiatric Nurses Association*, vol. 17, no. 6, pp. 393–403, 2011.

[108] K. Hoehn and E. N. Marieb, *Human Anatomy and Physiology*, Benjamin Cummings, San Francisco, Calif, USA, 2010.

[109] G. P. Chrousos and P. W. Gold, "The concepts of stress and stress system disorders: overview of physical and behavioral homeostasis," *Journal of the American Medical Association*, vol. 267, no. 9, pp. 1244–1252, 1992.

[110] S. J. Lupien, A. Fiocco, N. Wan et al., "Stress hormones and human memory function across the lifespan," *Psychoneuroendocrinology*, vol. 30, no. 3, pp. 225–242, 2005.

[111] B. K. Lee, T. A. Glass, M. J. McAtee et al., "Associations of salivary cortisol with cognitive function in the Baltimore memory study," *Archives of General Psychiatry*, vol. 64, no. 7, pp. 810–818, 2007.

[112] A. S. Karlamangla, B. H. Singer, J. Chodosh, B. S. McEwen, and T. E. Seeman, "Urinary cortisol excretion as a predictor of incident cognitive impairment," *Neurobiology of Aging*, vol. 26, pp. S80–S84, 2005.

[113] R. A. Shippy and S. E. Karpiak, "The aging HIV/AIDS population: fragile social networks," *Aging and Mental Health*, vol. 9, no. 3, pp. 246–254, 2005.

[114] C. Grov, S. A. Golub, J. T. Parsons, M. Brennan, and S. E. Karpiak, "Loneliness and HIV-related stigma explain depression among older HIV-positive adults," *AIDS Care*, vol. 22, no. 5, pp. 630–639, 2010.

[115] S. C. Kalichman, T. Heckman, A. Kochman, K. Sikkema, and J. Bergholte, "Depression and thoughts of suicide among middle-aged and older persons living with HIV-AIDS," *Psychiatric Services*, vol. 51, no. 7, pp. 903–907, 2000.

[116] A. Gonzalez, M. J. Mimiaga, J. Israel, C. A. Bedoya, and S. A. Safren, "Substance use predictors of poor medication adherence: the role of substance use coping among HIV-infected patients in opioid dependence treatment," *AIDS and Behavior*, vol. 17, no. 1, pp. 168–173, 2013.

[117] M. C. Hampton, P. N. Halkitis, and J. S. Mattis, "Coping, drug use, and religiosity/spirituality in relation to HIV serostatus among gay and bisexual men," *AIDS Education and Prevention*, vol. 22, no. 5, pp. 417–429, 2010.

[118] R. Schuster, M. Bornovalova, and E. Hunt, "The influence of depression on the progression of HIV: direct and indirect effects," *Behavior Modification*, vol. 36, no. 2, pp. 123–145, 2012.

[119] K. J. Anstey, "Alcohol exposure and cognitive development: an example of why we need a contextualized, dynamic life course approach to cognitive ageing—a mini-review," *Gerontology*, vol. 54, no. 5, pp. 283–291, 2008.

[120] V. Kumar and L. J. Kinsella, "Healthy brain aging: effect of head injury, alcohol and environmental toxins," *Clinics in Geriatric Medicine*, vol. 26, no. 1, pp. 29–44, 2010.

[121] D. R. Brown, "Role of microglia in age-related changes to the nervous system," *The Scientific World Journal*, vol. 9, pp. 1061–1071, 2009.

[122] K. L. Medina, A. D. Schweinsburg, M. Cohen-Zion, B. J. Nagel, and S. F. Tapert, "Effects of alcohol and combined marijuana and alcohol use during adolescence on hippocampal volume and asymmetry," *Neurotoxicology and Teratology*, vol. 29, no. 1, pp. 141–152, 2007.

[123] P. L. Fazeli, J. C. Marceux, D. E. Vance, L. Slater, and C. A. Long, "Predictors of cognition in adults with HIV: implications for nursing practice and research," *Journal of Neuroscience Nursing*, vol. 42, no. 1, pp. 36–50, 2011.

[124] T. Al-Khindi, K. K. Zakzanis, and W. G. van Gorp, "Does antiretroviral therapy improve HIV-associated cognitive impairment? A quantitative review of the literature," *Journal of the International Neuropsychological Society*, vol. 17, no. 6, pp. 956–969, 2011.

[125] T. D. Parsons, A. J. Braaten, C. D. Hall, and K. R. Robertson, "Better quality of life with neuropsychological improvement on HAART," *Health and Quality of Life Outcomes*, vol. 4, article 11, 2006.

[126] P. P. Koopmans, R. Ellis, B. M. Best, and S. Letendre, "Should antiretroviral therapy for HIV infection be tailored for intracerebral penetration?" *Netherlands Journal of Medicine*, vol. 67, no. 6, pp. 206–211, 2009.

[127] Y. O. Obiabo and O. A. Ogunrin, "Effects of highly active antiretroviral therapy on cognitive functions in severely immune-compromised HIV-seropositive patients," *Journal of the Neurological Sciences*, vol. 313, no. 1-2, pp. 115–122, 2012.

[128] S. Letendre, J. Marquie-Beck, E. Capparelli et al., "Validation of the CNS penetration-effectiveness rank for quantifying antiretroviral penetration into the central nervous system," *Archives of Neurology*, vol. 65, no. 1, pp. 65–70, 2008.

[129] A. A. Howard, J. H. Arnsten, Y. Lo et al., "A prospective study of adherence and viral load in a large multi-center cohort of HIV-infected women," *AIDS*, vol. 16, no. 16, pp. 2175–2182, 2002.

[130] J. L. Raper, "The medical managment of HIV disease," in *The Person with HIV/AIDS: Nursing Perspective*, J. D. Durham and F. R. Lashley4th, Eds., pp. 221–291, Springer, New York, NY, USA, 2010.

[131] M. L. Ettenhofer, J. Foley, S. A. Castellon, and C. H. Hinkin, "Reciprocal prediction of medication adherence and neurocognition in HIV/AIDS," *Neurology*, vol. 74, no. 15, pp. 1217–1222, 2010.

[132] M. L. Ettenhofer, C. H. Hinkin, S. A. Castellon et al., "Aging, neurocognition, and medication adherence in HIV infection," *American Journal of Geriatric Psychiatry*, vol. 17, no. 4, pp. 281–290, 2009.

[133] A. D. Thames, M. S. Kim, B. W. Becker et al., "Medication and finance management among HIV-infected adults: the impact of age and cognition," *Journal of Clinical and Experimental Neuropsychology*, vol. 33, no. 2, pp. 200–209, 2011.

[134] N. Ciccarelli, M. Fabbiani, S. Di Giambenedetto et al., "Efavirenz associated with cognitive disorders in otherwise asymptomatic HIV-infected patients," *Neurology*, vol. 76, no. 16, pp. 1403–1409, 2011.

[135] S. W. Perry, J. P. Norman, A. Litzburg, D. Zhang, S. Dewhurst, and H. A. Gelbard, "HIV-1 transactivator of transcription protein induces mitochondrial hyperpolarization and synaptic stress leading to apoptosis," *Journal of Immunology*, vol. 174, no. 7, pp. 4333–4344, 2005.

[136] G. Logroscino, J. H. Kang, and F. Grodstein, "Prospective study of type 2 diabetes and cognitive decline in women aged 70–81 years," *British Medical Journal*, vol. 328, no. 7439, pp. 548–551, 2004.

[137] P. C. Elwood, J. Pickering, A. Bayer, and J. E. J. Gallacher, "Vascular disease and cognitive function in older men in the Caerphilly cohort," *Age and Ageing*, vol. 31, no. 1, pp. 43–48, 2002.

[138] F. Harrington, B. K. Saxby, I. G. McKeith, K. Wesnes, and G. A. Ford, "Cognitive performance in hypertensive and normotensive older subjects," *Hypertension*, vol. 36, no. 6, pp. 1079–1082, 2000.

[139] Y. Yakushiji, T. Noguchi, M. Hara et al., "Distributional impact of brain microbleeds on global cognitive function in adults without neurological disorder," *Stroke*, vol. 43, no. 7, pp. 1800–1805, 2012.

[140] S. Viamonte, D. Vance, V. Wadley, D. Roenker, and K. Ball, "Driving-related cognitive performance in older adults with pharmacologically treated cardiovascular disease," *Clinical Gerontologist*, vol. 33, no. 2, pp. 109–123, 2010.

[141] R. Fogari, A. Mugellini, A. Zoppi et al., "Influence of losartan and atenolol on memory function in very elderly hypertensive

patients," *Journal of Human Hypertension*, vol. 17, no. 11, pp. 781–785, 2003.

[142] N. C. Li, A. Lee, R. A. Whitmer et al., "Use of angiotensin receptor blockers and risk of dementia in a predominantly male population: prospective cohort analysis," *British Medical Journal*, vol. 340, Article ID b5465, 2010.

[143] M. Braganca and A. Palha, "Depression and neurocognitive performance in Portuguese patients infected with HIV," *AIDS and Behavior*, vol. 15, no. 8, pp. 1879–1887, 2011.

[144] A. D. Thames, B. W. Becker, T. D. Marcotte et al., "Depression, cognition, and self-appraisal of functional abilities in HIV: an examination of subjective appraisal versus objective performance," *Clinical Neuropsychologist*, vol. 25, no. 2, pp. 224–243, 2011.

[145] D. E. Vance, J. E. Dodson, J. Watkins, B. H. Kennedy, and N. L. Keltner, "Neurological and psychiatric diseases and their unique cognitive profiles: implications for nursing practice and research," *Journal of Neuroscience Nursing*. In press.

[146] K. H. Claypoole, A. J. Elliott, K. K. Uldall et al., "Cognitive functions and complaints in HIV-1 individuals treated for depression," *Applied Neuropsychology*, vol. 5, no. 2, pp. 74–84, 1998.

[147] K. N. Devlin, A. Gongvatana, U. S. Clark et al., "Neurocognitive effects of HIV, hepatitis C, and substance use history," *Journal of the International Neuropsychological Society*, vol. 18, no. 1, pp. 68–78, 2012.

[148] C. S. Meade, N. A. Conn, L. M. Skalski, and S. A. Safren, "Neurocognitive impairment and medication adherence in HIV patients with and without cocaine dependence," *Journal of Behavioral Medicine*, vol. 34, no. 2, pp. 128–138, 2011.

[149] A. J. Applebaum, M. W. Otto, M. A. Richardson, and S. A. Safren, "Contributors to neuropsychological impairment in HIV-infected and HIV-uninfected opiate-dependent patients," *Journal of Clinical and Experimental Neuropsychology*, vol. 32, no. 6, pp. 579–589, 2010.

[150] M. Cherner, P. Suarez, C. Casey et al., "Methamphetamine use parameters do not predict neuropsychological impairment in currently abstinent dependent adults," *Drug and Alcohol Dependence*, vol. 106, no. 2-3, pp. 154–163, 2010.

[151] D. A. Byrd, R. P. Fellows, S. Morgello et al., "Neurocognitive impact of substance use in HIV infection," *Journal of Acquired Immune Deficiency Syndromes*, vol. 58, no. 2, pp. 154–162, 2011.

[152] J. E. Iudicello, S. P. Woods, O. Vigil et al., "Longer term improvement in neurocognitive functioning and affective distress among methamphetamine users who achieve stable abstinence," *Journal of Clinical and Experimental Neuropsychology*, vol. 32, no. 7, pp. 704–718, 2010.

[153] I. Grant, R. Reed, and K. M. Adams, "Diagnosis of intermediate-duration and subacute organic mental disorders in abstinent alcoholics," *Journal of Clinical Psychiatry*, vol. 48, no. 8, pp. 319–323, 1987.

[154] H. G. Pope, A. J. Gruber, J. I. Hudson, M. A. Huestis, and D. Yurgelun-Todd, "Neuropsychological performance in long-term cannabis users," *Archives of General Psychiatry*, vol. 58, no. 10, pp. 909–915, 2001.

[155] S. B. Rourke and I. Grant, "The interactive effects of age and length of abstinence on the recovery of neuropsychological functioning in chronic male alcoholics: a 2-year follow-up study," *Journal of the International Neuropsychological Society*, vol. 5, no. 3, pp. 234–246, 1999.

[156] W. W. Beatty, R. Tivis, H. D. Stott, S. J. Nixon, and O. A. Parsons, "Neuropsychological deficits in sober alcoholics: influences of chronicity and recent alcohol consumption," *Alcoholism*, vol. 24, no. 2, pp. 149–154, 2000.

[157] S. B. Rourke and I. Grant, "Neuropsychological correlates of alcoholism," in *Neuropsychological Assessment of Neuropsychiatric and Neuromedical Disorders*, I. Grant and K. M. Adams, Eds., pp. 398–454, Oxford Press, New York, NY, USA, 3rd edition, 2009.

[158] J. H. Atkins, S. L. Rubenstein, T. L. Sota, S. Rueda, H. Fenta, and J. Bacon, "Impact of social support on cognitive symptom burden in HIV/AIDS," *AIDS Care*, vol. 22, no. 7, pp. 793–802, 2010.

[159] J. T. Coyle, "Use it or lose it—do effortful mental activities protect against dementia?" *The New England Journal of Medicine*, vol. 348, no. 25, pp. 2489–2490, 2003.

[160] P. P. Foster, K. P. Rosenblatt, and O. R. Kuljiš, "Exercise-induced cognitive plasticity, implications for mild cognitive impairment and Alzheimer's disease," *Frontiers in Neurology*, vol. 2, no. 28, pp. 1–15, 2011.

[161] Y. Feng and X. Wang, "Antioxidant therapies for Alzheimer's disease," *Oxidative Medicine and Cellular Longevity*, vol. 2012, Article ID 472932, 17 pages, 2012.

[162] E. Kesse-Guyot, V. A. Andreeva, C. Jeandel, M. Ferry, S. Hercberg, and P. Galan, "A healthy dietary pattern in midlife is associated with subsequent cognitive performance," *The Journal of Nutrition*, vol. 142, no. 5, pp. 909–915, 2012.

[163] S. Schaffer, H. Assesburg, S. Kuntz, W. E. Muller, and G. P. Eckert, "Effects of polyphenols on brain ageing and Alzheimer's disease: focus on mitochondria," *Molecular Neurobiology*, vol. 46, no. 1, pp. 161–178, 2012.

[164] E. Rrapo, Y. Zhu, J. Tian et al., "Green tea-EGCG reduces GFAP associated neuronal loss in HIV-1 Tat transgenic mice," *American Journal of Translational Research*, vol. 1, no. 1, pp. 72–79, 2009.

[165] D. E. Vance, G. Eagerton, B. Harnish, P. McKie, and P. L. Fazeli, "Cognitive prescriptions: a nursing approach to increasing cognitive reserve," *Journal of Gerontological Nursing*, vol. 37, no. 4, pp. 22–29, 2011.

[166] S. Rollnick, W. R. Miller, and C. C. Butler, *Motivational Interviewing in Health Care: Helping Patients Change Behavior*, Guilford Press, New York, NY, USA, 2007.

[167] G. W. LaVigna and A. M. Donnellan, *Alternatives to Punishment: Solving Behavior Problems with non-Aversive Strategies*, Irvington, New York, NY, USA, 1986.

[168] D. E. Vance, K. Heaton, Y. Eaves, and P. L. Fazeli, "Sleep and cognition on everyday functioning in older adults: implications for nursing practice and research," *Journal of Neuroscience Nursing*, vol. 43, no. 5, pp. 261–273, 2011.

[169] H. Noice and T. Noice, "A theatrical intervention to improve cognition in intact residents of long term care facilities," *Clinical Gerontologist*, vol. 29, no. 3, pp. 59–76, 2006.

[170] D. E. Vance, M. A. Graham, P. L. Fazeli, K. Heaton, and L. Moneyham, "An overview of non-pathological geroneuropsychology: implications for nursing practice and research," *Journal of Neuroscience Nursing*, vol. 44, no. 1, pp. 43–53, 2012.

[171] D. Vance, J. Dawson, V. Wadley et al., "The accelerate study: the longitudinal effect of speed of processing training on cognitive performance of older adults," *Rehabilitation Psychology*, vol. 52, no. 1, pp. 89–96, 2007.

[172] T. D. Marcotte, R. K. Heaton, T. Wolfson et al., "The impact of HIV-related neuropsychological dysfunction on driving behavior," *Journal of the International Neuropsychological Society*, vol. 5, no. 7, pp. 579–592, 1999.

[173] J. M. Wood, A. Chaparro, P. Lacherez, and L. Hickson, "Useful field of view predicts driving in the presence of distractors," *Optometry and Vision Science*, vol. 89, no. 4, pp. 373–381, 2012.

[174] D. E. Vance, P. L. Fazeli, L. Ross, V. G. Wadley, and K. K. Ball, "Speed of processing training with middle-aged and older adults with HIV: a pilot study," *Journal of the Association of Nurses in AIDS Care*, vol. 23, no. 6, pp. 500–510, 2012.

[175] D. E. Vance, P. McNees, and K. Meneses, "Technology, cognitive remediation, and nursing: directions for successful cognitive aging," *Journal of Gerontological Nursing*, vol. 35, no. 2, pp. 50–56, 2009.

[176] M. S. George and G. Aston-Jones, "Noninvasive techniques for probing neurocircuitry and treating illness: vagus nerve stimulation (VNS), transcranial magnetic stimulation (TMS) and transcranial direct current stimulation (tDCS)," *Neuropsychopharmacology*, vol. 35, no. 1, pp. 301–316, 2010.

[177] C. Miniussi and G. Vallar, "Brain stimulation and behavioural cognitive rehabilitation: a new tool for neurorehabilitation?" *Neuropsychological Rehabilitation*, vol. 21, no. 5, pp. 553–559, 2011.

[178] V. Walsh and A. Pascual-Leone, *Transcranial Magnetic Stimulation: A Neurochronometrics of Mind*, The MIT Press, Cambridge, Mass, USA, 2003.

[179] L. M. Bullard, E. S. Browning, V. P. Clark et al., "Transcranial direct current stimulation's effect on novice versus experienced learning," *Experimental Brain Research*, vol. 213, no. 1, pp. 9–14, 2011.

[180] C. Cerruti and G. Schlaug, "Anodal transcranial direct current stimulation of the prefrontal cortex enhances complex verbal associative thought," *Journal of Cognitive Neuroscience*, vol. 21, no. 10, pp. 190–197, 2009.

[181] V. P. Clark, B. A. Coffman, A. R. Mayer et al., "TDCS guided using fMRI significantly accelerates learning to identify concealed objects," *Neuroimage*, vol. 59, no. 1, pp. 117–128, 2012.

[182] A. Flöel, W. Suttorp, O. Kohl et al., "Non-invasive brain stimulation improves object-location learning in the elderly," *Neurobiology of Aging*, vol. 33, no. 8, pp. 1682–1689, 2012.

[183] D. Fox, "Brain buzz," *Nature*, vol. 472, pp. 156–159, 2011.

[184] R. Lindenberg, V. Renga, L. L. Zhu, D. Nair, and G. Schlaug, "Bihemispheric brain stimulation facilitates motor recovery in chronic stroke patients," *Neurology*, vol. 75, no. 24, pp. 2176–2184, 2010.

[185] M. A. Nitsche, "Beyond the target area: remote effects of non-invasive brain stimulation in humans," *Journal of Physiology*, vol. 489, part 13, pp. 3053–3054, 2011.

[186] M. Rosedale, D. Malaspina, D. Malamud et al., "Developing patient-center treatment protocols in brain stimulation: a rationale for combining quantitative and qualitative approaches in persons with HIV," *Journal of the American Nurses Association*, vol. 18, no. 3, pp. 166–174, 2012.

[187] H. Knotkova, M. Rosedale, S. Strauss et al., "Using transcranial direct current stimulation to treat depression in HIV-infected persons: the outcomes of a feasibility study," *Frontiers in Psychiatry*, vol. 3, no. 59, pp. 1–8, 2012.

[188] D. E. Vance, T. Struzick, and K. Farr, "Spaced retrieval technique-a cognitive tool for social workers and their clients," *Journal of Gerontological Social Work*, vol. 53, no. 2, pp. 148–158, 2010.

[189] C. Haslam, K. I. Hodder, and P. J. Yates, "Errorless learning and spaced retrieval: how do these methods fare in healthy and clinical populations?" *Journal of Clinical and Experimental Neuropsychology*, vol. 33, no. 4, pp. 432–447, 2011.

[190] K. L. Morrow and J. Fridriksson, "Comparing fixed- and randomized-interval spaced retrieval in anomia treatment," *Journal of Communication Disorders*, vol. 39, no. 1, pp. 2–11, 2006.

[191] M. M. Neundorfer, C. J. Camp, M. M. Lee, M. J. Skrajner, M. L. Malone, and J. R. Carr, "Compensating for cognitive deficits in persons aged 50 and over with HIV/AIDS: a pilot study of a cognitive intervention," *Journal of HIV/AIDS and Social Services*, vol. 3, no. 1, pp. 79–97, 2004.

[192] D. E. Vance, N. M. Webb, J. C. Marceaux, S. M. Viamonte, A. W. Foote, and K. K. Ball, "Mental stimulation, neural plasticity, and aging: directions for nursing research and practice," *Journal of Neuroscience Nursing*, vol. 40, no. 4, pp. 241–249, 2008.

[193] J. Huntley, D. Bor, A. Hampshire, A. Wen, and R. Howard, "Working memory task performance and chunking in early Alzheimer's disease," *British Journal of Psychiatry*, vol. 198, no. 5, pp. 398–403, 2011.

[194] D. Tomasi, N. D. Volkow, G. J. Wang et al., "Methylphenidate enhances brain activation and deactivation responses to visual attention and working memory tasks in healthy controls," *NeuroImage*, vol. 54, no. 4, pp. 3101–3110, 2011.

[195] Y. Harel, N. Appleboim, M. Lavie, and A. Achiron, "Single dose of methylphenidate improves cognitive performance in multiple sclerosis patients with impaired attention process," *Journal of the Neurological Sciences*, vol. 276, no. 1-2, pp. 38–40, 2009.

[196] R. M. Julien, *A Primer of Drug Action*, W. H. Freeman and Company, New York, NY, USA, 1998.

[197] C. H. Hinkin, S. A. Castellon, D. J. Hardy, R. Farinpour, T. Newton, and E. Singer, "Methylphenidate improves HIV-1-associated cognitive slowing," *Journal of Neuropsychiatry and Clinical Neurosciences*, vol. 13, no. 2, pp. 248–254, 2001.

[198] J. R. Berger, M. Kumar, A. Kumar, J. B. Fernandez, and B. Levin, "Cerebrospinal fluid dopamine in HIV-1 infection," *AIDS*, vol. 8, no. 1, pp. 67–71, 1994.

[199] G. Charach, N. Kaysar, I. Grosskopf, A. Rabinovich, and M. Weintraub, "Methylphenidate has positive hypocholesterolemic and hypotrigylceridemic effects: new data," *Journal of Clinical Pharmacology*, vol. 49, no. 7, pp. 848–851, 2009.

[200] E. J. Wright, B. Grund, K. Robertson et al., "Cardiovascular risk associated with lower baseline cognitive performance in HIV-positive persons," *Neurology*, vol. 75, no. 10, pp. 864–873, 2010.

[201] D. C. Turner, L. Clark, J. Dowson, T. W. Robbins, and B. J. Sahakian, "Modafinil improves cognition and response inhibition in adult attention-deficit/hyperactivity disorder," *Biological Psychiatry*, vol. 55, no. 10, pp. 1031–1040, 2004.

[202] M. McElhiney, J. Rabkin, W. Van Gorp, and R. Rabkin, "Modafinil effects on cognitive function in HIV+ patients treated for fatigue: a placebo controlled study," *Journal of Clinical and Experimental Neuropsychology*, vol. 32, no. 5, pp. 474–480, 2010.

[203] J. A. Yesavage, L. Friedman, J. W. Ashford et al., "Acetylcholinesterase inhibitor in combination with cognitive training in older adults," *Journals of Gerontology B8*, vol. 63, no. 5, pp. P288–P294, 2008.

[204] H. E. Gorby, A. M. Brownawell, and M. C. Falk, "Do specific dietary constituents and supplements affect mental energy? Review of the evidence," *Nutrition Reviews*, vol. 68, no. 12, pp. 697–718, 2010.

[205] M. J. Serby, S. J. Burns, and D. M. Roane, "Treatment of memory loss with herbal remedies," *Current Treatment Options in Neurology*, vol. 13, no. 5, pp. 520–528, 2011.

[206] B. E. Snitz, E. S. O'Meara, M. C. Carlson et al., "Ginkgo biloba for preventing cognitive decline in older adults a randomized trial," *Journal of the American Medical Association*, vol. 302, no. 24, pp. 2663–2670, 2009.

[207] M. J. Serby, C. Yhap, and E. Y. Landron, "A study of herbal remedies for memory complaints," *Journal of Neuropsychiatry and Clinical Neurosciences*, vol. 22, no. 3, pp. 345–347, 2010.

[208] D. W. Luchtman and C. Song, "Cognitive enhancement by omega-3 fatty acids from child-hood to old age: findings from animal and clinical studies," *Neuropharmacology*, vol. 64, pp. 550–565, 2013.

[209] E. Leblanc, B. Chan, and H. D. Nelson, *Hormone Replacement Therapy and Cognition. U. S. Preventive Services Task Force Evidence Syntheses, Formerly Systematic Evidence Reviews*, Agency for Healthcare Research and Quality, Rockville, Md, USA, 2002.

[210] V. Sharma and P. Perros, "The management of hypogonadism in aging male patients," *Postgraduate Medicine*, vol. 121, no. 1, pp. 113–121, 2009.

[211] E. Hogervorst and S. Bandelow, "Sex steroids to maintain cognitive function in women after the menopause: a meta-analyses of treatment trials," *Maturitas*, vol. 66, no. 1, pp. 56–71, 2010.

[212] N. Mitsiades, D. Correa, C. P. Gross, A. Hurria, and S. F. Slovin, "Cognitive effects of hormonal therapy in older adults," *Seminars in Oncology*, vol. 35, no. 6, pp. 569–581, 2008.

[213] S. A. Shumaker, C. Legault, S. R. Rapp et al., "Estrogen plus progestin and the incidence of dementia and mild cognitive impairment in postmenopausal Women—the Women's Health Initiative Memory Study: a randomized controlled trial," *Journal of the American Medical Association*, vol. 289, no. 20, pp. 2651–2662, 2003.

[214] N. Bassil and J. E. Morley, "Late-life onset hypogonadism: a review," *Clinics in Geriatric Medicine*, vol. 26, no. 2, pp. 197–222, 2010.

[215] D. E. Vance, L. A. Ross, and C. A. Downs, "Self-reported cognitive ability and global cognitive performance in adults with HIV," *Journal of Neuroscience Nursing*, vol. 40, no. 1, pp. 6–13, 2008.

[216] M. F. Folstein, S. E. Folstein, and P. R. McHugh, "'Mini mental state'. a practical method for grading the cognitive state of patients for the clinician," *Journal of Psychiatric Research*, vol. 12, no. 3, pp. 189–198, 1975.

[217] Z. Nasreddine, "Montreal Cognitive Assessment (MoCA): administration and scoring instructions," 2012, http://www.mocatest.org/.

[218] D. E. Broadbent, P. F. Cooper, P. FitzGerald, and K. R. Parkes, "The cognitive failures questionnaire (CFQ) and its correlates," *British Journal of Clinical Psychology*, vol. 21, no. 1, pp. 1–16, 1982.

[219] D. E. Vance, "A review of metacognition in aging with HIV," *Perceptual and Motor Skills*, vol. 103, no. 3, pp. 693–696, 2006.

[220] D. E. Vance, K. F. Farr, and T. Struzick, "Assessing the clinical value of cognitive appraisal in adults aging with HIV," *Journal of Gerontological Nursing*, vol. 34, no. 1, pp. 36–41, 2008.

[221] C. H. Hinkin, W. G. Van Gorp, P. Satz et al., "Actual versus self-reported cognitive dysfunction in HIV-1 infection: memory-metamemory dissociations," *Journal of Clinical and Experimental Neuropsychology*, vol. 18, no. 3, pp. 431–443, 1996.

[222] I. Mocchetti, A. Bachis, and V. Avdoshina, "Neurotoxicity of human immunodeficiency virus-1: viral proteins and axonal transport," *Neurotoxicity Research*, vol. 21, no. 1, pp. 79–89, 2012.

[223] J. Chmielewski and C. Hrycyna, "Tools for eradicating HIV in the brain: prodrug dimeric inhibitors of P-gp," *Therapeutic Delivery*, vol. 3, no. 6, pp. 689–692, 2012.

[224] H. Dou, C. B. Grotepas, J. M. McMillan et al., "Macrophage delivery of nanoformulated antiretroviral drug to the brain in a murine model of NeuroAIDS," *Journal of Immunology*, vol. 183, no. 1, pp. 661–669, 2009.

[225] H. L. Wong, N. Chattopadhyay, X. Y. Wu, and R. Bendayan, "Nanotechnology applications for improved delivery of antiretroviral drugs to the brain," *Advanced Drug Delivery Reviews*, vol. 62, no. 4-5, pp. 503–517, 2010.

[226] L. R. Hanson and W. H. Frey, "Strategies for intranasal delivery of therapeutics for the prevention and treatment of neuroAIDS," *Journal of Neuroimmune Pharmacology*, vol. 2, no. 1, pp. 81–86, 2007.

[227] D. E. Vance, "Olfactory and psychomotor symptoms in HIV and aging: potential precursors to cognitive loss," *Medical Science Monitor*, vol. 13, no. 10, pp. 1–3, 2007.

[228] D. E. Vance and J. Burrace Jr., "Chemosenory declines in older adults with HIV: identifying interventions," *Journal of Gerontological Nursing*, vol. 32, no. 7, pp. 42–48, 2006.

[229] S. Craft, L. D. Baker, T. J. Montine et al., "Intranasal insulin therapy for Alzheimer disease and amnestic mild cognitive impairment: a pilot clinical trial," *Archives of Neurology*, vol. 69, no. 1, pp. 29–38, 2012.

[230] S. L. Letendre, S. P. Woods, R. J. Ellis et al., "Lithium improves HIV-associated neurocognitive impairment," *AIDS*, vol. 20, no. 14, pp. 1885–1888, 2006.

[231] G. Schifitto, J. Zhong, D. Gill et al., "Lithium therapy for human immunodeficiency virus type 1-associated neurocognitive impairment," *Journal of NeuroVirology*, vol. 15, no. 2, pp. 176–186, 2009.

[232] T. H. Shepard, R. L. Brent, J. M. Friedman et al., "Update on new developments in the study of human teratogens," *Teratology*, vol. 65, no. 4, pp. 153–161, 2002.

[233] J. F. M. Wetzels, J. D. Van Bergeijk, A. J. Hoitsma, F. T. M. Huysmans, and R. A. P. Koene, "Triamterene increases lithium excretion in healthy subjects: evidence for lithium transport in the cortical collecting tubule," *Nephrology Dialysis Transplantation*, vol. 4, no. 11, pp. 939–942, 1989.

[234] G. Schifitto, B. A. Navia, C. T. Yiannoutsos et al., "Memantine and HIV-associated cognitive impairment: a neuropsychological and proton magnetic resonance spectroscopy study," *AIDS*, vol. 21, no. 14, pp. 1877–1886, 2007.

[235] Y. Zhao, B. A. Navia, C. M. Marra et al., "Memantine for AIDS dementia complex: open-label report of actg 301," *HIV Clinical Trials*, vol. 11, no. 1, pp. 59–67, 2010.

[236] T. D. Marcotte, D. Lazzaretto, J. C. Scott et al., "Visual attention deficits are associated with driving accidents in cognitively-impaired HIV-infected individuals," *Journal of Clinical and Experimental Neuropsychology*, vol. 28, no. 1, pp. 13–28, 2006.

[237] K. Ball, J. D. Edwards, L. A. Ross, and G. McGwin Jr., "Cognitive training decreases motor vehicle collision involvement of older drivers," *Journal of the American Geriatrics Society*, vol. 58, no. 11, pp. 2107–2113, 2010.

[238] M. E. Berryhill and K. T. Jones, "tDCS selectively improves working memory in older adults with more education," *Neuroscience Letters*, vol. 521, no. 2, pp. 148–151, 2012.

8

Do High Frequency Ultrasound Images Support Clinical Skin Assessment?

Alison P. Porter-Armstrong,[1] Catherine Adams,[2,3] Anne S. Moorhead,[2,4] Jeannie Donnelly,[5] Jane Nixon,[6] Daniel L. Bader,[7,8] Courtney Lyder,[9] and May D. Stinson[1]

[1] *The Institute of Nursing and Health Research, School of Health Sciences, University of Ulster, Newtownabbey BT37 0QB, UK*
[2] *School of Health Sciences, Faculty of Life and Health Sciences, University of Ulster, Newtownabbey BT37 0QB, UK*
[3] *School of Sociology, Social Policy & Social Work, Queen's University Belfast, Belfast BT7 1LP, UK*
[4] *Institute for Research in Social Sciences, School of Communication, University of Ulster, Newtownabbey BT37 0QB, UK*
[5] *Tissue Viability, The Royal Hospital, Belfast Health and Social Care Trust, Belfast BT12 6BA, UK*
[6] *Clinical Trials Research Unit, University of Leeds, Leeds LS2 9JT, UK*
[7] *School of Engineering and Materials Science, Queen Mary University of London, London E1 4NS, UK*
[8] *Faculty of Health Sciences, University of Southampton, Southampton SO17 1BJ, UK*
[9] *School of Nursing, University of California Los Angeles, Los Angeles, CA 90095, USA*

Correspondence should be addressed to Alison P. Porter-Armstrong; a.porter@ulster.ac.uk

Academic Editors: N. M. C. Alexandre and B. Mandleco

High frequency ultrasound imaging has been reported as a potential method of identifying the suspected tissue damage in patients "at risk" of pressure ulceration. The aim of this study was to explore whether ultrasound images supported the clinical skin assessment in an inpatient population through identification of subcutaneous tissue damage. Skin on the heels and/or sacral coccygeal area of fifty vascular surgery inpatients was assessed clinically by tissue viability nurses and with ultrasound pre operatively and at least every other day until discharge. Images were compared to routine clinical skin assessment outcomes. Qualitative classification of ultrasound images did not match outcomes yielded through the clinical skin assessment. Images corresponding to 16 participants were classified as subgroup 3 damage at the heels (equivalent to grade 2 pressure ulceration); clinical skin assessment rated no heels as greater than grade 1a (blanching erythema). Conversely, all images captured of the sacral coccygeal area were classified as normal; the clinical skin assessment rated two participants as grade 1b (non-blanching erythema). Ultrasound imaging is a potentially useful adjunct to the clinical skin assessment in providing information about the underlying tissue. However, further longitudinal clinical assessment is required to characterise images against actual and "staged" pressure ulceration.

1. Introduction

A pressure ulcer is defined as an area of localised damage to the skin and the underlying tissue caused by prolonged mechanical loading involving a combination of pressure, shear, and/or friction [1] with costs to the individual including pain, embarrassment, social exclusion, and a reduced quality of life [2]. Financial costs to the NHS of this largely preventable condition have been estimated to range from £1.4 to £2.1 billion per annum [3]. One subset of pressure ulcers, known as deep tissue injuries, has been characterised by damage which is localised in tissues at the bone muscle fascia, and which progresses up through the tissues in the form of oedema until reaching the skin surface [4, 5]. These are not readily apparent to the eye, and thus, by the time the clinical signs of deep tissue injury are evident, the injury is often well established and its resulting prognosis is variable [6].

The need for the investigation into early detection of pressure ulcers so that timely healthcare interventions can occur has been recognised [7]. Early detection and prevention would greatly reduce the burden on the patient and the associated economic and social costs associated with this condition. A number of techniques capable of early detection have been proposed, including the ultrasonic visualisation of subcutaneous oedema [4, 7, 8]. High frequency ultrasound (HFUS), at a frequency of 20 MHz, allows the real-time two-dimensional imaging of internal structures in a noninvasive manner and has been shown to be a potentially valuable method for the assessment of subcutaneous tissue damage pertaining to numerous pathophysiologies including the evaluation of wounds [7, 9–11]. The potential it offers in establishing parameters associated with the echogenicity of the ultrasound image could provide earlier identification of tissue damage than that being achievable through clinical skin assessment or photography alone [7, 8].

The aim of this study was to explore whether ultrasound images supported clinical skin assessment in a cohort of vascular surgery hospital inpatients.

2. Materials and Methods

Full ethical approval for the study was gained through the Office of Research Ethics Committee Northern Ireland (ORECNI). Hospital inpatients were approached to participate in the study if they were admitted for elective vascular surgery, provided written informed consent, and had intact skin on one or more areas to be scanned (sacral coccygeal area and either/or both heels). A single exclusion criterion of existing pressure damage of greater than, or equal to, *grade two* pressure ulceration (partial thickness skin loss involving epidermis, dermis, or both) [1] visible on the skin (including blisters, abrasions, and ulcers, where skin loss is present) of either heels or sacral coccygeal area was applied.

Patients were provided with written information on the study at a preassessment clinic approximately one week prior to admission and written informed consent gained within 24 hours of admission. During the six-month data collection period, a total of 90 patients were preassessed for vascular surgery, of whom 60 agreed to provide consent and were recruited to the study. Two participants subsequently withdrew consent, and a further eight participants were excluded from the analysis due to incomplete data resulting in a total of 50 participants being reported upon. Consenting participants had clinical assessments and high frequency ultrasound scanning conducted at least every other day throughout their inpatient hospital stay.

2.1. Clinical Assessments. Baseline clinical assessment was conducted by one of three tissue viability clinical research nurses (CRNs) using a comprehensive clinical research record Form (CRRF). Baseline characteristics were recorded including a summary of medical history and a number of completed standardised assessments including the Braden Scale for pressure ulcer risk [13], the Charlson index for comorbidities [14], and the Malnutrition Universal Screening Tool (MUST) for nutrition [15]. A clinical skin assessment was conducted at baseline, postoperatively and at least every other day by the CRN until discharge using a standard skin assessment record incorporating the modified EPUAP classification scale of pressure ulceration (Table 1) [12].

Table 1: Modified European Pressure Ulcer Advisory Panel grading system [12].

Grade	Description
0	Intact skin with no visible erythema
1a	Blanchable erythema of intact skin
1b	Nonblanchable erythema of intact skin
2	Partial thickness skin loss involving epidermis, dermis, or both
3	Full thickness skin loss involving damage to or necrosis of subcutaneous tissue that may extend down to, but not through, the underlying fascia
4	Full thickness skin loss with extensive destruction, tissue necrosis, or damage to muscle, bone, or supporting structures

2.2. Instrumentation and Scanning Procedure. The EPISCAN I-200 high frequency ultrasound scanner (Longport Inc, USA) was used to capture the images in this study. All ultrasound assessments were conducted by two trained researchers. In order to minimize any participant discomfort caused by repeated moving and handling, images were recorded at the same time as clinical skin assessments being recorded by the CRN. Heels were scanned at the three areas of the greatest potential pressure, that is, lateral, posterior, and medial aspects as well as the bony prominences of the coccyx and right and left sacrums.

2.3. Qualitative Image Assessment. Qualitative image assessment was performed by two blinded raters. Images were classified into four distinct subgroups based upon categorisation used by Quintavalle et al. [4] (Table 2 and Figure 1).

Statistical analysis was performed using SPSS version 15. Data were found not to be normally distributed using the Kolmogorov-Smirnov test. An α level of $P < 0.05$ was set a priori for all the analyses. Friedman's tests were used to determine differences over time in the clinical skin assessments; Spearman's rank order correlations were applied to determine the relationship between the clinical skin assessment and the qualitative image analysis; and a weighted Kappa statistic was applied to the qualitative image analysis, results to determine the interobserver agreement.

3. Results

Eleven females and 39 males with a mean age of 65 years (SD 9.66 years) participated in the study with average weight of 82.57 kgs (SD 17.41 kg), height of 171.74 cms (SD 9.13 cm), and body mass index of 28.14 (SD 4.38) Kg/m^2. Whilst only three participants were considered to be "at risk" of pressure ulceration (Braden Scale score of 15–18) and 90% of participants were identified to be at low risk of malnutrition according to the "MUST" tool, more than half of the participants (56%) were within the high risk category of comorbidity as indicated by the Charlson index.

Of the 50 participants who completed the study, 32 had their heels and sacral coccygeal area scanned, 17 had heels only scanned, and one had only the sacral coccygeal area scanned. A total of 1492 ultrasound images were assessed by the two raters (Table 3).

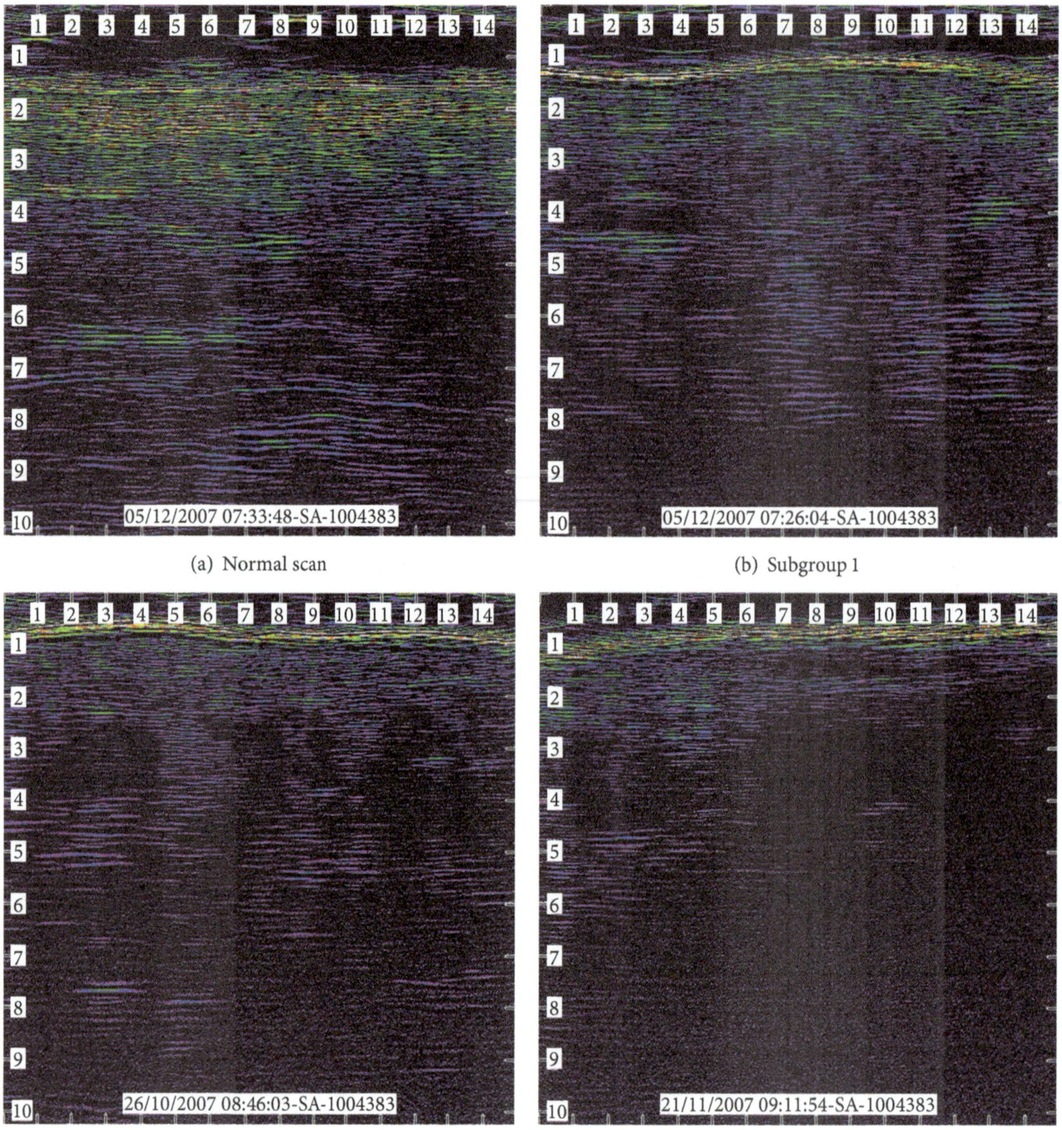

(a) Normal scan

(b) Subgroup 1

(c) Subgroup 2

(d) Subgroup 3

FIGURE 1: Examples of (a) "normal," (b) "subgroup 1," (c) "subgroup 2," and (d) "subgroup 3" images.

TABLE 2: Categories for the classification of high frequency ultrasound images [4].

Category	Description
0	Normal scan—no sign of PU development
Subgroup 1	Pockets of subcutaneous oedema
Subgroup 2	Strips of dermal damage and increased subcutaneous damage
Subgroup 3	Subepidermal inflammation, strips of dermal damage, and major subcutaneous damage
Ungraded	Unable to assess due to poor image quality

3.1. Clinical Assessment. No participants were clinically assessed as presenting with tissue changes greater than a grade 1b (nonblanching erythema of intact skin). Two participants were clinically assessed as showing signs of non-blanching erythema (*grade 1b*) on the marked skin sites on the coccyx, one of whom was also clinically assessed as showing signs of a *grade 1b* pressure ulcer on the left sacrum at a single time point postoperatively (Table 4). The two participants with nonblanching erythema had peripheral vascular disease and hypertension; however, neither of them were assessed as being "at risk" of developing pressure ulceration as per the Braden Scale [13].

Participants, heels were consistently clinically assessed as being either "normal" or presenting as no greater than a *grade 1a* (blanchable erythema of intact skin: see Table 4). Friedman's tests revealed no statistically significant changes over time.

3.2. Qualitative Image Assessment. Whilst clinical skin assessment identified the presence of non-blanching erythema on the coccyx in two participants and on the sacrum of one

Table 3: Clinical Skin Assessment.

	Grade 0 (%)	Grade 1a (%)	Grade 1b (%)
Left lateral heel	45 (90.00)	19 (38.00)	0 (0)
Left posterior heel	45 (90.00)	18 (36.00)	0 (0)
Left medial heel	40 (80.00)	20 (40.00)	0 (0)
Right lateral heel#	44 (89.80)	20 (40.82)	0 (0)
Right posterior heel#	44 (89.80)	18 (36.73)	0 (0)
Right medial heel#	44 (89.80)	20 (40.82)	0 (0)
Coccyx*	30 (90.91)	5 (15.15)	2 (6.06)
Right sacrum*	31 (93.94)	4 (12.12)	0 (0)
Left sacrum*	32 (96.97)	5 (15.15)	1 (3.03)

#Data available for 49 participants; 1 participant had right above knee amputation.
*Total of 33 participants.

Table 4: High frequency ultrasound image assessment of total 1492 images.

	Number of images		Number of participants	
	Rater 1	Rater 2	Rater 1	Rater 2
0 (normal)	748	808	49	48
Subgroup 1	375	291	46	43
Subgroup 2	285	265	34	39
Subgroup 3	69	121	16	18
Ungraded	15	7	6	5

participant, all ultrasound images of the coccyx and sacrum for all participants were assessed as being "normal" by both raters.

Conversely, 43 participants were assessed as having at least one heel image assessed by both raters as being *subgroup 1*, 34 having at least one heel image jointly assessed as being *subgroup 2*, and 16 having at least one heel image jointly assessed as being *subgroup 3* (Table 3). The Friedman test conducted on the entire data set, and on the subsample of participants presented with subgroup 3 images, revealed no statistically significant changes over time. The weighted kappa statistic applied to the qualitative image classifications revealed an overall agreement of 0.80, indicating a good level of agreement between the raters for all images.

4. Discussion

Increasing attention is being paid to the use of high frequency ultrasound scanning as a modality for wound and ulcer examination [9, 11] with some reports highlighting the potential application of high frequency ultrasound in imaging suspected subcutaneous oedema pertaining to pressure ulcers [7, 8, 10]. That is, in providing images of tissue damage below the skin surface that cannot be seen by the naked eye.

The present study investigated the use of high frequency ultrasound in supporting the clinical skin assessment by tissue viability nurses in the hospital inpatient setting. Two participants were clinically assessed as presenting with non-blanching erythema of intact skin (*grade 1b*) on the coccyx and for one individual on the sacrum. However, the images yielded by high frequency ultrasound for these participants were rated by both raters as being "normal." That is, the internal structures in the images of the sacral coccygeal areas appeared clear, accompanied by good definition of the epidermis, dermis, and subcutaneous tissues.

Conversely, the clinical skin assessment assessed no participant as presenting with skin damage greater than grade 1a (blanching erythema of intact skin) on any aspect of their heels, yet high frequency ultrasound revealed images concurrent with the suspected underlying tissue damage to the heels. The qualitative image analysis of this data set revealed 16 participants (32%) having at least one *subgroup 3* image. This incidence of *subgroup 3* category images, that is, sub-epidermal inflammation, strips of dermal damage, and major subcutaneous damage, infers the presence of clinical signs equivalent to *grade two* pressure ulceration and above. Such signs were not however assessed clinically. Due to the absence of any longer term followup following the discharge from the vascular surgery ward (average 5.8 days ± 3.38 days SD postadmission), it is unknown whether or not this suspected subcutaneous damage progressed into clinical signs of pressure ulceration. As the pathophysiology of the hypoechogenicity visualised in the *subgroup 3* images remains uncertain, and no correlation existed between the presence of those hypoechoic areas and the clinical assessment of pressure ulceration in this study, no firm conclusions can be drawn as to whether these images represented true deep tissue damage not visible to the eye through routine clinical skin assessment. With so little tissue damage clinically evident in this study, it remains unknown whether any areas of low echogenicity as visualised in the images equated to actual tissue damage.

5. Conclusion

Ultrasound imaging offers a potentially useful adjunct to the clinical skin assessment in providing information about the underlying tissue damage not seen by the naked eye. However, further longitudinal clinical work is required to scan "at risk" individuals over time to characterise the images yielded against manifest pressure ulcers and the various stages of skin breakdown, as well as against clinical skin assessment outcomes.

Acknowledgments

This study was funded by the University of Ulster, the Strategic Priority Fund, and the Department of Learning and Development, Northern Ireland. The authors would like to acknowledge Mr. Paul Wilson and Longport Inc for the loan of the ultrasound scanner, Mr. Paul Brannigan and Mr. Shay Deegan, Medical Physics Agency, Northern Ireland, and the Clinical Research Nurses and Mr. Paul Blair, Consultant Vascular Surgeon, Belfast Health and Social Care Trust in facilitating data collection, and Ms. Evie Gardner (formerly University of Ulster) for the statistical advice.

References

[1] European Pressure Ulcer Advisory Panel, "Pressure Ulcer Treatment Guidelines," 1999, www.epuap.org/gltreatment.html.

[2] K. Spilsbury, A. Nelson, N. Cullum, C. Iglesias, J. Nixon, and S. Mason, "Pressure ulcers and their treatment and effects on quality of life: hospital inpatient perspectives," *Journal of Advanced Nursing*, vol. 57, no. 5, pp. 494–504, 2007.

[3] G. Bennett, C. Dealey, and J. Posnett, "The cost of pressure ulcers in the UK," *Age and Ageing*, vol. 33, no. 3, pp. 230–235, 2004.

[4] P. R. Quintavalle, C. H. Lyder, P. J. Mertz, C. Phillips-Jones, and M. Dyson, "Use of high-resolution, high-frequency diagnostic ultrasound to investigate the pathogenesis of pressure ulcer development." *Advances in Skin & Wound Care*, vol. 19, no. 9, pp. 498–505, 2006.

[5] L. Agam and A. Gefen, "Pressure ulcers and deep tissue injury: a bioengineering perspective," *Journal of Wound Care*, vol. 16, no. 8, pp. 336–342, 2007.

[6] J. E. Grey, S. Enoch, and K. G. Harding, "ABC of wound healing: pressure Ulcers," *British Medical Journal*, vol. 332, no. 7539, pp. 472–475, 2006.

[7] E. S. Andersen and T. Karlsmark, "Evaluation of four non-invasive methods for examination and characterization of pressure ulcers," *Skin Research and Technology*, vol. 14, no. 3, pp. 270–276, 2008.

[8] K. Yabunaka, S. Iizaka, G. Nakagami et al., "Can ultrasonographic evaluation of subcutaneous fat predict pressure ulceration?" *Journal of Wound Care*, vol. 18, no. 5, pp. 192–196, 2009.

[9] M. Dyson, S. Moodley, L. Verjee, W. Verling, J. Weinman, and P. Wilson, "Wound healing assessment using 20 MHz ultrasound and photography," *Skin Research and Technology*, vol. 9, no. 2, pp. 116–121, 2003.

[10] N. Kanno, T. Nakamura, M. Yamanaka, K. Kouda, T. Nakamura, and F. Tajima, "Low-echoic lesions underneath the skin in subjects with spinal-cord injury," *Spinal Cord*, vol. 47, no. 3, pp. 225–229, 2009.

[11] M. Ueta, J. Sugama, C. Konya et al., "Use of ultrasound in assessment of necrotic tissue in pressure ulcers with adjacent undermining," *Journal of Wound Care*, vol. 20, no. 11, pp. 503–510, 2011.

[12] J. Nixon, H. Thorpe, H. Barrow et al., "Reliability of pressure ulcer classification and diagnosis," *Journal of Advanced Nursing*, vol. 50, no. 6, pp. 613–623, 2005.

[13] N. Bergstrom, B. J. Braden, A. Laguzza, and V. Holman, "The braden scale for predicting pressure sore risk," *Nursing Research*, vol. 36, no. 4, pp. 205–210, 1987.

[14] M. E. Charlson, P. Pompei, K. A. Ales, and C. R. MacKenzie, "A new method of classifying prognostic comorbidity in longitudinal studies: development and validation," *Journal of Chronic Diseases*, vol. 40, no. 5, pp. 373–383, 1987.

[15] Malnutrition Advisory Group, *The 'MUST' Report Nutritional Screening of Adults: A multidisciplinary Responsibility*, BAPEN, Redditch, UK, 2003.

9

Subjectively Evaluated Effects of Domestic Violence on Well-Being in Clinical Populations

Marika Poutiainen and Juha Holma

Department of Psychology, Psychotherapy Training and Research Center, University of Jyväskylä, P.O. Box 35, 40014 Jyväskylä, Finland

Correspondence should be addressed to Juha Holma; juha.m.holma@jyu.fi

Academic Editors: R. Constantino and P. J. Kelly

Effects of domestic violence are reflected in victims' physical, psychological, and sexual health as well as in victims' subjective evaluations of health or subjective well-being. The principal aim of this study was to study the extent to which the consequences of domestic violence are reflected in patients' subjectively evaluated well-being, life management, and sense of security in an emergency department, a maternity department, and a reception unit of a psychiatric hospital. A questionnaire on the effects of domestic violence was administered to 530 patients. 61 patients reported either current or previous domestic violence that affected their current well-being and life management. Domestic violence was reported to have an effect on subjective well-being and sense of security: the more recent or frequent the experience of violence was, the greater was considered its impact on well-being and sense of security. Routine inquiry can uncover hidden cases of abuse and hence would be of great benefit in the healthcare context. Early identification of abuse victims can prevent further harm caused by violence.

1. Introduction

Findings from previous studies suggest that violence increases the use of all health services [1, 2]. As a result, the prevalence of domestic violence is assumed to be higher in clinical settings than in the general population. A review of prevalence studies on domestic violence against women found high figures for violence in obstetrics and gynaecology, psychiatric, and emergency clinic settings [3]. Results for the same Finnish clinical populations as in this study [4] indicate moderate to high prevalence rates of both recent and lifetime domestic violence. In the maternity department, nearly 3% reported experiencing current abuse, whereas over 29% reported previous abuse. These prevalences mirror some previous findings [5], but are lower than others [6]. Among the emergency department respondents, 10% reported current domestic violence and over 20% past experience of abuse. Similar lifetime prevalences have been reported, for instance, by Boyle and Todd [7]. The highest incidence and lifetime prevalence rates were found among the patients in the psychiatric hospital: current domestic violence was reported by 29% and previous violence by 51% of these patients. These findings are also consistent with those found in other studies [8].

Although violence increases the use of all health services, studies have shown that victims of abuse often seek medical help for other health complications than abuse-related injuries [9]. Findings from previous studies suggest that female victims may delay seeking help until the abuse becomes extremely serious [10]. Two-fifths of the women killed by their intimate partner had sought medical care in the year prior to their murder [11]. Moreover, victims of abuse may be reluctant to discuss their experiences: evidence suggests that the disclosure of abuse is related to being directly asked about it [12, 13]. Such low rates of spontaneous disclosure suggest that the responsibility for the identification of domestic violence may lie with healthcare professionals. However, there is a tendency for health professionals to focus on fixing the injuries and consequences of domestic violence and bypassing violence as the cause of symptoms and injuries [14]. Routine inquiry may be of great benefit in such situations.

Routine inquiry—also referred to as universal screening—is defined as inquiry about domestic violence targeted at all patients in a given setting [15]. Not only does routine inquiry have many advantages [16], it is also accepted by the victims of abuse [17, 18]. Routine inquiry increases the detection of violence victims by uncovering hidden cases of abuse; it makes access to support services easier for victims and helps maintain the safety of the victim [16]. In addition, routine inquiry changes health professionals' knowledge and attitudes towards domestic violence. It is commonly suggested that healthcare services constitute an ideal setting for screening for domestic violence because of the frequent contact of personnel with possible violence victims.

2. The Consequences of Domestic Violence for Well-Being

Domestic violence has adverse effects on a victim's physical, psychological, and sexual health regardless of the type of violence experienced. Studies have shown that the consequences of domestic violence can last long after the violence has ended [19]. Injuries, stress, and fear caused by domestic violence can lead to more chronic health problems, such as chronic pain, recurring central nervous system symptoms, and differential gastrointestinal symptoms and disorders [20]. Among possible psychological conditions, Macy and colleagues [2] reported that domestic violence can result in depression, anxiety, and posttraumatic stress disorder (PTSD). Victims of abuse are also more likely to have co-occurring mental illnesses. Moreover, the previous research suggests that there is a significant relationship between child abuse and different adult psychological disorders, including psychosis [21].

Researchers suggest that the timing, frequency, and type of violence experienced affect the overall magnitude of the impact of domestic violence on the health of victims. For instance, Wijma et al. [22] concluded that the recency of violence is related to the frequency of PTSD symptoms among physically or sexually abused women. Similarly, Macy and associates [2] found that recent violence has a more detrimental effect on health compared to previous domestic violence. A study conducted by Tolman and Rosen [23], in turn, indicated that women who had experienced abuse recently (within the past 12 months) were more likely to have a mental health disorder than the past-victim group (women who have not been abused in the past 12 months) and also reported more health-related concerns than nonabused women. Thus, although the impact of violence can be enduring [19], studies have shown that its effects may diminish over time if the abuse is not repeated [23].

Different types of violence may also have different consequences on individual well-being. Sexual abuse in particular is considered to be detrimental for women's physical and psychological health [2]. Furthermore, the impact of victimization may be greater if the violence takes multiple forms [2, 20]. In addition, studies suggest that severe and chronic forms of violence have the most serious effect on individual well-being [24].

It has been suggested that men and women have different interpretations of domestic violence and its consequences. In a study conducted by R. P. Dobash and R. E. Dobash [25] the results indicated that men's violence toward women differs from women's violence toward men not only in terms of frequency, severity and, consequences, but also in terms of the victim's sense of safety and well-being. Most men in the study reported women's violence towards them to be "inconsequential," "not so serious," or "slightly serious" and indicated that the violence did not affect their sense of well-being and safety [25, page 343]. Differences between these interpretations may be caused by the fact that men's and women's experiences of domestic abuse differ qualitatively and quantitatively [26]. Violence against women appears to be more frequent and severe, and women are also at greater risk for sexual violence or coercion [25–27]. Accordingly, some studies have suggested that the physical and psychological consequences of domestic violence may be more severe for women than men [28].

3. Subjective Well-Being

Violence adversely affects the victim's quality of life along multiple dimensions [2, 20, 29]. The detrimental effects of violence are reflected not only in victims' physical, psychological, and sexual health, but also in victims' subjective evaluations of health or subjective well-being (SWB). Studies have shown abuse victims to report their current health as "poor" or "very poor" more often than individuals who did not report abuse [19, 24, 30].

According to Friedman et al. [31, page 189] subjective well-being (SWB) refers to "the psychological well-being of a person and how satisfying a person believes his or her life is." In other words, SWB is a person's global assessment of quality of life, as measured from that individual's personal perspective [32, 33]. SWB is comprised of cognitive and affective components, involving one's cognitive judgment of overall life satisfaction and positive and negative emotional reactions to one's life, respectively [32, 34].

Research has shown that in addition to factors such as age, gender, income, and mental and physical health, life events also have a significant influence on SWB [33, 35]. Whereas positive events seem to increase one's SWB, negative events have a decreasing or negative impact. It is important to note that one's perceived ability to control life events is related to the overall impact an event has on one's SWB [35]. This suggests that life management or the relatively stable belief that one has the ability to control one's life and the things that happen to one will also contribute to one's SWB by moderating the effects of different life events.

Previous studies suggest that subjectively rated health has a strong relationship with happiness and SWB, whereas the relationship between objectively evaluated health and SWB is substantially weaker (yet statistically significant) [35]. It can thus be argued that an individual's subjective evaluation of well-being offers an alternative approach to more objective health measures (such as symptom checklists or physician ratings) in examining the effects of domestic violence on health and well-being. Subjective evaluation of well-being represents a global evaluation of life satisfaction, involving both physical and psychological aspects of health and the subject's affective reactions to life events. Although subjective well-being has been widely researched in different contexts [33, 35], the question of the influence of domestic violence on subjectively evaluated well-being has not received much interest.

4. Objectives

In most cases, the consequences of domestic violence for physical and psychological health have been studied using survey questionnaire methods. A common approach to addressing the relationship between violence and adverse health consequences is to present victims with questions about their life-time experiences of violence and recurrent health problems. Only few studies to date have also included victims' subjective opinion of their current health (e.g., [19, 24, 30]).

Wijma and colleagues [22] used subjective evaluations in order to compare violence experiences of women with PTSD and women who did not suffer from PTSD. Using a Likert-type scale ranging from 0 to 10, they asked female abuse victims to mark the number that best corresponded to their experience of abuse, when it happened, and how much they had suffered from that abuse. The results led to the conclusion that the more traumatic the experience was appraised as being, the more suffering it caused and the greater the risk for developing PTSD. PTSD, in turn, was found to be associated with the amount and recency of the abuse. Unfortunately, the possible influences of timing, type, or frequency of violence on victims' evaluations were not examined. Evidence further suggests that there are individual differences among abuse victims in their interpretation of the consequences of violence. For instance, Wijma and colleagues [6] found that not all abuse victims report ill effects experienced as a result of the experience of violence. However, the possible influences behind these differences were not thoroughly addressed in this study either.

Given the gap in the literature pointed out above, this study focuses on subjective evaluations by the victims of domestic violence on its effects on their current well-being, life management, and sense of security. In particular, the overall objective of the study was to examine the factors influencing these subjective evaluations. It was hypothesized that these subjective evaluations would be moderated by the factors that influence the magnitude of the impact that violence has on health. These factors, which have been identified earlier, are the timing, frequency, and type of violence. The potential impact of gender differences and differences in the subjective evaluations between the three patient groups are also examined.

5. Methods

The effects of domestic violence were measured using a routine inquiry tool in the Violence Intervention in Specialist Healthcare (VISH) project. VISH is the first comprehensive project designed specifically for the social and healthcare sector in the Finnish context. It has been funded by the EU Daphne Programme in 2009-2010 and by Central Finland Health Care District (CFHCD). Its main objective is to improve early identification of and intervention in domestic violence in the District's hospitals by increasing the skills, ability, and willingness of the staff to ask about domestic violence and, if required, to intervene. In so doing, VISH will provide an evidence-based model for intervening in domestic violence in specialist healthcare settings and strengthen the channels for offering help to both the victims and perpetrators of violence and their families.

One of the specific research aims of the VISH project was to examine the prevalence, incidence, and nature of domestic violence in three pilot units: an emergency department (ED), a gynaecology department, and the acute unit of a psychiatric hospital. Data were collected during the VISH study, which focused on the identification of adult victims of violence, and further care assessments made by staff form the foundation for the present paper.

In the VISH project domestic violence is defined as abuse committed by current or former spouses, boy- or girlfriends, parents, step-parents, siblings, grandparents or other close relatives of the victim. The following types of violence are included: physical, emotional, sexual, religious/cultural, and economic violence, as well as neglect of care.

5.1. Measuring the Effects of Domestic Violence. The routine inquiry tool was developed on the basis of international screening instruments, such as the Abuse Assessment Screen (AAS) [36], the Hurt, Insult, Threaten and Scream (screening tool) scale (HITS) [37], the Partner Violence Screen (PVS) [38], and the Woman Abuse Screening Tool (WAST) [39]. Also considered in the design of the routine inquiry tool were the recommendations for data collection on domestic violence of The National Institute for Health and Welfare (THL) and The Council of European Member States. The documentation of domestic violence is recommended to at least include the following information: (1) age and (2) sex of the victim; (3) age and (4) sex of the perpetrator; (5) the relationship between the victim and the perpetrator; and (6) the type of violence (e.g., according to the International Classification of Diseases, ICD-10) [40].

The questionnaire includes both filter and mapping questions for healthcare professionals when interviewing patients about their domestic violence experiences. In the VISH study, questions were posed to respondents orally in a private space by members of the hospital staff, such as nurses or midwives. The filter questions addressed current or previous domestic violence experiences and their effect on the well-being and life management of the patient. Victims of abuse were asked to evaluate the effects of violence on their well-being, life management, and sense of security Respondents who reported that their well-being and life management were affected were invited to answer mapping questions, that is, more detailed questions about the violence they had experienced, and asked to estimate the extent to which this has affected both their current well-being and sense of security. The latter was assessed on an 11-point scale (0 = no effect, 10 = serious effect). The mapping questions also addressed the type of violence, perpetrator, latest time, and frequency, and whether or not children had witnessed the abuse. In addition, the healthcare professional conducting the interview was asked to evaluate whether the victim being interviewed was exposed to significant health risks in his or her current situation.

5.2. Setting and Subjects. The data collection was conducted during the Spring of 2010 among three VISH pilot units in the CFHCD. During set periods, patients from these pilot units were routinely questioned by means of a structured form about their experiences of domestic violence. Patients meeting the following excluding criteria were not included in the study: age under 18 years old; mother language other than Finnish or insufficient language skills in Finnish; disabled or handicapped; and resident outside the CFHCD.

Of the 530 patients presented with the filter questions, 61 patients indicated that current and/or previous domestic violence affected their current well-being and life management. These 61 individuals were further interviewed by means of the mapping questions.

5.3. Analysis. The analysis was conducted using the Predictive Analytics Software (PASW) Statistics 18.0 Package for Windows. This involved, first, comparisons of the different patient and gender groups based on respondents' verbal evaluations of the influence of domestic violence on their current well-being and life management. These comparisons were achieved by the means of the Pearson's Chi-Square (χ^2) test and the Fisher-Irwin Exact Test ($P < .01$). The Pearson's χ^2 was used where the relevant assumptions were satisfied (i.e., for all tables in which more than 25% of the expected counts were greater than five), and in all other cases the Fisher-Irwin Exact Test was used.

The comparison between patient groups with regard to their numerical evaluations of the influence of domestic violence on both well-being and sense of security was conducted using the Kruskal-Wallis one-way Analysis of Variance (ANOVA). The variables of interest were not normally distributed, and therefore this nonparametric test was used (as opposed to the parametric ANOVA). Pairwise comparisons were conducted using the Mann-Whitney *U* test.

Finally, the relationship between respondents' subjective evaluations and the specified background variables was studied using cross-tabulation and correlation coefficients, namely, the Pearson's Product-Moment Correlation Coefficient and the Spearman Rank Order Correlation Coefficient. Where sample sizes and the scale of the variables precluded the use of the parametric Pearson's correlation, these were computed solely to determine whether the Spearman coefficients resembled them sufficiently to justify the use of Regression Analysis.

Hierarchical Regression Analysis (RA) was used to enable the identification of the relative importance of each independent variable in accounting for the observed variance in the independent variables.

6. Results

Nearly all of the victims of current violence (21/22) reported that the most recent experience of abuse influenced their current well-being and life management. Patients in the ED were not presented with the question as during tests of the tool in the psychiatric hospital and the maternity department; it was found that current abuse was reported to have an effect on well-being and life management in nearly in all cases. However, only 38% (59/155) of the victims of previous violence (ED patients included) reported that these past experiences influenced their current well-being. The percentage difference between the impact of recent versus past experiences on well-being and life management was statistically significant ($z = 5{,}08$; $P < .001$). Thus, experiences of abuse were more often evaluated as impacting on the well-being and life management of victims of current violence than victims of previous violence.

6.1. Subjective Evaluations of the Effects of Domestic Violence. Although within each patient group small percentage differences were observed with regard to the number of victims who evaluated previous domestic violence as influencing their well-being and life management, no statistically significant differences were found between the three patient groups ($\chi^2(2) = .19$, $P > 0.99$).

Gender comparisons were conducted between the ED and the psychiatric hospital. In the ED, only one male victim of previous domestic violence reported current ill effects from this abuse. The corresponding rate for females was 41% (7/17). However, no statistically significant gender differences were found among the ED patients ($P = .61$, Fisher's Exact Test).

In the psychiatric hospital, in turn, 25% (3/12) of male victims and 56% (5/9) of female victims reported that previously experienced domestic violence influenced their current well-being and life management. In spite of the percentage difference, no statistically significant difference was found. Male and female patients in the psychiatric hospital did not differ in their evaluations of whether or not previously experienced violence affects their current well-being and life management ($P = .20$, Fisher's Exact Test).

During the mapping questions, victims who had stated that their experience of abuse, current or previous, had impacted on their current well-being and life management were asked to estimate on an 11-point scale (0 = no effect, 10 = serious effect) the extent to which the abuse has affected both their current well-being and sense of security. The medians of victims' subjective evaluations were 3 maternity patients, 9 psychiatric patients, and 10 ED patients.

The Kruskal-Wallis test showed significant differences between the patient groups' numerical subjective evaluations of the effects of domestic violence on well-being ($\chi^2(2) =$

15.6, $P < .001$). Further analysis through pairwise comparisons showed significant differences between the maternity department and the ED ($U = 61,5$, $P = .005$) as well as the maternity department and the psychiatric hospital ($U = 100,5$, $P = .001$). No differences were found between the subjective evaluations of the ED and psychiatric patients ($U = 46,5$, $P = .70$). The effects of domestic violence on well-being and life management were evaluated more negatively by the ED and psychiatric patients than maternity patients. Finally, no differences were found between the patient groups in their subjective evaluations of the effect of domestic violence on sense of security ($\chi^2(2) = .92$, $P = .63$).

6.2. Variables Influencing Subjective Evaluations. The subjective evaluations of the impact of domestic violence on well-being or sense of security were influenced by only one type of violence, namely, neglect of care. Only one participant did not report experiencing emotional abuse.

A significant association was found between the well-being evaluation and the security evaluation ($\rho = .55$, $P < .01$). With regard to the other background variables, the subjective evaluation of the effects of violence on well-being was found to be negatively correlated to the recency ($\rho = -.53$, $P < .01$) and frequency of violence ($\rho = -.40$, $P < .01$). This finding suggests that victims considered violence to have a higher impact on well-being if it was more recent or frequent. The subjective evaluations of the effect of violence on sense of security were also influenced by the most recent experience of violence ($\rho = -.51$, $P < .01$) and frequency of violence ($\rho = -.29$, $P < .05$).

As is apparent from Table 1 , the nonparametric correlation coefficients resembled the parametric coefficients sufficiently, and thus RA was conducted. Here, a hierarchical regression model was conducted, first for the sense of security evaluation. The reasoning behind this decision was based on the strong association between the two subjective evaluations and the possibility that the sense of security evaluation (which can also indicate fear) has an impact on the well-being evaluation. Variables were entered into models based on correlations.

The most recent experience of violence served as a significant predictor of the security evaluation ($\beta = -.59, t(59) = -5,57, P < .001$) and explained 34,5% of the variance in these evaluations ($F(1,59) = 31,04$, $P < .001$). When the effect of the most recent experience of abuse was accounted for, the frequency of violence did not significantly increase the proportion of the variance explained ($\Delta R^2 = .003$, $F(1,58) = .25$, $P = .62$). Consequently, this variable was excluded from the final model. Similarly, neglect of care was not included in the model, because one of the correlation coefficients was statistically significant.

The variables entered into the regression model for the well-being evaluation were the security assessment, most recent experience of violence, frequency of violence, and neglect of care. The analysis indicated that when frequency of violence was entered into the model as a second predictor, more variance was predicted ($\Delta R^2 = .06$) than when the most recent experience of violence was entered ($\Delta R^2 = .045$, ns). Thus, the final regression model included the sense of security evaluation ($\beta = .44, t(57) = 4,25, P < .001$), frequency of violence ($\beta = -.31, t(57) = -3,10, P = .003$), and neglect of care ($\beta = .28, t(57) = 2,78, P = .007$). This model explained a significant proportion (50%) of the variance of the well-being evaluation.

7. Discussion

The consequences of domestic violence were clearly reflected in victims' subjective evaluations. Moreover, nearly all the victims of current domestic violence reported the abuse to influence their current SWB and life management. Previous results have suggested that some types of domestic violence, especially sexual abuse, may have more detrimental consequences than others for the health of the victim [2]. However, in the present study, subjective evaluations of both well-being and sense of security were influenced by only one type of violence, namely, neglect of care. Thus, no significant association was found between sexual violence and the subjective evaluations. A possible explanation for this finding is that most of the victims of sexual violence reported the most recent experience of abuse to be earlier in adulthood or in their childhood, whereas over one-half of the victims of neglect of care reported experiencing violence within the past 24 hours, week, or month. As previous research has indicated, the traumatic consequences of abuse may diminish if the violence is not repeated [23]. For instance, victims of previous abuse may have already received help and treatment in their situation [6].

As already suggested above, the recency of violence was related to the subjective evaluations of both well-being and sense of security. Experiences of abuse were more often evaluated as impacting on their well-being and life management by victims of current domestic violence than victims of previous abuse. This finding is in accordance with findings from previous research which have suggested an association between the most recent experience of violence and its consequences for health [2, 6, 22, 23]. In addition, significant associations were found between both of the numerical subjective evaluations and the frequency of violence. This finding is also in accordance with previous research, which has indicated that the effects of violence may be more severe if the violence experienced is chronic [24]. Together these results lead to the conclusion that the more recent or frequent the violence was, the higher its impact on SWB and sense of security was perceived to be. In this regard, a significant relationship was also found between the two different subjective evaluations. A possible explanation for this finding is that the fear caused by violence influences the victim's sense of security, which in turn has an effect on overall SWB.

Finally, when the relative importance of each associated variable (the type, timing, and frequency of violence) and the relationship between the subjective evaluations were controlled, the results indicated that the subjectively evaluated effects of domestic violence on sense of security were mostly influenced by the most recent experience of violence. This

TABLE 1: Summary of Spearman and Pearson's correlations for scores on well-being, security, recency, frequency, and neglect of care.

Measure	1	2	3	4	5
(1) Well-being	—				
(2) Security	.549** (.609**)	—			
(3) Recency	−.534** (−.530**)	−.511** (−.587**)	—		
(4) Frequency	−.404** (−.418**)	−.279* (−.291*)	.623** (.569**)	—	
(5) Neglect of care	.380** (.386**)	.244 (.293*)	−.314* (−.356**)	.068 (.058)	—

Significance level: * $P < .05$, ** $P < .01$
Pearson's correlations are presented in parenthesis.

explained more than a third of the variance in the dependent variable. SWB, in turn, was influenced by the sense of security evaluation, the frequency of violence, and experiences of neglect of care. Together, these variables accounted for over 50% of the variance in SWB.

This study also examined possible differences with regard to the subjective evaluations by gender and patient group. In the patient groups, the effects of domestic violence on SWB were evaluated more negatively by the ED and psychiatric patients than maternity patients. One possible explanation for this finding is that most of the maternity patients reported experiencing violence earlier in adulthood or childhood, whereas for most of the ED and psychiatric patients the last experience of abuse was more recent. No significant gender differences were found.

For example, the present routine inquiry targeted at victims of domestic violence was comprehensive and aimed at reaching as many abuse victims as possible. The focus was not only on intimate partner violence (IPV, i.e., abuse committed by current or former spouses), but also on abuse committed by parents, step-parents, siblings, grandparents, or other close relatives. In addition, a wide variety of violent acts were screened for unlike several other studies, which have concentrated on the most common forms of abuse (i.e., psychological, physical, and sexual), this study also focused on victims of neglect of care, religious or cultural and economic violence. Finally, the abuse experiences of both sexes were examined, as previous studies have suggested that domestic violence affects both men and women.

8. Limitations and Strengths

The number of participants answering the mapping questions was small ($n = 61$), and the comparisons between the gender and patient groups were done for even smaller subgroups. Although a significant difference was found between the patient groups in their subjective well-being evaluations, these results must be interpreted with caution.

The data collection has some potential limitations. For instance, the answers given by the participants may have been influenced by the style in which the screening was conducted. Whereas in the present paper the questions were presented to the participants orally, some studies have suggested that victims of violence prefer self-administered questionnaires over face-to-face interviews [41]. However, this matter is controversial, since other studies have reported higher detection rates with verbal screening compared to self-administered written screening [42]. Also, since the data collected in this study rely solely on self-reports, the general unwillingness to disclose violence, possible recall bias, or suppression of traumatic memories may have influenced the findings [6, 43]. In the case of maternity patients, for example, mothers often fear that talking about domestic violence may cause them to lose custody of their children [10, 44, 45].

Despite the possible weaknesses mentioned above, this study also had a number of strengths worthy of consideration.

9. Conclusions

This study adds to the literature by indicating the presence of high incidence and lifetime prevalence rates of domestic violence among clinical populations. Most of these incidences, current or past, would have remained concealed had this study not been conducted. It may therefore be concluded that routine inquiry into abuse experiences may be of great benefit in the healthcare context. As the previous literature has suggested, routine inquiry uncovers hidden cases of violence, changes perceptions of the acceptability of domestic violence, and makes support services more accessible to victims, while at the same time assisting in maintaining their safety [16].

This study also addressed a specific gap in the previous research, namely, the relationship between violence and subjective well-being. The results of this study indicated that the consequences of abuse are strongly reflected in the subjectively evaluated well-being, life management, and sense of security of the victim. The more recent and frequent the abuse was, the higher its impact on well-being and sense of security was evaluated to be. Although intervention at any point can be regarded as effective, since the effects of the abuse can be enduring [29], the results of this study underline the importance of early detection of victims of domestic violence. Such early detection can prevent violence from escalating in severity and causing its victims further harm.

References

[1] B. Bergman and B. Brismar, "A 5-year follow-up study of 117 battered women," *American Journal of Public Health*, vol. 81, no. 11, pp. 1486–1489, 1991.

[2] R. J. Macy, J. Ferron, and C. Crosby, "Partner violence and survivors' chronic health problems: Informing social work practice," *Social Work*, vol. 54, no. 1, pp. 29–43, 2009.

[3] S. Alhabib, U. Nur, and R. Jones, "Domestic violence against women: systematic review of prevalence studies," *Journal of Family Violence*, vol. 25, no. 4, pp. 369–382, 2010.

[4] M. Notko, J. Holma, M. Husso et al., "Lähisuhdeväkivallan tunnistaminen erikoissairaanhoidossa. English summary: identifying domestic violence within specialized care," *Duodecim*, vol. 127, no. 15, pp. 1599–1606, 2011.

[5] L. W. Hedin, H. Grimstad, A. Möller, B. Schei, and P. O. Janson, "Prevalence of physical and sexual abuse before and during pregnancy among Swedish couples," *Acta Obstetricia et Gynecologica Scandinavica*, vol. 78, no. 4, pp. 310–315, 1999.

[6] B. Wijma, B. Schei, K. Swahnberg et al., "Emotional, physical, and sexual abuse in patients visiting gynaecology clinics: a Nordic cross-sectional study," *The Lancet*, vol. 361, pp. 2107–2113, 2003.

[7] A. A. Boyle and C. Todd, "Incidence and prevalence of domestic violence in a UK emergency deparment," *Emergency Medicine Journal*, vol. 20, no. 5, pp. 438–442, 2003.

[8] L. M. Howard, K. Trevillion, H. Khalifeh, A. Woodall, R. Agnew-Davies, and G. Feder, "Domestic violence and severe psychiatric disorders: prevalence and interventions," *Psychological Medicine*, vol. 40, no. 6, pp. 881–893, 2010.

[9] M. C. Wadman and R. L. Muelleman, "Domestic violence homicides: ED use before victimization," *American Journal of Emergency Medicine*, vol. 17, no. 7, pp. 689–691, 1999.

[10] S. Peckover, "I could have just done with a little more help: an analysis of women's help-seeking from health visitors in the context of domestic violence," *Health and Social Care in the Community*, vol. 11, no. 3, pp. 275–282, 2003.

[11] P. W. Sharps, J. Koziol-McLain, J. Campbell, J. McFarlane, C. Sachs, and X. Xu, "Health care providers' missed opportunities for preventing femicide," *Preventive Medicine*, vol. 33, no. 5, pp. 373–380, 2001.

[12] S. R. Hayden, E. D. Barton, and M. Hayden, "Domestic violence in the emergency department: How do women prefer to disclose and discuss the issues?" *Journal of Emergency Medicine*, vol. 15, no. 4, pp. 447–451, 1997.

[13] J. Read and A. Fraser, "Abuse histories of psychiatric lnpatients: to ask or not to ask?" *Psychiatric Services*, vol. 49, no. 3, pp. 355–359, 1998.

[14] M. Husso, T. Virkki, M. Notko, J. Holma, A. Laitila, and M. Mäntysaari, "Making sense of domestic violence interventions in professional health care," *Health and Social Care in the Community*, vol. 20, no. 4, pp. 347–355, 2012.

[15] C. H. Chuang and J. M. Liebshutz, "Screening for intimate partner violence in the primary care setting: a critical review," *Journal of Clinical Outcomes Management*, vol. 9, no. 10, pp. 565–571, 2002.

[16] A. Taket, J. Nurse, K. Smith et al., "Routinely asking women about domestic violence in health settings," *British Medical Journal*, vol. 327, no. 7416, pp. 673–676, 2003.

[17] K. F. Hurley, T. Brown-Maher, S. G. Campbell, T. Wallace, R. Venugopal, and D. Baggs, "Emergency department patients' opinions of screening for intimate partner violence among women," *Emergency Medicine Journal*, vol. 22, no. 2, pp. 97–98, 2005.

[18] D. Sethi, S. Watts, A. Zwi, J. Watson, and C. McCarthy, "Experience of domestic violence by women attending an inner city accident and emergency department," *Emergency Medicine Journal*, vol. 21, no. 2, pp. 180–184, 2004.

[19] M. Ellsberg, H. F. M. Jansen, L. Heise, C. H. Watts, and C. Garcia-Moreno, "Intimate partner violence and women's physical and mental health in the WHO multi-country study on women's health and domestic violence: an observational study," *The Lancet*, vol. 371, no. 9619, pp. 1165–1172, 2008.

[20] J. C. Campbell, "Health consequences of intimate partner violence," *The Lancet*, vol. 359, no. 9314, pp. 1331–1336, 2002.

[21] J. Read, J. van Os, A. P. Morrison, and C. A. Ross, "Childhood trauma, psychosis and schizophrenia: a literature review with theoretical and clinical implications," *Acta Psychiatrica Scandinavica*, vol. 112, no. 5, pp. 330–350, 2005.

[22] K. Wijma, J. Söderquist, I. Björklund, and B. Wijma, "Prevalence of post-traumatic stress disorder among gynecological patients with a history of sexual and physical abuse," *Journal of Interpersonal Violence*, vol. 15, no. 9, pp. 944–958, 2000.

[23] R. M. Tolman and D. Rosen, "Domestic violence in the lives of women receiving welfare," *Violence Against Women*, vol. 7, no. 2, pp. 141–158, 2001.

[24] A. L. Coker, K. E. Davis, I. Arias et al., "Physical and mental health effects of intimate partner violence for men and women," *American Journal of Preventive Medicine*, vol. 23, no. 4, pp. 260–268, 2002.

[25] R. P. Dobash and R. E. Dobash, "Women's violence to men in intimate relationships: working on a puzzle," *British Journal of Criminology*, vol. 44, no. 3, pp. 324–349, 2004.

[26] P. Tjaden and N. Thoennes, "Prevalence and consequences of male-to-female and female-to-male intimate partner violence as measured by the national violence against women survey," *Violence Against Women*, vol. 6, no. 2, pp. 142–161, 2000.

[27] S. C. Swan and D. L. Snow, "A typology of women's use of violence in intimate relationships," *Violence Against Women*, vol. 8, no. 3, pp. 286–319, 2002.

[28] D. G. Saunders, "Are physical assaults by wives and girlfriends a major social problem?—A review of the literature," *Violence Against Women*, vol. 8, no. 12, pp. 1424–1448, 2002.

[29] A. L. Coker, P. H. Smith, L. Bethea, M. R. King, and R. E. McKeown, "Physical health consequences of physical and psychological intimate partner violence," *Archives of Family Medicine*, vol. 9, no. 5, pp. 451–457, 2000.

[30] U. Pikarinen, T. Saisto, B. Schei, K. Swahnberg, and E. Halmesmäki, "Experiences of physical and sexual abuse and their implications for current health," *Obstetrics and Gynecology*, vol. 109, no. 5, pp. 1116–1122, 2007.

[31] H. S. Friedman, M. L. Kern, and C. A. Reynolds, "Personality and health, subjective well-being, and longevity," *Journal of Personality*, vol. 78, no. 1, pp. 179–216, 2010.

[32] M. A. Busseri and S. W. Sadava, "A review of the tripartite structure of subjective well-being: Implications for conceptualization, operationalization, analysis, and synthesis," *Personality and Social Psychology Review*, vol. 15, no. 3, pp. 290–314, 2011.

[33] A. Lee and M. O. Browne, "Subjective well-being, sociodemographic factors, mental and physical health of rural residents," *Australian Journal of Rural Health*, vol. 16, no. 5, pp. 290–296, 2008.

[34] E. Diener and C. Diener, "Most people are happy," *Psychological Science*, vol. 7, no. 3, pp. 181–185, 1996.

[35] E. Diener, "Subjective well-being," *Psychological Bulletin*, vol. 95, no. 3, pp. 542–575, 1984.

[36] J. McFarlane, B. Parker, K. Soeken, and L. Bullock, "Assessing for abuse during pregnancy: severity and frequency of injuries and associated entry into prenatal care," *Journal of the American Medical Association*, vol. 267, no. 23, pp. 3176–3178, 1992.

[37] K. M. Sherin, J. M. Sinacore, X. Q. Li, R. E. Zitter, and A. Shakil, "Hits: a short domestic violence screening tool for use in a family practice setting," *Family Medicine*, vol. 30, no. 7, pp. 508–512, 1998.

[38] K. M. Feldhaus, J. Koziol-McLain, H. L. Amsbury, I. M. Norton, S. R. Lowenstein, and J. T. Abbott, "Accuracy of 3 brief screening questions for detecting partner violence in the emergency department," *Journal of the American Medical Association*, vol. 277, no. 17, pp. 1357–1361, 1997.

[39] J. B. Brown, B. Lent, G. Schmidt, and G. Sas, "Application of the Woman Abuse Screening Tool (WAST) and WAST-short in the family practice setting," *Journal of Family Practice*, vol. 49, no. 10, pp. 896–903, 2000.

[40] E. Ruuskanen and K. Aromaa, Administrative data collection on domestic violence in Council of Europe member states. European Institute for Crime Prevention and Control, affiliated with the United Nations (HEUNI). Directorate General of Human Rights and Legal Affairs Council 28 of Europe. Strasbourg, 2008.

[41] H. L. MacMillan, C. N. Wathen, E. Jamieson et al., "Approaches to screening for intimate partner violence in health care settings: a randomized trial," *Journal of the American Medical Association*, vol. 296, no. 5, pp. 530–536, 2006.

[42] J. McFarlane, K. Christoffel, L. Bateman, V. Miller, and L. Bullock, "Assessing for abuse: self-report versus nurse interview," *Public Health Nursing*, vol. 8, no. 4, pp. 245–250, 1991.

[43] D. Houry, K. V. Rhodes, R. S. Kemball et al., "Differences in female and male victims and perpetrators of partner violence with respect to WEB scores," *Journal of Interpersonal Violence*, vol. 23, no. 8, pp. 1041–1055, 2008.

[44] C. García-Moreno, H. A. Jansen, M. Ellsberg, L. Heise, and C. H. Watts, "Prevalence of intimate partner violence: findings from the WHO multi-country study on women's health and domestic violence," *The Lancet*, vol. 368, no. 9543, pp. 1260–1269, 2006.

[45] D. Rose, K. Trevillion, A. Woodall, C. Morgan, G. Feder, and L. Howard, "Barriers and facilitators of disclosures of domestic violence by mental health service users: qualitative study," *British Journal of Psychiatry*, vol. 198, no. 3, pp. 189–194, 2011.

10

Light Reduction Capabilities of Homemade and Commercial Incubator Covers in NICU

Susan M. Ludington-Hoe[1] and Amel Abouelfettoh[2,3]

[1] *Frances Payne School of Nursing, Case Western Reserve University, Cleveland, OH 44120, USA*
[2] *Faculty of Nursing, Cairo University, Cairo, Egypt*
[3] *College of Nursing, King Saud bin Abdulaziz University for Health Sciences, Al Ahsa 31982, Saudi Arabia*

Correspondence should be addressed to Amel Abouelfettoh; amelmoataz@hotmail.com

Academic Editors: L. W. Lam and D. Whitehead

Reduction of high-risk neonates' exposure to aversive light stimulation is an important component of developmentally supportive care. In neonatal intensive care unit (NICU), usually light is reduced by reducing the room's light level or by using incubator covers. Many types of incubator covers are in use, including homemade and commercial covers. A comparative study was used to determine the light reducing capabilities of 19 homemade incubator covers, 2 commercial covers, and 1 receiving blanket. The covers were tested by covering and uncovering an incubator and an oxygen hood in the NICU during daytime and nighttime lightings. The light reducing capabilities value was determined for each cover using an Extech light dosimeter when the cover was placed over and removed from an oxyhood, and an incubator. The study showed that the light reducing capability of the commercial covers was 91.2%, the homemade covers capability was 72.1%, and the receiving blankets capability was 55.1%. A significant difference between the commercial and homemade covers was found ($F = 452.50$, $P < 0.00$). Commercial incubator covers are the most effective covers to achieve light reduction; homemade covers can be effective if made large enough so that they completely cover all sides of the incubator.

1. Introduction

Reduction of the exposure of high-risk neonates to aversive light stimulation is an important component of developmentally supportive care [1–3]. Neonatal intensive care units (NICUs) usually reduce light by reducing the room's light level or by using incubator covers [4, 5]. Many types of incubator covers are in use, including homemade and commercial covers. Homemade covers are not standardized, and only one report of their light reducing capability during daytime and evening time could be found [6], and that report was based on a simulated level of light created in a windowless nursing school skills because reports of light reduction capability of homemade incubator covers in an actual NICU could not be found.

The lighting in nurseries is known to be relatively constant [1, 5, 7], but light levels really are quite variable [8]. Two measures of light are referenced in the study presented here. A footcandle (ftc) is defined as a unit of illumination on a surface that is one foot from a point source of one candle; lux is defined as a unit of illumination that is equal to the direct illumination on a surface that is one meter from a uniform point source of one candle intensity or equal to one lumen per square meter (lumen/m^2). The amount of light received by any infant varies from 15 to 2500 ftc (foot candles) or from 1.5 to 250 luxes, depending on his or her location in the nursery, the time of day, and the amount of sunlight present [9–11].

The light level that is appropriate for an NICU is still controversial [8] and may account for the persistently high levels of light in NICUs (Table 1). 9-10 luxes are thought to be needed to allow evaluation of infant skin color and perfusion [12]. The most recent Illuminating Engineering Society recommendations suggest ambient light levels of 1-2 luxes (10–20 ftc) with individual rheostat controls providing temporary increases in illumination for assessments and procedures [13]. Individual lighting creates a substantial change in ambient light, as does the use of halogen spot lights instead of fluorescent overhead lighting [12]. Light intensity is also reduced by 10% on average with double-walled incubators during normal nighttime electric hospital lighting [14].

Infants in the NICU spend weeks or months exposed to the NICU's light level. Research with animals has established the hazards of exposure to light at intensities similar to those found in the nursery [8, 15]. The effects of light on preterm infants have been reviewed extensively elsewhere [2, 16–18]. Exposure to fluorescent lighting greater than 60 ftc for preterm infants weighing less than 1000 gms has been associated with more retinopathy of prematurity (ROP) than exposure to 25 ftc or less [19]. The finding of increased retinopathy was not replicated in Ackerman and colleagues' study [20]. However, current thought is that high light levels do not affect ROP [21]. Altered visual functioning and arrested eye growth are important considerations for infants less than 750 grams, as these infants are experiencing a marked increase in ROP [22].

Oxygen saturation remained stable with light reduction from 100 ftc to 5 ftc, and 22% of infants experienced a significant oxygen saturation decrease when light was increased from 5 ftc to 100 ftc [23]. Slevin and colleagues found that when NICU light was reduced during quite periods (switching off all the lights and pulling down all the blinds), infants' oxygen saturations increased by 0.25, and diastolic blood pressures and mean arterial pressures were significantly reduced by 2 mmHg [24]. Suppression of melatonin is associated with high illumination levels [25]. Sleep is also adversely affected by high levels of light [26]. In contrast, reduced light levels (using blindfolds for 10 hours per night) have been associated with increased alertness and improved respiratory stability [27] and a 75% reduction in infant movements and a 2 mmHg reduction in blood pressure [24]. Reducing visible light by wearing goggles has failed to improve weight gain, duration of oxygen therapy, duration of mechanical ventilation, or length of hospital stay in preterm infants [28], and covering incubators has failed to improve neurological and mental development or growth at 1 and 2 years after birth in a 32-week gestation preterm infants [29].

The incentive to reduce ambient light to foster sleep now exists. Preterm infants exhibited much more quiet sleep when ambient light levels were lowered by turning off several lights for 2-3 hours than when all lights in a room were left on [30]. When light reduction occurs regularly over part of the twenty-four hours of the day, the lighting condition is referred to as "cycled light." Cycled lighting during lower lighting periods has been associated with decreased heart rate, decreased activity [31], decreased respiratory rate [32], improved sleep patterns, weight gain, and early establishment of rest-activity patterns that are in phase with the 24-hour light-dark cycle [26, 33]. Day-night cycling of light was found to increase sleep, decrease feeding time, and improve weight gain in 21 infants randomly assigned to a cycled light group when compared to 20 infants in a noncycled light group. Differences were still evident at 3 months after expected date of delivery [26].

Incubator covers have been identified as a means of cutting light but are disparaged for their "ill-fitting and unprofessional appearance" and for being made of fabrics that may prevent accurate evaluation of skin color [39]. Initially, infant flannel blankets were used in NICU to cover incubators. This practice expanded to the use of homemade covers of varying fabrics and size. Lee and colleges [6] evaluated the light reducing capacity of homemade quilted incubator covers by comparing the light level in the middle of an incubator in a nursing school skills laboratory when the covers were over the incubator and removed from the incubator. Quilted covers reduced the light by 37% when the incubator was covered. Light reductions in NICU were not measured nor were measurements taken during daytime and nighttime lighting conditions. Several commercial incubator covers are currently available. Some cover the entire incubator while others cover the top, sides, and back. Additionally, commercial covers come in different colors and are made of a variety of materials. Although these commercial covers are advertised as being able to "block out all excess light" and to "dim light," no studies that examined the light reducing properties of commercial incubator covers or receiving blankets could be located.

The current study was conducted to determine the light reducing capabilities of homemade crocheted, quilted, and flannel covers of a receiving blanket and of commercial incubator covers during daytime and evening time light levels

TABLE 1: Light levels in NICU and with different types of lighting.

Year	Light levels	Source of data
1960s	10 foot candles (100 luxes)	Glass et al., 1985 [19]
1980s	90 foot candles (900 luxes)	Glass et al., 1985 [19]
1981	Mean = 53 foot candles (530 luxes) Range = 34–140 foot candles (344–1400 luxes)	Gottfried et al., 1981 [34]
1990s	19–148 foot candles (192–1488 luxes)	Glotzbach et al., 1993 [35, 36], Robinson et al., 1990
1998	During day: mean = 29 foot candles (290 luxes) During evening: mean = 34 foot candles (340 luxes) During night: mean = 22 foot candles (220 luxes)	Gray et al., 1998 [37]
2001	Individual lighting decreases daytime ambient light level from 20 foot candles (200 luxes) to 1.5 foot candles (15 luxes) Fluorescent lights provide 19 foot candles (193 luxes) Halogen spot light on "maximum" provides 19-20 candles (193–202 luxes) Halogen spot light on default provides 1.2 foot candles (12 luxes)	Walsh-Sukys et al., 2001 [12]
2002	>646 luxes (60 footcandles)	American Academy of Pediatrics (2006) [38]

in the NICU and to compare the light-reducing capabilities of homemade covers and a receiving blanket to commercial incubator covers during daytime and evening time light levels in a NICU.

2. Materials and Methods

A comparative, repeated measures study was conducted in a six-bed nursery (three to a side) in a tertiary care NICU in the first week of September in Northeast Ohio. The nursery has fluorescent lighting and one large external window with thin aluminum blinds; the window faces South onto a walkway between two tall buildings, and the NICU is on the second floor. For daytime lighting conditions, blinds were entirely open, 2 overhead fluorescent lights in the middle of the room were on, and six soffit lights over the wall-hugging counter (and directed away from the incubators) were on, providing an ambient lighting level of 628 luxes on the window side of the incubator used for testing. For nighttime conditions, the blinds were also open, overhead lights were turned off, and only two of six soffit lights over the counters were on, providing an overall ambient light level of 29 luxes on the window side of the one incubator used for testing. Reduced lighting conditions are commonly encountered during night, defined as 8:00 pm to 5:00 am for the purposes of this investigation. During the day of data collection, no quiet time was scheduled because quiet times are associated with large reductions in light (i.e., from 254 luxes to 3.0 luxes [24]).

Placement of the incubator in the nursery and the position of the oxyhood and researcher were standardized to prevent inconsistent shadowing and lighting. The unoccupied incubator was placed in the closest bed spot to the window. All light recordings were taken within the incubator, where the infant's head would be positioned on the side of the incubator towards the center of the nursery.

2.1. Research Questions. The study reported here examined the light-reducing effects of commercial and homemade incubator covers and addressed the following research questions.

Q1: What is the percent of light reduction with homemade covers, a receiving blanket, and two commercial covers that are placed over an Ohmeda Ohio Care Plus incubator during daytime and nighttime?

Q2: What difference, if any, exists in percent of light reduction between homemade covers, a receiving blanket, and commercially available incubator covers?

Q3: What is the percent of light reduction with homemade, receiving blanket, and commercial incubator covers that completely occlude an oxygen hood during daytime and nighttime?

2.2. Instruments. The Extech light dosimeter has a light sensor connected by a 3-foot cable to the digital display. The light sensor sat in the center of the oxygen hood and inside the incubator with the cable extending outside so readings could be taken without disturbing the placement of the covers to get the reading. The light dosimeter (a photometer) was autocalibrated each time; it was turned on, requiring a two-minute warm-up period (five minutes was given to prevent measurement drift) and was given a fifteen-second interval between different lighting conditions to insure accurate readings. A switch on the front of the dosimeter permitted the value to be digitally displayed as lux or foot candles; lux was chosen. The dosimeter has been approved for medical purposes and has reliability greater than 90% established by the manufacturer. The sensitivity of the dosimeter is ± 0.10 lumen/ft^2. One researcher read the light levels as another recorded them after repeating the value to the reader, a measure taken to insure recording accuracy.

Incubator Covers. Ten homemade crocheted covers of varying sizes, nine three-layered homemade quilts, three homemade flannel covers, one commercial single-layer flannel receiving blanket (16% polyester, 84% cotton of 35×29 inches and white with 3 light blue stripes of 1 inch width interspersed between six 1/4 inch light pink and blue strips at one end of the blanket), and two commercial incubator covers (white with 1/4 inch diameter light purple, aqua, and pink hearts randomly spaced across the entire surface) (Children's Medical Ventures Incubator Cover Models, Boston, Mass, USA) were evaluated. The commercial incubator covers differed in that one (Model 6812315) did not cover the portholes and incorporated Velcro closures; the other (Model C100/450XL Incubator) had no open porthole areas (no flaps at all only a solid cover) and snaps for closure. Both commercial covers were quilted incubator covers.

2.3. Outcome Measures

2.3.1. Light Reducing Capability. Lighting was measured in lux as lumen/m^2 [40]. The level of light is called illuminance and was measured by the light dosimeter. Light reducing capability was defined as the percent of light reduced by the covers (covered light level/uncovered light level) measured in lux.

2.3.2. Procedure. The study was conducted from 11:30 am to 5 pm for daytime assessment and from 8:00 pm to 12 midnight for nighttime assessment. Data were collected in one day.

Homemade covers were collected from the large bin in the NICU. Detailed descriptions and measurements of each cover were recorded (Tables 2(a), 2(b), and 2(c)). The covers were taken to an incubator next to the window in one room of the NICU nursery. As most covers did not completely cover the incubator, determination of light-filtering abilities value over an oxyhood, which could be completely covered, was first performed. The oxygen hood was placed inside the unoccupied incubator described previously, at the place where an infant's head would be. The Extech light dosimeter (Model no. 401025; Extech Instruments, Waltham, MA, USA) was warmed up for five minutes with the light sensor in the center of the uncovered oxygen hood. Next, ten baseline measurements 15 seconds apart were taken from the center of the oxygen hood to determine mean ambient light. The hood was

TABLE 2: (a) Description of crochet (open weave) incubator and oxyhood covers by length, width, total area, weight, and color. (b) Description of 3 layer quilts (closed weave) over incubator and oxyhood covers by length, width, total area, weight, and color. (c) Description of commercial blanket covers over incubator and oxyhood covers by length, width, total area, weight, and color. (d) Description of flannel covers and receiving blanket cover over incubator and oxyhood covers by length, width, total area, weight, and color.

(a)

Cover crochet	Length (inches)	Width (inches)	Total area (inches)	Weight (Kg)	Color side 1 (1), side 2 (2)
1	18.60	17.00	316.20	.100	Solid royal blue
2	19.10	17.20	328.52	.115	5 stripessolid navy blue royal blue, grey, and hunter green
3	18.30	17.40	318.42	.135	Solid light beige
4	35.60	23.40	833.04	.300	5 stripesrust, salmon, dark brown, cream, and dark green
5	20.00	18.00	360.00	.140	Solid sage and grey stripes
6	18.70	16.50	308.55	.105	Solid royal blue
7	18.60	18.40	342.24	.130	Solid red, rose, and brown stripes
8	20.20	16.40	331.28	.130	Solid heather and light beige stripes
9	20.70	17.50	362.25	.150	Solid sage
10	19.20	17.00	326.40	.100	Solid royal blue
Mean	20.90	17.88	382.70	.141	
SD	5.22	2.03	159.20	.059	

(b)

Cover quilt	Length (inches)	Width (inches)	Total area (inches)	Weight (Kg)	Color side 1 (1), side 2 (2)
1	42.60	40.10	1708.30	.295	(1) Lime green, (2) lime green, mustard, white, and brown in floral pattern
2	42.00	34.00	1428	.500	(1), (2) Pink/red/hunter green/yellow patchwork with yellow and white flowers on white with fringed edge
3	34.00	33.00	1122	.900	(1) White, (2) snoopy figures on cream background
4	41.00	34.00	1394	.280	(1) Rust with small, white dots, (2) rose and green flowers
5	36.60	36.30	1328.60	.340	(1) Beige/cream check (2) Beige, beige/cream squares
6	36.50	36.20	1321.30	.295	(1) Pink with small white stars (2) alternating squares of pink, star fabric, and solid light pink
7	44.70	40.50	1810.40	.495	(1) Light blue/white stripes (2) Same as side 1 with strawberry shortcake circles
8	43.60	34.10	1486.80	.280	(1) White with pink/green/blue alphabet and angels (2) Squares of pink/green/blue letters
9	42.00	41.60	1747.20	.350	(1) White with pink/blue hearts/stars (2) Pink/yellow/blue clouds-white/lavender background
Mean	40.20	36.50	1474.80	.329	
SD	4.00	3.40	243.30	.068	

(c)

Cover	Length (inches)	Width (inches)	Total area (inches)	Weight (Kg)	Color side 1 (1), side 2 (2)
			Commercialclosed wave		
1-new	C = 37.70 R = 18.70 L = 19.10	C = 35.30 R =16.60 L = 16.70	C = 1330.81 R = 310.42 L = 318.97	.680	(1) Light grey (2) White with small purple, blue, purple, and pink hearts
2worn	C = 31.86 R = 16.37 L = 16.50	C = 37.13 R = 19.99 L = 20.25	C = 1182.96 R = 327.24 L = 334.13	.495	(1) Light grey (2) White with small purple, blue, purple, and pink hearts

(c) Continued.

Cover	Length (inches)	Width (inches)	Total area (inches)	Weight (Kg)	Color side 1 (1), side 2 (2)
Mean	MC = 34.78* MR = 17.54** ML = 17.8***	MC = 36.22 MR = 18.30 ML = 18.47	MC = 1256.89 MR = 318.83 ML = 326.55	.588	
Total mean				1902.27	
Total SD				±57.94	

*MC: mean area of incubator that is covered. **MR: mean area of right end wall of incubator that is covered. ***ML: mean area of left end wall of incubator that is covered. C: center of incubator cover. R: right side cover of incubator cover. L: left side cover of incubator.

(d)

Cover	Length (inches)	Width (inches)	Total area (inches)	Weight (Kg)	Color side 1 (1), side 2 (2)
			Flannelclosed weave		
1	42.50	33.50	1423.80	.340	(1) Aqua, (2) yellow squares on green/white checked background
2	36.25	31.00	1123.75	.170	(1), (2) Small pink/white checks with yellow pony
3	4.37	34.13	1173.05	.360	(1) White, (2) random squares of pink, aqua, blue white, green, and bright yellow
Mean			1340.20		
SD			±122.40		
			Receiving blanketopen weave		
1	34.88	28.5	994.08	.125	White with varying width pink and light blue stripes at one edge

then completely enclosed by one of the covers, and after waiting 15 seconds for the meter to recalibrate, one light reading was taken. The hood was then uncovered, and the procedure with the same cover was repeated nine times more to obtain a mean light-filtering value based on ten readings for each cover. After data collection for the first cover was complete the procedure was repeated for each additional cover.

Next, the light reducing capability of the covers over an incubator was determined using the same procedure to acquire 10 baseline measurements of ambient light level inside the incubator (the meter was placed where the infant's head would be in the Ohmeda Incubator Plus double-walled incubator). A cover was then placed over the top edge at the "head side" of the incubator, and the light level was recorded. The incubator cover was then removed and immediately replaced and the light level was recorded. This procedure occurred ten times for each cover with 15-second intervals between each measurement. After determining light reduction of each homemade cover, two commercial incubator covers were put through the same procedure as was in one hospital receiving blanket.

3. Results

Each of the covers was qualitatively described and measured (Tables 2(a), 2(b), and 2(c)). The area of each cover was also calculated. All covers varied in color hue, predominant color (dark colors did not predominate, the light colors did), length, width, density of the weave or material, and in their dimensions, reflecting possible variation when multiple people are engaged in producing quilts and when guidelines for the quilt's production are not given. The majority of the crocheted covers were too small to occlude any porthole and/or incubator side as they were the smallest of all the covers, and the crochet weave was loose in all of them. Most of the quilts were able to cover the nearest porthole the infant's head but did not go down the sides of the incubators nor simultaneously cover any other porthole. All of the homemade covers were smaller than the commercial covers and therefore did not cover the incubator as completely as the commercial covers. Thus, the area covered, in descending order, was 1902.27 (±57.94) inches by commercial incubator covers, 1474.80 (±243.30) inches by quilts, 1240.20 (±122.40) inches by flannels, 994.08 inches by the one commercial receiving blanket, and 382.70 (±159.20) inches by the crocheted covers. However, there was one crocheted cover that was larger than the others (no. 4), and when this outlier was removed, the mean area covered by crocheted blankets was reduced to 332.65 ± 14.79 inches.

Ten recordings were obtained of ambient light level for daytime and nighttime lighting when the oxygen hood and incubator were covered and then uncovered, yielding ten values of percent of light reduction for each cover. Percent of light reduction for each cover over an incubator under day and nighttime conditions is conveyed in Table 3. Commercial incubator covers reduced light by 83%, followed closely by quilted (69%) and flannel (67%) covers. The receiving blanket reduced light by 47%, and crocheted covers reduced the least amount of light (44%). Light reduction capabilities over an incubator during night time were similar (Table 3).

Light reducing capabilities over the oxygen hood are reported in Table 4 for daytime and night time conditions.

Table 3: Percent of light reduced over incubator under daytime and nighttime conditions of all cover types.

Cover	Day				Night			
	N	Mean	SD	Range	N	Mean	SD	Range
Crochet	10	43.74	8.96	36–68	10	20.07	17.78	9–70
Quilt	9	69.28	11.45	57–86	9	65.34	16.94	45–90
Flannel	3	66.64	4.33	64–72	3	62.03	8.34	54–70
Receiving blanket	1	47.80			1	34.71		
Commercial covers	2	83.07	0.36	82-83	2	83.68	12.84	75–93

Table 4: Percent of light reduced over oxygen hood under daytime and nighttime conditions of all cover types and differences in light reduction between covers.

Cover	Day				Night			
	N	Mean	SD	Range	N	Mean	SD	Range
Crochet	10	92.60	2.05	89–95	10	71.56	13.38	53–94
Quilt†	9	87.20	9.31	75–99	9	82.04	10.84	68–95
Flannel‡	3	88.31	6.55	81–92	3	85.77	8.12	76–90
Receiving blanket*	1	61.56			1	57.69		
Commercial covers±	2	98.91	0.40	98-99	2	95.39	0.34	95.15–95.63

*Comparison not available because only one receiving blanket was tested, and no mean is available.
†Crochet versus quilt: daytime: $F = 16.69$, $P = 0.000$; nighttime: $F = 5.32$, $P = 0.23$.
‡Crochet versus flannel: daytime: $F = 13.31$, $P = 0.008$; nighttime: $F = 7.62$, $P = 0.28$.
±Crochet versus commercial: daytime: $F = 15.71$. $P = 0.000$; nighttime: $F = 8.97$, $P = 0.07$.

During the daytime, commercial incubator covers reduced light by 99%, crocheted by 93%, flannels and quilts by 88%, and the receiving blanket by 62%. Light reducing capabilities over the oxygen hood changed with night time conditions: commercial incubator covers reduced light by 95%, flannels by 86%, quilts by 82%, crocheted by 72%, and commercial receiving blanket by 58%.

Differences between the types of covers were analyzed using ANOVA and Tukey post hoc tests. The data from the one receiving blanket was removed from the ANOVA calculation. During daytime, percent of light reduction was significantly different between the covers when placed over an incubator ($F = 16.99$; $P = 0.00$), but it was not significantly different when placed over an oxygen hood ($F = 2.43$, $P = 0.10$). Commercial incubator covers reduced incubator daytime lighting significantly more than crocheted ($P = 0.000$); quilted covers reduced light more than crocheted ($P = 0.000$); flannels reduced light more than crocheted ($P = 0.008$); and crocheted covers reduced significantly less light than all other covers ($P < 0.01$).

Under night time conditions, covers differed significantly in the ability to reduce lighting over an incubator ($F = 16.69$; $P = 0.00$) and over an oxygen hood ($F = 3.26$; $P = 0.04$). Crocheted covers reduced lighting less than quilted ($P = 0.00$), flannel ($P = 0.01$), and commercial incubator covers ($P = 0.00$) over an incubator. The difference in oxygen hood light reduction was between crocheted and commercial incubator covers, but the difference only approached statistical significance ($P = 0.07$).

3.1. Open Weave versus Closed Weave. Two-tailed t-tests were conducted to determine light reducing difference between the translucent "open weave" crocheted covers (plus the receiving blanket which was quite thin and translucent too) and the flannel and quilted "closed weave" covers (Table 5). Closed weave covers reduced significantly more light than open weave covers in both daytime and night time conditions for the incubator and in night time conditions for the oxygen hood.

Table 5: Percent of light reduced over incubator and oxyhood by open weave and closed weave covers under daytime and nighttime conditions.

Source	n	Mean	SD	df	t	P
			Incubator			
Daytime				20	−6.06	0.00*
Open	10	43.74	8.96			
Closed	12	68.62	10.01			
Nighttime				20	−6.37	0.00*
Open	10	20.07	17.78			
Closed	12	64.51	14.95			
			Oxyhood			
Daytime				20	2.03	0.06
Open	10	92.6	2.05			
Closed	12	68.62	10.01			
Nighttime				20	−2.29	0.03*
Open	10	71.56	13.38			
Closed	12	82.97	10.01			

*$P < .05$.

4. Discussion

The endpoints of the study were to determine the light reducing capabilities of homemade incubator covers and compare those capabilities to those of commercial incubator covers and a receiving blanket. Three types of homemade covers were assessed, crocheted, quilted, and flannel covers made by volunteers for a metropolitan, university-based neonatal intensive care unit. Crocheted covers reduced significantly less light than all other covers when they were palced over an incubator under day and night time conditions. The receiving blanket performed nearly as badly as the crocheted covers. Quilted and flannel covers performed relatively similarly to each other. Commercial incubator covers reduced the most light as compared to homemade covers and receiving blanket, but the difference in light reduction between commercial incubator covers and quilted and flannel covers failed to reach statistical significance. The data lead us to speculate that it is not the quality (weave or opacity) of the cover that reduced lighting, but the cover's size. Covers with an area equal to or greater than 1200 inches (30 × 40 inches) covered enough of the incubator to make them as effective in light reduction as commercial covers. The flannel and quilted covers were sufficiently large to meet this critical area. The receiving blanket's area was less than 1000 inches, and its light reducing capabilities were close to those of the poorest performing crocheted covers under daytime and night time conditions.

The data derived from testing the covers over an oxygen hood also support the proposition that the area that is covered determines light reducing capability better than the quality of the cover. All covers were able to occlude the oxygen hood completely, increasing the amount of light reduction of each cover. The light reducing capabilities of all covers when placed over an oxygen hood did not differ significantly, even though crocheted covers were loosely woven and had light penetrating holes in them. The data suggest that when the item can be completely covered by the homemade cover, open weave homemade covers are as effective as close weave homemade covers.

The incentive to cut light to improve developmental outcome of premature infants and to reduce ROP is a matter of question. A reduction in light and persistent nesting did not affect neurological and developmental outcomes at one and two years after birth in infants born at <32-week gestation [29]. In relation to ROP, a Cochrane review of randomized controlled trials of early light reduction (within seven days following birth) on the incidence of acute or poor outcomes of retinopathy of prematurity (ROP) in very low birth weight infants revealed no reduction in the incidence of ROP [41]. Yet, mechanisms by which light exposure can be detrimental exist. The pathophysiology of ROP in premature infants is understood to start with the injury to the incomplete developing of retinal capillaries. Damage could potentially occur before or during birth, but it is thought to primarily occur in the days following delivery when ambient light may reach the retina. Once the developing vessels have been damaged, it is hypothesized that the retina responds by producing vascular growth factors that stimulate new vascularization [41]. Oxygen free radicals are considered one cause of the injury of developing retinal capillaries in the premature infant [42]. Energy from light striking the retina may induce or increase the number of oxygen free radicals in the retina, particularly in the face of high levels of tissue oxygen. Numerous animal studies have demonstrated retinal injury from light, but these injuries have been due to other parts of the retina than the blood vessels (as is the case of infants) [42, 43]. Using incubator covers to decrease retinal ambient light exposure in premature infants to reduce the incidence of ROP is not supported by the existing evidence.

Further research is needed to examine the influence of color and hue intensity on light reduction capabilities, as well as the effect of multiple washings. Confirmation by research is also needed to determine the effect of long-term use of incubator covers on infant development, especially regarding to visual development which matures rapidly as the infant approaches term age. Whether covers should be used continuously or intermittently should also be investigated, as continuous reduction of light and other sensory input may make it more difficult for the preterm infant to establish circadian rhythms [44]. Light reduction is still a major part of individualized developmental care for premature infants [5, 8, 45], and in concert with other elements of developmental care—that is, minimal interruptions, individualized caregiving based on infant organization, and skin-to-skin contact—may have a positive influence on the need for respiratory support, motor development, weight gain, and length of hospital stay [44]. Based on the findings reported here, commercial incubator covers are the most effective covers to achieve light reduction; homemade covers can be effective if made large enough so they completely cover all sides of the incubator. Closed weave covers will be more effective than open weave covers.

Acknowledgments

The study was funded in part by 5RO1 NR 04926-0IAI and Ohio Nurse Foundation Grant 423059 to the first author. The authors would like to thank Ms. Karen Ishler, for her programming assistance.

References

[1] S. N. Graven, "Early neurosensory visual development of the fetus and newborn," *Clinics in Perinatology*, vol. 31, no. 2, pp. 199–216, 2004.

[2] T. T. Lai and C. F. Bearer, "Iatrogenic environmental hazards in the neonatal intensive care unit," *Clinics in Perinatology*, vol. 35, no. 1, pp. 163–181, 2008.

[3] A. Symington and J. Pinelli, "Developmental care for promoting development and preventing morbidity in preterm infants," *Cochrane Database of Systematic Reviews*, no. 2, Article ID CD001814, 2006.

[4] M.-S. Roy, C. Caramelli, J. Orquin, J. Uleckas, P. Hardy, and S. Chemtob, "Effects of early reduced light exposure on central visual development in preterm infants," *Acta Paediatrica*, vol. 88, no. 4, pp. 459–461, 1999.

[5] R. D. White, "Lighting design in the neonatal intensive care unit: practical applications of scientific principles," *Clinics in Perinatology*, vol. 31, no. 2, pp. 323–330, 2004.

[6] Y. L. Lee, N. Malakooti, and M. J. Lotas, "A comparison of the light-reduction capacity of commonly used incubator covers," *Neonatal Network*, vol. 24, no. 2, pp. 37–44, 2005.

[7] S. N. Graven, "Clinical research data illuminating the relationship between the physical environment and patient medical outcomes," *Journal of Healthcare Design*, vol. 9, pp. 15–24, 1997.

[8] D. C. Stevens, M. Akram Khan, D. P. Munson, E. J. Reid, C. C. Helseth, and J. Buggy, "The impact of architectural design upon the environmental sound and light exposure of neonates who require intensive care: an evaluation of the Boekelheide Neonatal Intensive Care Nursery," *Journal of Perinatology*, vol. 27, supplement 2, pp. S20–S28, 2007.

[9] P. Mac Leod and L. Stern, "Natural variations in environmental illumination in a newborn nursery," *Pediatrics*, vol. 50, no. 1, pp. 131–133, 1972.

[10] R. D. White, "Recommended standards for the newborn ICU," *Journal of Perinatology*, vol. 27, supplement 2, pp. S4–S19, 2007.

[11] R. D. White and G. I. Marin, "New standards for newborn intensive care unit (NICU) design," *Journal of Perinatology*, vol. 26, pp. S2–S18, 2006.

[12] M. Walsh-Sukys, A. Reitenbach, D. Hudson-Barr, and P. DePompei, "Reducing light and sound in the neonatal intensive care unit: an evaluation of patient safety, staff satisfaction and costs," *Journal of Perinatology*, vol. 21, no. 4, pp. 230–235, 2001.

[13] M. S. Rea, *IESNA Lighting Handbook: Reference and Application*, Illumination Engineering Society of North America, New York, NY, USA, 9th edition, 2000.

[14] G. Sjors, K. Hammarlund, P.-A. Oberg, and G. Sedin, "An evaluation of environment and climate control in seven infant incubators. The investigated incubators differ sharply in their performance characteristics," *Biomedical Instrumentation and Technology*, vol. 26, no. 4, pp. 294–301, 1992.

[15] S. Böse-O'Reilly, U. Heudorf, T. Lob-Corzilius, K. E. V. Mühlendahl, M. Otto, and S. Schmidt, "Children's environment in Central Europe: threats and chances," *International Journal of Hygiene and Environmental Health*, vol. 210, no. 5, pp. 503–507, 2007.

[16] S. Blackburn, "Environmental impact of the NICU on developmental outcomes," *Journal of Pediatric Nursing*, vol. 13, no. 5, pp. 279–289, 1998.

[17] A. DiBiasie, "Evidence-based review of retinopathy of prematurity prevention in VLBW and ELBW infants," *Neonatal Network*, vol. 25, no. 6, pp. 393–403, 2006.

[18] M. J. Lotas and M. Walden, "Individualized developmental care for very low-birth-weight infants: a critical review," *Journal of Obstetrical and Neonatal Nursing*, vol. 25, no. 8, pp. 681–687, 1996.

[19] P. Glass, G. B. Avery, and K. N. Siva Subramanian, "Effect of bright light in the hospital nursery on the incidence of retinopathy of prematurity," *New England Journal of Medicine*, vol. 313, no. 7, pp. 401–404, 1985.

[20] B. Ackerman, E. Sherwonit, and J. Williams, "Reduced incidental light exposure: effect on the development of retinopathy of prematurity in low birth weight infants," *Pediatrics*, vol. 83, no. 6, pp. 958–962, 1989.

[21] A. R. Fielder and M. J. Moseley, "Environmental light and the preterm infant," *Seminars in Perinatology*, vol. 24, no. 4, pp. 291–298, 2000.

[22] M. T. O'Connor, B. R. Vohr, R. Tucker, and W. Cashore, "Is retinopathy of prematurity increasing among infants less than 1250 g birth weight?" *Journal of Perinatology*, vol. 23, no. 8, pp. 673–678, 2003.

[23] M. Shogan and L. L. Schumann, "The effect of environmental lighting on the oxygen saturation of preterm infants in the NICU," *Neonatal Network*, vol. 12, no. 5, pp. 7–13, 1993.

[24] M. Slevin, N. Farrington, G. Duffy, L. Daly, and J. F. A. Murphy, "Altering the NICU and measuring infants' responses," *Acta Paediatrica*, vol. 89, no. 5, pp. 577–581, 2000.

[25] J. Bullough, M. S. Rea, and R. G. Stevens, "Light and magnetic fields in a neonatal intensive care unit," *Bioelectromagnetics*, vol. 17, no. 5, pp. 396–405, 1996.

[26] N. P. Mann, R. Haddow, and L. Stokes, "Effect of night and day on preterm infants in a newborn nursery: randomised trial," *British Medical Journal*, vol. 293, no. 6557, pp. 1265–1267, 1986.

[27] Y. Shiroiwa, Y. Kamiya, S. Uchiboi et al., "Activity, cardiac and respiratory responses of blindfold preterm infants in a neonatal intensive care unit," *Early Human Development*, vol. 14, no. 3-4, pp. 259–265, 1986.

[28] K. A. Kennedy, A. R. Fielder, R. J. Hardy, B. Tung, D. C. Gordon, and J. D. Reynolds, "Reduced lighting does not improve medical outcomes in very low birth weight infants," *Journal of Pediatrics*, vol. 139, no. 4, pp. 527–531, 2001.

[29] C. M. Maguire, F. J. Walther, P. H. T. Van Zwieten, S. Le Cessie, J. M. Wit, and S. Veen, "No change in developmental outcome with incubator covers and nesting for very preterm infants in a randomised controlled trial," *Archives of Disease in Childhood*, vol. 94, no. 2, pp. F92–F97, 2009.

[30] S. M. Ludington-Hoe, M. W. Johnson, K. Morgan et al., "Neurophysiologic assessment of neonatal sleep organization: preliminary results of a randomized, controlled trial of skin contact with preterm infants," *Pediatrics*, vol. 117, no. 5, pp. e909–e923, 2006.

[31] I. S. Jung, "Effects of cycled lighting on body weight, physiological variables and behavioral states in low birth weight infants," *Taehan Kanho Hakhoe chi*, vol. 35, no. 1, pp. 143–153, 2005.

[32] M. J. Lotas, "Effects of light and sound in the neonatal intensive care unit environment on the low-birth-weight infant," *NAACOG's Clinical Issues in Perinatal and Women's Health Nursing*, vol. 3, no. 1, pp. 34–44, 1992.

[33] D. H. Brandon, D. Holditch-Davis, and M. Belyea, "Preterm infants born at less than 31 weeks' gestation have improved growth in cycled light compared with continuous near darkness," *Journal of Pediatrics*, vol. 140, no. 2, pp. 192–199, 2002.

[34] A. W. Gottfried, P. Wallace-Lande, and S. Sherman-Brown, "Physical and social environment of newborn infants in special care units," *Science*, vol. 214, no. 4521, pp. 673–675, 1981.

[35] S. F. Glotzbach, E. A. Rowlett, D. M. Edgar, R. J. Moffat, and R. L. Ariagno, "Light variability in the modern neonatal nursery: chronobiologic issues," *Medical Hypotheses*, vol. 41, no. 3, pp. 217–224, 1993.

[36] J. Robinson, M. J. Mosely, and A. R. Fielder, "Illuminance of neonatal units," *Archives of Disease in Childhood*, vol. 65, no. 7, pp. 679–682, 1990.

[37] K. Gray, S. Dostal, C. Ternullo-Retta, and M. A. Armstrong, "Developmentally supportive care in a neonatal intensive care unit: a research utilization project," *Neonatal Network*, vol. 17, no. 2, pp. 33–38, 1998.

[38] American Academy of Pediatrics, *American College of Obstetricians and Gynecologists. Guidelines for Perinatal Care*, American Academy of Pediatrics, Elk Grove Village, Ill, USA, 5th edition, 2002.

[39] L. S. Treas, "Incubator covers: health or hazard?" *Neonatal Network*, vol. 12, no. 8, pp. 50–51, 1993.

[40] H. H. Seliger and W. D. Mc Elroy, *Light: Physical and Biologic Action*, Academic Press, New York, NY, USA, 1965.

[41] D. L. Phelps and J. L. Watts, "Early light reduction for preventing retinopathy of prematurity in very low birth weight infants," Cochrane Review, Issue 2, 2013, http://www.nichd.nih.gov/Cochrane/Phelps/Phelps.HTM.

[42] E. Wesolowski and L. E. H. Smith, "Effect of light on oxygen-induced retinopathy in the mouse," *Investigative Ophthalmology and Visual Science*, vol. 35, no. 1, pp. 112–119, 1994.

[43] J. S. Penn, B. L. Tolman, L. A. Lowery, and C. A. Koutz, "Oxygen-induced retinopathy in the rat: hemorrhages and dysplasias may lead to retinal detachment," *Current Eye Research*, vol. 11, no. 10, pp. 939–953, 1992.

[44] S. Aucott, P. K. Donohue, E. Atkins, and M. C. Allen, "Neurodevelopmental care in the NICU," *Mental Retardation and Developmental Disabilities Research Reviews*, vol. 8, no. 4, pp. 298–308, 2002.

[45] K. A. VandenBerg, "Individualized developmental care for high risk newborns in the NICU: a practice guideline," *Early Human Development*, vol. 83, no. 7, pp. 433–442, 2007.

11

Reasons for Nonattendance across the Hepatitis C Disease Course

Gail Butt,[1] Liza McGuinness,[1] Terri Buller-Taylor,[1] and Sandi Mitchell[2]

[1] *UBC/BCCDC, 655 West 12th Avenue, Vancouver, BC, Canada V5Z 4R4*
[2] *BC Centre for Disease Control, 655 West 12th Avenue, Vancouver, BC, Canada V5Z 4R4*

Correspondence should be addressed to Gail Butt; gail.butt@bccdc.ca

Academic Editors: A. Kenny and H. Rhee

This descriptive qualitative study examined the patient, provider, and institutional factors contributing to nonattendance for hepatitis C (HCV) care throughout the disease course. Eighty-four patients and health and social care providers were interviewed. Thematic analysis of the data yielded 6 interrelated nonattendance themes: self-protection, determining the benefits, competing priorities, knowledge gaps, access to services, and restrictive policies. Factors within the themes varied with the disease course, type of provider/service, and patient context. Nonattendance could span months to years and most frequently began at diagnosis where providers either advised that followup was not necessary or did not recommend any followup. The way services were organized (low barrier access) and delivered (nonjudgmental approach) and higher HCV knowledge levels of patients and providers encouraged attendance. This is the first study to explore the reasons for nonattendance for HCV care throughout the disease course and validate them from multiple perspectives. There are missed opportunities for providers to encourage attendance throughout the disease course beginning at diagnosis. Interventions required include development of integrated health and social service delivery models; mechanisms to improve knowledge dissemination of the disease, its management, and treatment; and implementation of standardized followup protocols for liver disease monitoring in primary care.

1. Introduction

We report the findings from qualitative research to ascertain the patient, provider, and institutional factors that contribute to nonattendance for care for hepatitis C virus (HCV) infection at various points along the disease course.

HCV is a chronic infectious disease, spread through blood to blood contact that affects 170 million worldwide, including approximately 250,000 Canadians [1]. Because HCV has a heterogeneous presentation and a slow, unpredictable course of liver inflammation that spans decades, patients require long-term monitoring for signs of progressive liver disease and associated issues such as cirrhosis, end-stage liver disease, liver cancer, HIV coinfection, fatty liver disease, and alcohol overuse [2–8].

Patients receive diagnostic and most followup services in primary care due to the large number affected and the relative shortage of specialists [9]. Specialists provide complex disease management for those with advanced disease including the provision of a 24- to 48-week course of antiviral therapy for those eligible, consenting, and able to tolerate it. Treatment uptake has been historically low, even though antiviral therapy can permanently arrest viral replication (initially in 10% but presently in 70% of cases) [10], improve quality of life and liver function, decrease the likelihood of developing liver cancer, and improve survival [11, 12].

Disease management, whether in primary or specialist settings, can assist patients to manage symptoms and prevent liver disease acceleration [13]. Despite these benefits, patient nonattendance rates range from 28 to 80% [14–16], and little is known about the reasons for this. Nonattendance results in wasted clinician time and health care resources, but a more critical issue is the delay in presentation and lack of monitoring and management that can predispose the patient to complications unnecessarily.

Gaps in HCV care have been noted to result from patient and provider actions. Many patients begin HCV testing but do not return to obtain their results or complete the diagnostic testing process [16–18]. Other gaps occur when patients with a history of nonattendance in primary care are not offered a specialist referral by their provider [14, 19, 20]. Of those who are referred, many fail to attend the specialist appointment. A small study that looked at reasons why patients referred to a specialist clinic who did not attend found fear of the unknown precipitated nonattendance, for example, fear of being asked to undergo a liver biopsy, or being told that they had advanced disease or were going to die [21]. The research did not include factors such as whether patient preparation at the primary care level affects nonattendance for specialist assessment. For those under specialist care, studies have identified patient factors specific to the decision to decline or defer antiviral therapy which include concern over side effects, inconvenient time to start, belief that the disease is not serious enough to need intervention, disbelief in treatment efficacy, ongoing drug or alcohol use, and chaotic lifestyles [22–26].

Nonattendance has been noted as an outcome of HCV stigma from health care provider and institutional policies/practices. For example, policies that restrict eligibility for HCV treatment and agencies that give preference to patients with certain characteristics are viewed by patients as stigmatizing and result in nonattendance [27]. HCV stigma is thought to be rooted in a lack of knowledge of HCV and its association with injection drug use [27, 28].

HCV nonattendance research, although sparse, is consistent with findings from other chronic diseases which indicate that the factors affecting nonattendance are complex and involve the patient, the provider, and the health care system [29]. As a first step towards enhancing our understanding of the HCV nonattendance issues, we report the findings of descriptive research to identify, analyse, and describe patient, provider, and institutional factors contributing to nonattendance throughout the disease course [30]. The purpose of this paper is to describe the breadth of the nonattendance issue and identify areas for action.

2. Methods

A descriptive design was used to answer the research question, what are the reasons individuals with HCV do not attend for HCV care? Nonattendance was defined as instances when patients did not attend appointments and when patients delayed or deferred care. To extend our understanding of the perceived contributing factors, patients and HCV providers from multiple contexts were engaged in the research.

2.1. Ethics. Ethics approval was granted from two required review boards. Prior to interviews, written and oral information was given to all participants to ensure informed consent. To maximize confidentiality and accessibility, patient participants were interviewed by phone on a toll-free line with the exception of four patients who requested in-person interviews. To facilitate participation by patients without phones, community support agencies provided a private space and telephone. Data confidentiality was maintained using codes in place of personal identifiers and restricting transcript and data access to the research team. Participants received a $40 honorarium for their time and incidental costs.

2.2. Data Collection, Management, and Analysis. Purposeful sampling techniques were used to obtain a varied sample of "patient" and "provider" participants [31]. Patients were recruited through advertising by staff in health promotion, harm reduction, health, and social service programs and through snowballing, where participants recruit others directly or through postings on their blogs or online groups. Providers who were experienced in hepatitis C care were recruited through advertisements circulated by the research team and their provider networks.

Patient interviews lasted 45 to 90 minutes. Three trained interviewers used standard questions to collect demographic data followed by broad open-ended queries that led to more individual-focused questions to elicit the patient's experiences with HCV care and specifically instances of nonattendance. An interview guide, based on our previous work and input from an expert advisory committee of patients and providers, was used to facilitate exploration and enrich the data [32]. Ninety-minute interviews were conducted in-person with groups of 6 to 9 providers by the principle investigator (PI) (GB) for consistency [31]. All interviews were audio-recorded, transcribed verbatim, and thematically analyzed. Analysis occurred concurrent with data collection to facilitate identification of new questions and areas for further exploration or clarification [30].

Data were managed through NVivo 9 software which enabled separation of patient and provider data, data interrogation, refinement of the coding structure, and themes. The first five transcripts were read, reread, and manually coded by the PI (GB). The other team members (LM, SM) subsequently read, reread, and coded the same transcripts. The team then produced an inclusive list of codes through consensus. The coding structure was refined at weekly team meetings. Notes were kept to record thoughts, interpretations, questions, and decisions, about the data and its interpretation. Thematic analysis allowed for the data to be interpreted and organized into themes through inductive coding and systematic classification. For example, codes that described the issues considered by patients when deciding whether to attend for care were grouped under the theme "determining the benefits." Recruitment ceased shortly after no new codes or themes were identified.

2.3. Sample Characteristics. Participants included 55 patients with self-reported HCV and 29 HCV health and social care providers from 5 provinces: Nova Scotia, Quebec, Ontario, Manitoba, and British Columbia. Patient demographic data in Table 1 reveals that although patients tended to be over 40 years (73%) and well educated (69% had 12 or more years of formal education), most required income support (76%), a need they attributed to their poor health status. Patients reported difficulty determining which symptoms to ascribe to HCV as they had a mean of 4 other coexisting conditions (range 1 to 9) including arthritis, diabetes, digestive problems, chronic pain, addictions, anxiety, and depression. Their

Table 1: Characteristics of patient participants (n = 55).

Variable	N (%)
Gender	
Male	30 (55)
Female	25 (45)
Age	
19–29	3 (5)
30–39	12 (22)
40–49	12 (22)
50+	28 (51)
Province	
BC	35 (64)
MB	1 (2)
ON	8 (15)
NS	10 (18)
NB	1 (2)
Education	
Elementary/some high school	17 (31)
Completed high school	12 (22)
Postsecondary	26 (47)
Source of income	
Disability/social assistance	42 (76)
Employed full or part time	13 (24)
Living arrangements	
Live alone	23 (42)
Live with family/others	32 (58)
Years since diagnosis	
<1	1 (2)
1–10	25 (45)
11–19	21 (38)
20+	8 (15)

mean number of medications was 3 (range 0 to 15), with methadone, antidepressants, sleeping pills, analgesics, and antihypertensives being the most frequently reported.

Years since HCV diagnosis ranged from 1 to more than 20. Four (7%) had cleared the virus spontaneously. Of the 22 (40%) patients who had experienced antiviral therapy, 13 (59%) attained viral clearance, while 2 were currently on therapy.

The 29 providers represented a range of agencies including public health (8), prison health (3), street outreach (1), community clinics (4), community support agencies (7), and specialist clinics (6). Mean years experience working with HCV patients was 8.5 (range <1 to 15+ years; n = 20/29).

3. Results

Patient and provider data, although analysed separately, revealed the same six themes, evidencing congruence between patient perspectives and that of providers that specialize in working with HCV patients. The six themes were self-protection; determining the benefits; competing priorities; knowledge gaps; access to services; and restrictive policies. The first four themes center around the patient and provider at the individual and interpersonal levels, while the final two themes align with the institutional (system) level. The results are presented using examples where it enhances the explanation or description.

3.1. Self-Protection. This theme represents nonattendance as a self-protective response precipitated by the perception of being negatively judged or treated differently by providers on patient disclosure of HCV infection. Providers echoed the powerful and pervasive patient accounts. The participants perceived that negative provider behaviours were closely linked to a lack of HCV knowledge and the association of HCV with injection drug use. Patients described strong emotional responses to negative experiences in primary care, emergency care, and to a lesser extent specialty care. The emotional response and the need to prevent further negative events were so strong that many patients not only avoided disclosing their status to potential sources of support but also described periods of up to several years in which they did not attend care or changed providers.

In primary care settings, patients relayed that, beginning at HCV diagnosis, they felt that they were unfairly judged or treated as a "drug user." A few patients described delaying diagnostic testing to keep their HCV status a secret in order to protect themselves from anticipated negative experiences. Patients described many instances in which they felt obliged to disclose their HCV status resulting in a "go to the back of the line" experience or providers indicating, implicitly or explicitly, that they were "not worthy of care." Implications of disclosure were magnified in patient accounts from small, rural, and remote communities as confidentiality is difficult to maintain and there are few choices of where to receive services. Other difficulties arose if providers occupied additional roles such as cultural or religious leader. In one example, the patient's physician was also a religious leader, so the patient felt conflicted as disclosure of the behaviour that led to HCV infection was in opposition to religious norms. The possibility that diagnosis or disclosure could lead to service termination by the practitioner created a patient dilemma.

Many participants described care in emergency departments as "rude" and "judgmental." Patients described being treated "like a dog" or "like dirt." In some cases they were accused of drug seeking and/or discharged without assessment for their presenting problem. Many participants pointed out that women found emergency room experiences particularly difficult and that they refused to seek emergency services. One participant related that his partner delayed attending for so long she died within hours of entering hospital:

> *cuz they treated her like she was a dog ... she'd go out and get dope, you know, four blocks from the hospital but she wouldn't go to the hospital, you know, and she basically they uh, one day the ambulance picked her up, took her to the hospital and she was dead by midnight.*

In contrast, walk-in clinics were frequented, and when explored further, it was perceived that the way clinics are run, for example, no appointments were required and approachable staff created a comfortable atmosphere. Patients explained that walk-in clinic staff had more experience working with people with HCV and were more knowledgeable about the disease.

Although disclosure avoidance was rarely mentioned in relation to specialist care, some patients expressed discomfort with sitting in waiting rooms because of judgments they perceived other patients might make about them. Providers recounted that patients delay or defer treatment because they fear that someone they know will guess their diagnosis if they are seen attending hepatitis clinics or have visible symptoms during treatment. One provider recounted a particular client who struggled with the decision to start treatment: "she did not want to go to be treated, because she said everybody knows me, I'm well known in this city ... if I come here to visit you and to see you they'll know what I'm here for."

Patients who received intensive phone support during treatment were appreciative as it was easily accessed and more anonymous than an office visit. Providers also noted that flexibility and willingness to provide phone support could act as an attendance facilitator. Some questioned the effectiveness of strict requirements for frequent in-person visits during treatment citing clients' expressions of difficulty, especially when they were ill from the treatment effects.

Patients and providers expressed concern that an unintended consequence of disclosure avoidance is that few patients speak out about the issues they face or lobby for the type of services they need to improve their care. Examples of needed support services included peer and group support programs, volunteer driver programs, HCV chronic illness management education groups, and home support and volunteer visitor services for those on antiviral therapy.

3.2. Determining the Benefits of Attendance. Patients described a decision process of determining or weighing the benefits of attending for care. Patients readily identified benefits in primary care related to attending for diagnosis, acute episodic care, and obtaining a specialist referral. Specialty care was circumscribed with benefits focused on issues surrounding treatment with a course of antiviral therapy or, in a few instances, management of advanced liver disease when treatment was not an option.

Most patients did not report attendance for planned HCV monitoring in primary care. Those that reported planned care were being monitored for troublesome HCV symptoms or other conditions. For example, patients who reported regular laboratory monitoring of liver function in primary care relayed that these tests were required for methadone or HIV monitoring. Several explanations ensued regarding the absence of monitoring.

Early in the disease course patients did not attend largely because of the absence of provider guidance on the need for monitoring following diagnosis. Patients relayed being advised to "live healthy," eat a healthy diet, get exercise, and avoid alcohol. Provider participants confirmed this finding and said that youth were particularly at risk of not receiving any HCV followup. Providers explained that the lack of monitoring in primary care was linked to a knowledge gap and the paucity of detailed guidelines on long-term monitoring requirements in primary care.

Patients made assumptions regarding the lack of followup advice. Some assumed that because of their addiction experiences they were not offered followup:

> *I think that some of the physicians think because like I'm an ex drug addict, and I think they think that people that are drug addicts, I dunno, they figure that we're not going to pursue the treatment or you know we're not going to stick with it because we have addictions and everything and that's not the case ... Like, maybe I wasn't told about it cuz maybe they saw it well like you know she has an addiction problem.*

Others assumed that followup was not advised because treatment was unavailable or they were ineligible. For example, a participant, diagnosed for four years, was surprised to learn about available treatments through the study.

Several patients said that they began to consider the need for monitoring when they learned more about HCV and observed HCV complications among their peers or experienced symptoms. In contrast, a few patients noted that, with increased knowledge, they were less likely to attend, "I knew as much as him, I did not see why I should go and use up that time."

Many patients reported that they did not attend for HCV care for years because they "felt fine" or had increased feelings of well-being after recovery from addictions. A few believed that the virus was "dormant" or not causing damage because they were taking care of themselves. However, others said they feared that the disease was a death sentence and thought that followup was futile: "it scared the crap out of me, I did not know anything about it. I thought that it was a disease that was gonna just progress so fast that, I actually thought I was gonna die from it, right?"

With respect to treatment, many patients relayed that they sought treatment after they considered information from their peers, pamphlets, or the internet. Most patients said that they had to initiate the request for referral for treatment and be very assertive and persistent to obtain treatment:

> *I've always known that it was my right to get healthcare even though I know certain nurses or doctors how they can treat you. You know I, I know that I have a right to healthcare just as much as anybody else you know whatever kind of coverage they have. I knew I had a right to it. So I, I never let that stop me.*

While some expressed a strong and urgent desire to undertake treatment, many spoke of weighing the risks and benefits. In preparation for therapy, fear of the risks from the required liver biopsy caused some to withdraw from care. One individual recalled how on three separate occasions he participated in the pretreatment workup until a liver biopsy was required:

> *I've been doing this for many years now where I get to the point where I go in, I get an ultrasound*

done, I do my blood tests, I get my ultrasound done and then I'm supposed to get a biopsy on my liver and I usually, every time, I've chickened out and that's when I've relapsed and then I have to wait again.

Providers relayed that the liver biopsy requirement can also affect future treatment opportunities:

I have a case I remember, a patient is positive for hep C, has cancelled four times a liver biopsy, and that usually with our doctor we work for its strike three, strike four and that's it end of story.

Other patients identified weighing the positive outcomes of antiviral therapy versus the difficult to tolerate side effects: "the point of treating something that's not bothering me at this point in time and make myself sick for the next six months, well, it does not make a lot of sense to me."

For those who had experience with injection drug use, there were additional considerations:

the other thing that scares me is being sick all the time because I, you know, being a, a junkie, when I was, or an addict or whatever, you know, you use that needle to make yourself better, you know, not to make yourself feel sick, right?

Some decided to avoid experiencing treatment because the side effects would be "like going through withdrawal." Others said that knowledge of rigours of treatment caused them to reject treatment until they could establish a more stable lifestyle and stronger support system. Others decided that the antiviral therapy success rates were too low and the personal costs too high, preferring to wait for newer improved therapies to emerge:

some of the things I've seen people go through while on treatment and then come out at the end worse than they were when they started it, so that's one of the reasons I don't seek treatment until they get it right.

Many expressed concerns about the mental and emotional impacts of antiviral therapy including the effects on their significant others. They were concerned that therapy would trigger a depression or volatile emotions that they often termed "ribo-rage." Many said that they delayed HCV treatment because of what they heard from others who had experienced treatment, including opinions that regardless of the success rate they would not attempt treatment again. A participant who had prior experience with cancer chemotherapy recounted:

I was very unwell . . . I went for chemotherapy for four years, I was in the palliative wing, I was very unwell and I survived that and I found this [HCV antiviral treatment] tougher. I found this tougher because it took away all of my fight, it took away because of the mental [impact], this was new territory for me. I've been near sick and dying before, I can do that—this was worse.

A few said that they rejected treatment in the belief that "it is not a cure" or because they "felt pushed" by an emphasis on treatment at the specialist clinic.

3.3. Competing Priorities. The competing priorities theme illuminates the place that HCV is given when patients have multiple and sometimes conflicting priorities in the other aspects of their life such as other health, work, or social needs.

A number of patients described competing priorities of their work or family caregiver obligations. As one woman said, concern about HCV was supplanted by the needs of her sick husband:

he was my number one thing to look after and my life and my health took a back seat to his because he was very, very sick and when he came home from the hospital he needed more aftercare . . . and he took up a lot of my time, you know and it, it just went by the wayside.

Several patients said that they did not attend for care when they were actively using drugs. They described addictions as a "black hole" that absorbed them. A provider described youth who were addicted to crack as especially hard to engage because their lives were so chaotic. Related to drug use were disruptions in attendance for care on admittance to or release from prison. For example, treatment begun in prison would be interrupted on release until the person could access alternate resources in the community. Many said that prison release led to nonattendance for care because of other obstacles such as resumption of drug use or unstable living conditions.

Social service providers identified that many of their clients with HCV have unstable income and living conditions, for various reasons, and those issues absorb their time and energy:

I don't even know that some of the people that we work with who are homeless, who are street involved, whose lives are pretty chaotic, that they're even at a point where they feel that they have a choice, you know, because there are so many things that need to kind of get into place before the choice of treatment even enters their thinking about hep C.

Patients spoke of needing to give time and priority to managing other coexisting conditions. One said "I got so much things wrong with me I, just like, oh, like it's my arthritis or whatever, like, I completely forgot I had hep C." They also described not having the time to deal with HCV because the lack of an integrated approach required them to travel to a different provider for each condition, making their health management more complex.

Many examples dealt with taking time out to realign life plans that patients described as necessary before accessing HCV treatment. It was a common belief that it was necessary to be recovered from addictions in order to access therapy, but there were other associated goals. For example, a young woman who used illicit drugs said that she was motivated to "get clean," so she could access HCV treatment and be cured of the disease. She said her ultimate goal was to be healthy enough to "get her children back." Other patient goals identified were to be healthy enough to start a family, protect family members or future sexual partners from the risk of transmission, be free from stigma, and prevent worse outcomes.

For those with advanced liver disease, competing priorities were managing symptoms like fatigue and memory loss. Nonattendance resulted from not having enough energy to travel or simply forgetting about appointments.

3.4. Knowledge Gaps. Gaps in patient and provider knowledge represent a prevalent theme in participant interviews. Knowledge gaps arose from a lack of knowledge, lack of understanding of information, misinterpretation of information, misinformation, and difficulty appraising information.

Patients said that they obtained information through family, social and peer-networks, the internet, pamphlets, support groups, service providers, and community agencies such as drop-in centres. Information obtained focused on how HCV is acquired, prevention of transmission, and treatment with antiviral therapy. Patients described a lack of information that would help them sort out which of their symptoms were related to HCV, how often they should be monitored by a health care provider, what monitoring should involve, and how to most effectively self-manage their disease. This was especially relevant for those who did not or could not access antiviral therapy or for those who had not cleared their infection through therapy. Providers said that they were not aware of any standard recommendations for the type and frequency of monitoring for advancing liver disease in primary care, unlike specialty care where patient monitoring is individualized and based on specialist recommendations.

Providers pointed out connections between the lack of monitoring and missed opportunities for patient education in primary care:

> *we get a lot of calls about people asking if it's too late for treatment, if they've missed their chance for treatment and they're just people who maybe had hep C often for just a few years. So I think that also is a sign of these missed opportunities for conversations and ... I think that's a sign that monitoring is not there because if people were going for monitoring they'd know, they would hopefully have a better sense of whether treatment is an option for them at this time.*

In addition, gaps in provider knowledge resulted in missed opportunities for patients to access services like testing and treatment. One provider said, "on the helpline, I receive calls from people from all over ... and the first information they receive is from a doctor who ... says that it cannot be treated."

Participants relayed examples of omissions in diagnostic testing perceived to be related to inadequate provider knowledge. Two consecutive tests, a HCV antibody test followed by a HCV RNA test, are required to determine a chronic HCV infection, and yet many individuals have been told they had HCV, based solely on the antibody test, only to find out years later that this was not the case.

A number of patients believed that gaps in provider knowledge resulted from the low profile assigned to HCV in training and education programs. For example, one patient recounted, "there's this street nurse that we have in [our small] town, she knows a bit about hepatitis but not that much because they did not give them a lot of training."

There were other missed opportunities for education when patients were diagnosed that impacted decisions to attend care. One woman said, "I found out in jail. They just gave me a pamphlet and I went back to my cell crying, cuz like, no education, I thought it was like, next thing to AIDS, yeah, no education."

Patients relayed that many individuals make the decision not to attend for antiviral therapy based on misinformation or the absence of information. For example, a reason for treatment deferral was a common belief within the drug using community that one had to be "clean" or off drugs and alcohol for at least six months prior to requesting treatment. A patient deferred treatment because he believed that he could not manage the 48-week treatment course. Had he known his HCV genotype required a 24-week treatment course, he would not have delayed.

Many patients explained they frequently came across conflicting information requiring them to make decisions about which information to trust. Many privileged personal experience. For example, one patient said that the treatment information pamphlets did not correspond accurately with what he had seen friends endure. Nurse participants working in HCV treatment clinics said that they spend several sessions during the treatment preparation period assisting clients sort out "the myths and facts" and filling in knowledge gaps. They pointed out the dilemma of trying to establish a trusting relationship when patients disagree with or do not trust the accuracy of provider information. Providers identified the first few visits as critical to engaging patients and maintaining attendance for the duration of therapy.

Sometimes patients felt overwhelmed by the complexity of information:

> *I can't keep straight in my mind what tests I need to get from who and what blood work I need to get when. And what will happen to my body if I don't take these tests and get the blood works done. Also it would be good to know what the tests actually do and what they mean.*

Others had difficulties understanding HCV information such as the medical terms used by providers and were not comfortable exposing these difficulties. For example, many patients described their hepatitis as "dormant" or "resolved" but said that they were unsure what that meant. Others expressed problems wading through and understanding written information preferring to learn through other means:

> *I really don't know nothing about hep C, I really like, it's um, it's just a word to me ... because I don't have no information. I try to read it online, I read some but I couldn't understand it, like I needed to,*

for me to read something like that um, I couldn't understand but if somebody could explain it to me maybe I'd understand better.

3.5. Access to Services. This theme encompasses the institutional (system) contributors that lead to nonattendance because services were either difficult to access or inaccessible. Issues include poverty, provider shortages, long wait times, few integrated or culturally appropriate services, and difficulty scheduling appointments.

Poverty or limited financial resources were an important contributor to nonattendance. Participants provided detailed examples of deferred or delayed care because patients did not have the financial resources for such things as drugs, transportation (which for specialist appointments often required travel to a large centre with high parking fees), phone calls, and childcare. Travel from rural/remote areas for specialist care was particularly difficult if the person needed to pay for a caregiver to accompany them or a hotel stay.

Provider shortages in primary and specialist care and long wait times restricted access resulting in nonattendance. Those in rural settings without family doctors said walk-in clinics were unavailable, leaving the hospital emergency the only option, which many would not access because of past negative experiences. A lack of local providers precipitated decisions not to access treatment, because treatment requires a local provider for managing urgent issues when patients live far from specialist clinics. Participants noted that there was a general shortage of specialists and supports such as social work, mental health, and addictions services. Where services existed, there were long wait times, which patients said deterred attendance. A provider from a large urban centre explained that "up to 50% of people referred to HCV specialists do not attend, and most of those are no shows."

In contrast, availability of integrated and culturally appropriate services (youth, Aboriginal, and immigrant) positively impacted attendance. Participants and providers said that patients were more likely to attend appointments if services were fully integrated, colocated, or organized as a one-stop-shop through a case manager. The types of services frequently mentioned for inclusion in integrated approaches included primary care, hepatitis specialty services, mental health, addictions, housing, and social services:

they tried to do as much as they could for, for me in the appointment, right? And they had everybody in that one building so you know . . . the nurses and the psychiatrist and the doctors and, you know, um, yeah, that helped a lot, being able to just go to one spot.

Providers confirmed that to improve attendance, patients need services based on the social determinants of health to "meet them where they are at." This approach would ensure attention to such things as the contextual and cultural needs for youth, Aboriginal, and immigrant populations.

The time it takes to attend appointments and the frequency of appointments contributed to nonattendance. For example, the time spent in waiting rooms, sometimes for more than two hours, was a deterrent. The frequency of appointments required in preparation for a course of antiviral therapy complicated patients' life plans prompting nonattendance. For example, several patients spoke of making changes in their life plans that they thought necessary in anticipation of the six months to one year on therapy. They explained that these plans were disrupted by a long pre-treatment preparation time which included several months of waiting for and attending for various tests and consultations with multiple specialists prior to treatment initiation:

. . . it's just been a long process and, and, and, you know, I wish when the doctor says you'd be starting it then that's when you start it, you don't get thrown all these other obstacles to get there which is, very, you know, cause you get all ready to do it and then you're like oh, now I have to do that and that's going to take three months, like that's wrong, right? You get yourself ready for it and then it's not happening.

Providers confirmed that the time required for the pre-treatment evaluation is not widely communicated, even though it is essential to ensure the patient is fit to withstand the rigors of treatment.

3.6. Restrictive Policies. Restrictive policies, the other institutional (system) level theme identified, impacted patients' ability to attend and engage with HCV care. Policies that impacted attendance ranged from local office policies to provincial system level requirements including requirements for a doctor's referral to a specialist; abstinence before consideration for treatment at some clinics; treatment eligibility criteria in many provinces; frequency of required clinic visits for treatment monitoring; and practices that restricted how or when services could be accessed.

Policies at the agency level that deterred attendance included limited calling times for making appointments, financial penalties, or service withdrawal for missed appointments and segregated appointment times or waiting rooms for those who used illicit drugs. Some patients pointed out that because of restrictive policies they dropped out of care and received only episodic care through drop-in clinics.

Many spoke of system level policies that affected their ability to access treatment. The requirement for doctor's referral to a hepatitis specialist was difficult to meet especially in areas with family physician shortages. In some provinces, treatment eligibility policies such as the requirement to demonstrate liver damage through repeated lab tests or liver biopsy acted as a deterrent.

Participants reported that those with addictions who needed to be enrolled in a methadone program prior to HCV therapy reported difficulties normalizing their life while complying with the program regulations because of daily reporting requirements, restricted dispensing times, and drug effects. Obtaining "carries" such as a three-day methadone supply allowed some freedom, but that privilege depended on the degree of adherence, length of time in the program, and the methadone prescriber:

the methadone program the way it is set up in this province does not make somebody's life more livable because you gotta go to the pharmacy every couple of days, you gotta go to doctors appointments, you gotta go for mandated urine tests whether you're working or not, right, if you're out on a fishing boat you've gotta come in every three days to pick up your juice at the pharmacy, right?

4. Discussion and Implications

This study explored the reasons for nonattendance for HCV care and identified factors affecting attendance at various points along the disease course: on diagnosis, postdiagnosis monitoring for disease progression, during preparation for and treatment with antiviral therapy once the disease had progressed, and in managing the disease when treatment was not an option. Analysis revealed nonattendance issues arise from the individual (patient or provider), patient/provider interactions, and institution (systemic) practices. The issues are contained within six interrelated themes: self-protection, competing priorities, determining the benefits, knowledge gaps, access to services, and restrictive policies. The findings from patients and HCV providers working in a variety of health and social service settings were congruent, confirming the work of Stewart who found concordance between patient, HCV specialist provider, and counsellor perspectives regarding HCV help-seeking and coping [33].

The study has several limitations. Participants were provided a small honorarium which may have influenced decisions to participate. In order to obtain a breadth and diversity of views, the participants were purposefully recruited, limiting the generalizeability of the findings. The results are based on participant recall which can be influenced by time and circumstances; for example, events in the present may be remembered with more clarity than distant events. However, the study's feedback loops during concurrent data collection and analysis provided opportunities to confirm, expand, or refute the points raised with subsequent participants.

The issues identified in the self-protection theme extend the HCV stigma literature by describing the impact on care engagement when patients anticipate or experience being negatively judged or treated poorly. It confirms the association of HCV with illicit drug use and describes issues arising from the lack of provider HCV knowledge [27, 28, 34]. In accordance with Paterson et al., emergency room care was a context that elicited particularly strong negative patient responses and in this study led to nonattendance even at great personal health risk [27]. Drop-in clinics and integrated service centres were contexts where patients were more likely to have positive experiences.

Determining the benefits of care, a recurrent theme throughout the disease course was of particular relevance on diagnosis as the absence of advice for monitoring or followup accounted for lengthy periods of nonattendance. Although there are specific guidelines for HCV assessment in primary care, they do not provide specifics for followup monitoring [35]. Closing the gap is crucial to improve secondary prevention of advanced liver disease and prevent premature deaths. As mortality studies have pointed out, interventions early in the course of the disease could prevent deaths from issues associated with HCV acquisition such as illicit drug use [36–38].

While the theme knowledge gaps confirmed previously identified HCV knowledge deficits among primary care providers, it clearly identifies consequences for patients [39]. In accordance with the findings of Holman and Lorig, participants identified needs for accurate information and self-care education to cope with and adjust to their chronic illness [40]. The findings revealed that patients rely on knowledge gained outside the health system to make care decisions but were limited in their ability to access comprehensive information, fully understand medical terminology, or appraise the accuracy of information. For example, active drug use was cited as a reason for patients not accessing treatment and for providers not discussing treatment options with patients even though evidence supports treatment provision both from a clinical and cost-effectiveness stand point [41, 42]. In addition, decisions to undergo treatment are often made in the absence of a discussion with a health care provider, and the patient literature is silent on pretreatment workup requirements, which for some took up to a year and precipitated nonattendance.

Competing priorities highlights the need to consider important aspects of lifestyle and other social determinants of health as well as disease specific aspects such as transmission and prevention, stages of illness, symptoms, prevention of progression, and options for antiviral therapy. This finding supports others who have identified the need for models of care that are patient-centered and integrate health and social care [9, 43]. Primary health care models that address complex health and social service needs similar to those of patients with chronic HCV have been shown to improve health outcomes [13, 44, 45].

The themes access to services and restrictive policies encompass multiple systemic obstacles faced by patients that impact care attendance such as lack of public transportation, provider shortages, long wait times, and the absence of culturally appropriate services. Restrictive policies were identified at single provider, agency, and provincial levels. These findings point to the need for system (policy) changes to improve service uptake such as: expanding specialist referral options to include self-referral and referral from allied health professionals; replicating approaches that improve access to specialists and reduce the need to travel to major centres by electronically linking medical specialists with generalist physicians in rural areas and nurse-led models of HCV prevention and care that include specialist consultation and have been shown to increase reach and access to care [18, 46, 47].

These results point to the need for clinical practice and system (policy) changes to increase engagement and retention in HCV care. Changes that would ensure patients are attended to in a respectful manner no matter what their background and that primary care providers have the knowledge and supports to provide patients with accurate and timely HCV information. Development and implementation of postdiagnosis monitoring protocols and mechanisms to improve knowledge dissemination in particular for nurses and physicians in primary care are recommended.

5. Conclusion

This is the first study to explore the reasons for nonattendance for HCV care throughout the disease course and validate the findings from multiple perspectives. It uncovered reasons for nonattendance, many of which are amenable through the provision of low barrier, nonjudgmental, and integrated services. It underscores the importance of provider and patient education that includes an emphasis on the psychological and sociocultural needs of the populations affected. This research can inform interventions, particularly in primary care, that are urgently required to engage and retain patients across the continuum of care, so that patients can realize the human and health system benefits of HCV care and emerging therapies that have the potential to cure 90–95% of those infected.

Acknowledgments

Special thanks are due to all project participants for their enthusiastic support of this research and for trusting the authors to tell their story. The authors are very grateful to their Advisory Committee whose commitment and contributions made this a truly national effort. And finally, the authors would like to acknowledge role of the Public Health Agency of Canada in providing the funding that made this project possible.

References

[1] R. Remis, "Modelling the incidence and prevalence of hepatitis C infection and its sequelae in Canada," Final Report, Public Health Agency of Canada, Ottawa, Canada, 2007.

[2] L. B. Seeff and J. H. Hoofnagle, "National Institutes of Health consensus development conference: management of hepatitis C: 2002," *Hepatology*, vol. 36, supplement 1, pp. S1–S2, 2002.

[3] L. B. Seeff, R. N. Miller, C. S. Rabkin et al., "45-year followup of hepatitis C virus infection in healthy young adults," *Annals of Internal Medicine*, vol. 132, no. 2, pp. 105–111, 2000.

[4] J. García-Samaniego, M. Rodríguez, J. Berenguer et al., "Hepatocellular carcinoma in HIV-infected patients with chronic hepatitis C," *American Journal of Gastroenterology*, vol. 96, no. 1, pp. 179–183, 2001.

[5] M. V. Ragni, C. G. Moore, K. Soadwa et al., "Impact of HIV on liver fibrosis in men with hepatitis C infection and haemophilia," *Haemophilia*, vol. 17, no. 1, pp. 103–111, 2011.

[6] L. E. Adinolfi, M. Gambardella, A. Andreana, M. Tripodi, R. Utili, and G. Ruggiero, "Steatosis accelerates the progression of liver damage of chronic hepatitis C patients and correlates with specific HCV genotype and visceral obesity," *Hepatology*, vol. 33, no. 6, pp. 1358–1364, 2001.

[7] G. Corrao and S. Arico, "Independent and combined action of hepatitis C virus infection and alcohol consumption on the risk of symptomatic liver cirrhosis," *Hepatology*, vol. 27, no. 4, pp. 914–919, 1998.

[8] F. Pessione, F. Degos, P. Marcellin et al., "Effect of alcohol consumption on serum hepatitis C virus RNA and histological lesions in chronic hepatitis C," *Hepatology*, vol. 27, no. 6, pp. 1717–1722, 1998.

[9] B. Zevin, "Managing chronic hepatitis C in primary-care settings: more than antiviral therapy," *Public Health Reports*, vol. 122, no. 2, pp. 78–82, 2007.

[10] T. J. Liang and M. G. Ghany, "Current and future therapies for hepatitis C virus infection," *The New England Journal of Medicine*, vol. 368, no. 20, pp. 1907–1917, 2013.

[11] C.-H. Hung, C.-M. Lee, S.-N. Lu et al., "Long-term effect of interferon alpha-2b plus ribavirin therapy on incidence of hepatocellular carcinoma in patients with hepatitis C virus-related cirrhosis," *Journal of Viral Hepatitis*, vol. 13, no. 6, pp. 409–414, 2006.

[12] H. Yoshida, Y. Arakawa, M. Sata et al., "Interferon therapy prolonged life expectancy among chronic hepatitis C patients," *Gastroenterology*, vol. 123, no. 2, pp. 483–491, 2002.

[13] S. B. Ho, E. Groessl, A. Dollarhide, S. Robinson, D. Kravetz, and E. Dieperink, "Management of chronic hepatitis C in veterans: the potential of integrated care models," *American Journal of Gastroenterology*, vol. 103, no. 7, pp. 1810–1823, 2008.

[14] H. Groom, E. Dieperink, D. B. Nelson et al., "Outcomes of a hepatitis C screening program at a large urban VA medical center," *Journal of Clinical Gastroenterology*, vol. 42, no. 1, pp. 97–106, 2008.

[15] R. A. Gunn, M. A. Lee, D. B. Callahan, P. Gonzales, P. J. Murray, and H. S. Margolis, "Integrating hepatitis, STD, and HIV services into a drug rehabilitation program," *American Journal of Preventive Medicine*, vol. 29, no. 1, pp. 27–33, 2005.

[16] J. Subiadur, J. L. Harris, and C. A. Rietmeijer, "Integrating viral hepatitis prevention services into an urban STD clinic: Denver, Colorado," *Public Health Reports*, vol. 122, no. 2, pp. 12–17, 2007.

[17] G. L. Armstrong, "Commentary: modelling the epidemiology of hepatitis C and its complications," *International Journal of Epidemiology*, vol. 32, no. 5, pp. 725–726, 2003.

[18] G. Butt, *Partnership and population outcome relationships in four nurse-led hepatitis C integrated prevention and care projects [Doctoral dissertation]*, McMaster University, Hamilton, Canada, 2009.

[19] A. A. Butt, M. Wagener, A. O. Shakil, and J. Ahmad, "Reasons for non-treatment of hepatitis C in veterans in care," *Journal of Viral Hepatitis*, vol. 12, no. 1, pp. 81–85, 2005.

[20] C. H. Cawthorne, K. R. Rudat, M. S. Burton et al., "Limited success of HCV antiviral therapy in United States veterans," *American Journal of Gastroenterology*, vol. 97, no. 1, pp. 149–155, 2002.

[21] L. Tiffen and S. Sheridan, "Improving take-up of hepatitis C services," *Nursing Times*, vol. 98, no. 43, pp. 30–32, 2002.

[22] S. L. Jowett, K. Agarwal, B. C. Smith et al., "Managing chronic hepatitis C acquired through intravenous drug use," *Quarterly Journal of Mathematics*, vol. 94, no. 3, pp. 153–158, 2001.

[23] H. F. Gidding, M. G. Law, J. Amin et al., "Predictors of deferral of treatment for hepatitis C infection in Australian clinics," *Medical Journal of Australia*, vol. 194, no. 8, pp. 398–402, 2012.

[24] J. Parkes, P. Roderick, B. Bennett-Lloyd, and W. Rosenberg, "Variation in hepatitis C services may lead to inequity of heath-care provision: a survey of the organisation and delivery of services in the United Kingdom," *BMC Public Health*, vol. 6, no. 1, article 3, 2006.

[25] C. E. Munoz-Plaza, S. Strauss, J. Astone-Twerell et al., "Exploring drug users' attitudes and decisions regarding hepatitis C (HCV) treatment in the U.S," *International Journal of Drug Policy*, vol. 19, no. 1, pp. 71–78, 2008.

[26] O. S. Khokhar and J. H. Lewis, "Reasons why patients infected with chronic hepatitis C virus choose to defer treatment: do they alter their decision with time?" *Digestive Diseases and Sciences*, vol. 52, no. 5, pp. 1168–1176, 2007.

[27] B. L. Paterson, M. Backmund, G. Hirsch, and C. Yim, "The depiction of stigmatization in research about hepatitis C," *International Journal of Drug Policy*, vol. 18, no. 5, pp. 364–373, 2007.

[28] G. Butt, "Stigma in the context of hepatitis C: concept analysis," *Journal of Advanced Nursing*, vol. 62, no. 6, pp. 712–724, 2008.

[29] B. L. Paterson, P. Charlton, and S. Richard, "Non-attendance in chronic disease clinics: a matter of non-compliance?" *Journal of Nursing and Healthcare of Chronic Illness*, vol. 2, no. 1, pp. 63–74, 2010.

[30] M. Sandelowski, "Focus on research methods: whatever happened to qualitative description?" *Research in Nursing and Health*, vol. 23, no. 4, pp. 334–340, 2000.

[31] M. Patton, *Qualitative Evaluation and Research Methods*, Sage, Thousand Oaks, Calif, USA, 1990.

[32] J. A. Smith, "Semi-structured interviewing and qualitative analysis," in *Rethinking Methods in Psychology*, pp. 9–26, Sage, Thousand Oaks, Calif, USA, 1995.

[33] B. J. Stewart, A. A. Mikocka-Walus, H. Harley, and J. M. Andrews, "Help-seeking and coping with the psychosocial burden of chronic hepatitis C: a qualitative study of patient, hepatologist, and counsellor perspectives," *International Journal of Nursing Studies*, vol. 49, no. 5, pp. 560–569, 2012.

[34] G. Butt, B. L. Paterson, and L. K. McGuinness, "Living with the stigma of hepatitis C," *Western Journal of Nursing Research*, vol. 30, no. 2, pp. 204–221, 2008.

[35] G. Pinette, J. Cox, J. Heathcote, L. Moore, K. Adamowski, and G. Riehl, *Primary Care Management of Chronic Hepatitis C: Professional Desk Reference*, Public Health Agency of Canada, Ottawa, Canada, 2009.

[36] L. I. Backus, D. B. Boothroyd, B. R. Phillips, P. Belperio, J. Halloran, and L. A. Mole, "Liver, pancreas, and biliary tract," *Clinical Gastroenterology and Hepatology*, vol. 9, no. 6, pp. 509–516, 2011.

[37] M. Krajden, M. Kuo, B. Zagorski, M. Alvarez, A. Yu, and M. Krahn, "Health care costs associated with hepatitis C: a longitudinal cohort study," *Canadian Journal of Gastroenterology*, vol. 24, no. 12, pp. 717–726, 2010.

[38] A. Yu, J. Spinelli, D. Cook, J. Buxton, and M. Krajden, "Mortality among British Columbians testing for hepatitis C antibody," *BMC Public Health*, vol. 13, article 291, no. 291, 10 pages, 2013.

[39] J. Cox, L. Graves, E. Marks et al., "Knowledge, attitudes and behaviours associated with the provision of hepatitis C care by Canadian family physicians," *Journal of Viral Hepatitis*, vol. 18, no. 7, pp. e332–e340, 2011.

[40] H. Holman and K. Lorig, "Patient self-management: a key to effectiveness and efficiency in care of chronic disease," *Public Health Reports*, vol. 119, no. 3, pp. 239–243, 2004.

[41] N. K. Martin, P. Vickerman, A. Miners et al., "Cost-effectiveness of hepatitis C virus antiviral treatment for injection drug user populations," *Hepatology*, vol. 55, no. 1, pp. 49–57, 2012.

[42] P. Higgs, R. Sacks-Davis, J. Gold, and M. Hellard, "Barriers to receiving hepatitis C treatment for people who inject drugs myths and evidence," *Hepatitis Monthly*, vol. 11, no. 7, pp. 513–518, 2011.

[43] F. Naffah, "Patients with hepatitis C are best managed by a specialist in liver diseases. CON: the management of hepatitis C in a community-based practice," *The American Journal of Gastroenterology*, vol. 102, no. 9, pp. 1839–1841, 2007.

[44] A. H. Litwin, I. Soloway, and M. N. Gourevitch, "Integrating services for injection drug users infected with hepatitis C virus with methadone maintenance treatment: challenges and opportunities," *Clinical Infectious Diseases*, vol. 40, supplement 5, pp. S339–S345, 2005.

[45] R. Saitz, M. J. Larson, C. Labelle, J. Richardson, and J. H. Samet, "The case for chronic disease management for addiction," *Journal of Addiction Medicine*, vol. 2, no. 2, pp. 55–65, 2008.

[46] K. Doucette, V. Robson, S. Shafran, and D. Kunimoto, "Improving access to care by allowing self-referral to a hepatitis C clinic," *Canadian Journal of Gastroenterology*, vol. 23, no. 6, pp. 421–424, 2009.

[47] S. Arora, K. Thornton, S. M. Jenkusky, B. Parish, and J. V. Scaletti, "Project ECHO: linking university specialists with rural and prison-based clinicians to improve care for people with chronic hepatitis C in New Mexico," *Public Health Reports*, vol. 122, supplement 2, pp. 74–77, 2007.

12

What Factors Facilitate Good Learning Experiences in Clinical Studies in Nursing: Bachelor Students' Perceptions

Bjørg Dale, Arne Leland, and Jan Gunnar Dale

Faculty of Health and Sport Sciences, University of Agder, Postboks 509, 4898 Grimstad, Norway

Correspondence should be addressed to Bjørg Dale; bjorg.dale@uia.no

Academic Editors: H. Rhee and D. M. Wilson

Clinical studies constitute 50% of the bachelor program in nursing education in Norway, and the quality of these studies may be decisive for the students' opportunities to learn and develop their professional competences. The aim of this study was to explore what bachelor students' in nursing perceived to be important for having good learning experiences in clinical studies. Data was collected in a focus group interview with eight nursing students who were in the last year of the educational program. The interview was transcribed verbatim, and qualitative content analysis was used for exploring and interpreting the content of the interview text. One main theme emerged from the analysis: "being in a vulnerable and exposed position characterized by conflicting needs." Four categories were found: "aspects related to the clinical setting", "aspects related to the nurse supervisor," "aspects related to the student," and "aspects related to the student-supervisor relationship". The findings revealed that the students' learning experiences and motivation were related to individual, relational, and organizational aspects. The students highlighted their own as well as their supervisors' attitudes and competences and the importance of positive relationships. In addition, feeling welcomed, included, and valued in the ward improved their motivation, self-confidence, and self-respect.

1. Introduction

Organizing a good learning arena in clinical settings is crucial for bachelor students in nursing because a major part of their studies and training take place in that context. The quality of the clinical studies has, therefore, a great impact on the quality of the studies as a whole. Our impression is that the students' experiences and how they perceive the quality of their clinical studies vary a lot.

Clinical studies in nursing education are reported to represent the most stressful parts for the students, particularly in the initial periods due to lacking competence and knowledge [1, 2]. A decisive aspect for having positive learning experiences is described to be the relationship between the student and the nurse supervisor [1, 3–7]. Regular feedback, reflections, and practical advice from the supervisor are important factors for improving the students' practical competence, confidence, motivation, and self-esteem [8]. The nurses may represent a positive role figure for the students in clinical training [3]. Having regular reflections and dialogue with their clinical supervisors are, therefore, among the most important ways for the students to learn [9]. Despite this, it has been shown that the nurses' awareness of the importance of such dialogues may be absent [9]. Furthermore, this relationship may also make the students vulnerable because they are dependent on the supervisors' assessment and judgment [7].

Webb and Shakespeare [4], describe that students often strive to convince the supervisors that they are "good students" in terms of attitudes as clinical competence.

Recently, a new standardized evaluation form was introduced at the university where the current study was conducted. The evaluation form includes assessment of the nursing students' competences in hospital studies related to knowledge, skills, and attitudes. At the same time, the students' responsibility for self-evaluation is more emphasized compared with previous procedures. They need to assess their level of competence and fill out the form, and the supervisors perform their own assessment correspondently. These assessments together constitute a basis for discussion and conversation in the evaluation meeting conducted with the university teacher present. Preliminary experiences and informal feedback from students indicate that the new assessment procedure may affect several aspects related to the students' clinical training in general and the student-supervisor relationship. Therefore, the aim of the present study was to explore what bachelor students' in nursing perceived to be important for having good learning experiences in clinical studies in hospital wards after a new evaluation form was introduced.

In the presentation of the present study, the terms "supervisor" and "mentor" will be used interchangeably, and refer to the ward nurses who are responsible for supervising and assessing the students in their clinical studies. These nurses have responsibility for the student guidance and patient care at the same time; that is, they are "working nurse mentors."

2. Materials and Methods

2.1. Participants and Data Collection. The data was collected by the second and last authors in a focus group interview performed with a group of students who were in the final year of their education. Focus group interview is described to be an appropriate qualitative data collection method for exploring experiences, attitudes, and viewpoints regarding phenomena that are common in a group of informants [10]. A purposeful sampling method was used in the recruitment of the participants [10]. Seven students who had completed their clinical studies in medical and surgical wards at the local public hospital were invited and agreed to participate in the study. It was emphasized to recruit participants who ranged in age and had experiences from different hospital wards. In addition, it was desirable that both sexes were represented. Seven students with an age ranging from 22 to 37 years constituted the group. One of the participants was male. Their previous experiences with health care varied from no experience at all to several years of experience as licensed practical nurse. A semistructured interview guide directed the interview, containing six questions about what they empathized for having good learning experiences in the clinical settings. The questions were particularly concerned with the student-supervisor relationships. The audiotaped interview lasted for one hour, and it was transcribed verbatim.

2.2. Data Analysis. Qualitative content analysis was used for exploring and interpreting the content of the interview text in this study. Graneheim and Lundman [11] describe this method to include both manifest and latent content of a text. The manifest content analysis concerns the description of the text as it is expressed by the informant and includes meaning units in the original text, condensation of the meaning units, and the creation of common categories. The latent content refers to the interpretation of the text and includes, according to Graneheim and Lundman [11], creation of the themes which emerge as an underlying meaning of the condensed meaning units and categories. The text was read and reread several times, moving backwards and forwards between the whole and the parts, to grasp the meaning of the phenomenon that was investigated. All authors were involved in the analysis.

In the analysis, the transcribed interview text was broken down to condensed meaning units, to grasp the manifest content of the message. In this stage, the meaning units were expressed in a language close to the interviewees' original articulations. Subsequently, the condensed meaning units were categorized, and further gathered into a main theme representing the latent content, which refers to the underlying meaning or what the text really talks about.

2.3. Ethical Considerations. The Norwegian Social Science Data Service (NSD) was consulted for advice regarding the obligation to report the study. They confirmed that reporting was not necessary if all personal identifying information was removed from the data set and the audiotaped interview was not downloaded on a computer. We acted in accordance with this advice and the interview was transcribed directly from the tape recorder.

In addition to the written informed consent, information about the study was repeated, and voluntariness and confidentiality were assured regarding the informants legal rights prior to each interviews [12]. Their right to withdraw at any time in the research process until publication of the study was also assured before the interview was performed.

3. Findings

One main theme, four categories and nine subcategories emerged from the analyses of the interview text. An overview is shown in Table 1.

In the following, the categories with their respective subcategories are presented, and some examples from the interview text are used to demonstrate the findings.

3.1. Aspects Related to the Clinical Setting

3.1.1. Feeling Welcomed and Waited. Many of the informants emphasized the importance of being waited and feeling welcomed in the clinical ward for having a positive start. Some of them had experienced being met with an attitude characterized by surprise, unpreparedness, or even negative reactions the first day in the ward. In this sense, an important prerequisite was that the nurse leader and the staff in general were sufficiently and appropriately informed about the actual practice period, which means that information sent from the university was picked up. Knowing the students' name and educational level was important and made them feel welcomed, and, particularly, that the supervisor was informed in advance.

3.1.2. A Student-Friendly Attitude and Atmosphere. While the former subcategory was mainly related to the first day or initial phase of their practice period, the informants also talked about how important it was that the ward in general had a student-friendly atmosphere. Although they appreciated to be included as a member of the staff, it was important that they were allowed to be students and use some time for their own reflections and studies. Some of them raised the problem of being (mis)used as labor resource and at the same

Table 1: Overview of the main theme, categories, and associated subcategories.

Main theme Being in a vulnerable and exposed position characterized by conflicting needs			
Category 1	Category 2	Category 3	Category 4
Aspects related to the clinical setting	Aspects related to the nurse supervisor	Aspects related to the student	Aspect related to the student-supervisor relationship
Subcategories	Subcategories	Subcategories	Subcategories
Feeling welcomed and waited	The supervisor's preparedness and expectations	The student's expectations and readiness to learn	Mutual respect and trust
A student-friendly attitude and atmosphere	The supervisor's motivations and attitude	The student's competences and confidence level	An open and inviting communication
	The supervisor's competence		

time being in a vulnerable position regarding sanctions if they complained or avoided to do what they were told. The "evaluation ghost" was constantly present. In addition, the advantage to have two supplemental nurse supervisors was emphasized, mainly for having back-up for holidays or sick leaves. Although a lack of continuity and divergence could be a problem when having two supervisors, it was mostly pointed out as an advantage. Another important concern related to the ward was the prioritizing of time and facilities for student supervision and reflections. Although this was mainly the supervisor's responsibility, it was important that the ward and the ward manager emphasized and arranged for it.

3.2. Aspects Related to the Nurse Supervisor

3.2.1. The Supervisor's Preparedness and Expectations. Some of the informants talked about difficult situations and experiences regarding the supervisor's lack of information and preparedness before they started the practice studies. Some of them were limited or not at all updated about the curricula or other important documents delivered from the university, for example, the composition of actual assessment form and how to make appropriate judgment of the individual student. Quite often they were not informed about the educational level of the actual student group, and they had not made themselves familiar with the students' names. Such details could influence the students' well-being and motivation.

3.2.2. The Supervisor's Motivations and Attitude. The majority of the students highlighted the importance of the supervisor's motivation and their engagement regarding the mentorship. One of the informants said that

> *"When I came to the ward I was allocated to a nurse who clearly expressed that she had asked to be released from the supervision duties several times-without success. She clearly expressed in many ways that that she felt discomfort and considered me as a burden"*

Another informant put it this way:

> *"...they (the supervisors) always receive a folder from the university with written information and documents, but I believe that less than 20% of them read it. We experience all the time that they say that they have not been prepared or informed about the mentorship-and that they do not want it. They are obviously not motivated at all..."*

The supervisor's ability to be open, friendly, including, and willing to adjust if necessary were qualifications also mentioned by the students. Positive experiences improved their own motivation for learning and their self-confidence, and, on the contrary, difficult or bad situations could result in a negative perception of the clinical studies as a whole. One informant told about a comment she had caught from a newly graduated nurse in the ward: "... and then I heard she (the nurse) said that she looked forward to be a supervisor now so she could get her own back..." Another interviewee responded to that experience in this way: "... so I think ... soon I will be a nurse myself, and then I will like to be a supervisor, and I will never treat the students the way they (the supervisors) treated me."

3.2.3. The Supervisor's Competence. When the students talked about the supervisor's competences they referred to professional competence as well as pedagogical skills. They underlined the significance of professional nursing qualifications as a decisive prerequisite for being a good mentor and a good role model. In this sense, they narrated positive as well as negative experiences. Some of the informants told about positive experiences when their supervisor prioritized to have regular appointments for supervising and time for reflections. They appreciated when the mentors challenged them and in general they felt flattered when the nurses trusted them for performing challenging tasks. However, feeling the safety of an companying mentor was expressed as one of the most important aspects for learning and developing in clinical studies. Other experiences included frustrations about the supervisors' lack of interest for updating own knowledge, and how they went in the defence if their skills were challenged. This was particularly true of the nurses who were trained years ago. One of the informants expressed:

> *"Many of them (the nurses) are narrow-minded! What they learned twenty-five years ago is still*

the right thing for them. What we (the students) learn today ... this you can just not give a damn"

In addition to professional nursing competences the informants talked just as much about the nurses' pedagogical or supervising competences. They were critical about the lack of pedagogical skills requirement and that the allocation of mentors seemed to happen rather by chance. Some informants underlined how important it is that clinical mentors have some pedagogical education or training. One of them expressed:

> *"It should be a mandatory demand from the school that all clinical supervisors should complete some kind of supervision training. Does the school really know how variable and coincidental the mentors' competences are?"*

Some of the informants expressed that they had positive experiences of having two mentors, and the advantages of how they could complement each other. This was viewed as a safety net if one of the mentors was absent for holidays, day offs, or sick leaves. Other aspects were the benefits from more than one mentor's competences and experiences, and it could work as an additional protection if the chemistry between the student and the mentor was not right.

3.3. Aspects Related to the Student

3.3.1. The Student's Expectations and Readiness to Learn. The students' own preparedness and expectations regarding focus and learning outcomes in the actual practice period was mentioned by some of the students as an important assumption for having optimal learning benefits during the clinical studies. Furthermore, to clarify and formulate their expectations to themselves as well as to their mentors from the very start of the practice period, preferably in a written document, was clearly viewed as an advantage. One of them said:

> *"It was very important for me to write down what I expected of myself and the supervisor—and what I expected from the academic teacher. I think that it is important that my supervisors know what the best way to learn for me is."*

Another informant said:

> *"I told them what I expected, and then I said that I like to be independent and take responsibilities for my own learning, so I hope that you will show me confidence and facilitate independence—within certain limits, of course. So having an open conversation from the very start about my expectations is important."*

They acknowledged that having success regarding the achievement of the learning outcomes was largely dependent on their own efforts, engagement, curiosity, and willingness to seek and attend new learning situations. Therefore, they clearly expressed their own responsibility for having positive learning experiences.

3.3.2. The Student's Competence and Confidence Level. The students' professional background and former practice experiences influenced their actual level of competence as well as the degree of self-confidence. Some of them shared stories about situations where they had been shown confidence in challenging patient situation, and how these experiences had influenced their personal and professional growth. Although information about their professional background before they started the university studies were registered in the present study, it is not unusual that nursing students have several years of former working experiences as health personnel. On the other hand, some of the students told stories about situations where they had been thrown into stressful and challenging situations without feeling comfortable and ready for it. If they failed in such situations, it could easily influence their courage and self-confidence in similar situations later. Consequently, the balance between their actual competences and experience, and their need for further instructions and training, appeared to vary a lot. Openness about their individual competences and guidance needs seemed to be a decisive factor in this sense.

Making regular diary and reflection notes were mentioned as very helpful and important tools to drive awareness of and formulate their own level of competence.

3.4. The Student-Mentor Relationship

3.4.1. Mutual Respect and Trust. An evident thread through the entire interview was the importance of the relationship between the students and their mentors. The mutual respect included the students' understanding and respect regarding the nurses' need to share out their time and to first and foremost prioritize patient care. On the other side, it also involved the nurses' understanding and respect for the student's need for instruction and for being included, seen, and heard. Making regular appointments for reflection and feedback improved the mutual understanding, and prevented unwanted and unpredictable situations. Several stories were told about uncomfortable, unexpected, and threatening evaluation episodes caused by the lack of continuous feedback, discrepant understanding regarding the evaluation form, and disagreement about the students actual competence level. They also told about tough experiences related to an imbalanced relationship where the mentor had used their power in an unfavorable way, like some kind of punishment. Such situations could result in the students' reluctance to be open about their own insecurity or to raise questions. One of the informants said:

> *"I think that many students are left with bad experiences associated with their mentors, and, you know, the consequences are that you quite*

simply do not dare to raise any question at all. This is not good and right!"

To assess their own competences was obviously a stressful task for many of the informants, particularly when their own opinions and self-perceptions were considerably different from the mentor's assessment. Some of the students had experienced that the mentor gave them higher marks than they had expected. When they commented on this, even with gratitude and humbleness, they had experienced comments like "ok, then we put the mark as you perceive it." Consequently, they felt that they were punished for being humble and they blamed themselves for not being brave enough to describe what they really felt and meant. On the other side, they also expressed disappointment and skepticism in relation to the supervisor's ability to perform an accurate assessment grounded on realistic and convincing perceptions and arguments.

3.4.2. An Open and Inviting Communication. According to the students, the relationship between the student and their mentor should also be characterized by a mutual openness and a constructive, respectful, and supportive dialogue. In this respect, they pointed out their own responsibility for establishing a fruitful relationship, and they viewed their own openness and attitude just as decisive as the mentor's attitude. By continually communicating and sharing their mutual experiences, good and bad, praise and criticism, they facilitated an open atmosphere. However, corrections and criticism should be given in a constructive and supportive way and demonstrate well-meaning.

The relationship should also, according to the students, be characterized by an including communication by inviting them to share their experiences, thoughts and opinions, and by appreciating them as valuable and equal staff members.

4. Discussion

This study aimed to explore what bachelor students' in nursing perceived to be important for having good learning experiences in clinical studies. The overall theme that recurred throughout the interview as a red line was that the students perceived that they were in a vulnerable and exposed position. They had to continuously balance their own needs for appropriate learning experiences and respect for the nurses' lack of time to provide as much guidance as they wanted. Being constantly controlled and evaluated made them vulnerable because they wanted to make a positive impression and they were reluctant to take up things that could be perceived negatively. In addition, to find the balance between taking challenges and to express uncertainty in unfamiliar situations made them vulnerable and exposed.

Almost all the informants talked about the importance of having a positive start when they started their studies in a new ward. Experiences from earlier practice periods could vary a lot and influence their expectations and confidence level, but they often felt stressed and a bit anxious before the first meeting. Thus, feeling waited and welcomed, and being met with friendliness from the very beginning, seemed to be decisive for their further motivation and confidence level. In their study, Courtney-Pratt et al. [13] found that students in general felt welcomed, belonging, and accepted in the ward. On the other hand, Sharif and Masoumi [1] describe that the initial phase of clinical placement represented an anxious and stressful phase for the students. They are particularly afraid of making mistakes when performing patient procedures, and for harming the patients because they lack experience and knowledge [1, 14].

The aspect of balancing the appreciation of being included and valued as a staff member and being (mis)used as merely a pair of hands during their clinical studies was another concern mentioned by many of the informants. This balancing act, which can often be difficult, is also outlined in other studies [5, 15]. On one side, students appreciate being valued as a team member [16], but on the other side, they may feel uncomfortable when they are used solely as work force rather than being valued as learners [5]. One factor that made this balancing act even harder was that they would be judged and evaluated. Experiences of being ignored and (mis)used as health care assistants or purely work force is shown to cause a great deal of "emotional labor" for students in clinical settings [4]. On the contrary, the feeling of being seen, heard and valued as individuals as well as students is described as an important prerequisite for experiencing good learning situations [5, 17]. In this sense, facilitating for good learning experiences does not solely rely on the mentor, but it is an organizational matter as well.

Many of the interviewees thought it was an advantage to have two supervisors who supplemented each other. One explanation to this finding may be the problems related to the mentors' absence, leaving the students being without supervision, and feedback, which also in another study is shown to cause frustration and insecurity [8]. On the other hand, studies have also shown that the allocation of students to more than one mentor has been recognized as a stressful factor for the students, and it may result in weakened feelings of belonging [13, 18]. Thus, although a risk for conflicting situations due to the mentors' different attitudes and pedagogical approach, the students may experience a copartner mentorship as favorable. The advantage of having two supervisors with different expertise and experience, and thus complement each other, is also reported by Webb and Shakespeare [4].

Several aspects related to the nurse mentor were described by the informants as crucial for their learning experiences during their clinical studies. One of these aspects was the mentors' motivation for supervising students, which also included that they were prepared and that they had acquired the necessary information about the curricula and the assessment form. The mentors' motivation for supervision is often reflected in their attitudes towards the students, and their willingness to teach them and share their knowledge with them [4, 19]. Although the students were aware of and respected that the nurses' primary duties were related to patient care, they also expected that the supervisors facilitated and allocated time for talks, reflection, and guidance. Good learning experiences in practice are shown to be clearly related to perceiving support, friendliness, and having mentors who stand by in new and stressful practice situations

[3, 4]. The findings also indicate that the students' experiences of negative or bad attitudes from the mentors can result in learning. The consequence of such experiences can be that the students take an opposite stance and they condemn such attitudes when they shall have the supervisor role in the future. In this way, negative experiences may be turned into learning opportunities by deciding how not to act in similar situations [3].

In addition to being supportive and encouraging, the students also emphasized their mentors' professional and pedagogical competences. While the former is well documented in earlier studies [3, 6, 17, 20], the literature focusing on the latter is more infrequent. Webb and Shakespeare [4] who found that well experienced nurses brought a well of knowledge and skills into the mentorship, which provided the students with a lot of learning opportunities. Well experienced and trained nurses may demonstrate nursing practice of eminent quality, be exemplary role models, and facilitate the students' self-confidence when used in appropriate ways. Nurses who are comfortable with their mentor role and possess sufficient educational qualifications may also affect students' learning outcomes in positive ways. The informants in the present study expressed criticism and skepticism to the lack of supervising skills they had experienced from some of the mentors. Problems related to the nurse mentor's lack of appropriate qualifications for supervising students may affect the students' possibility to improve their clinical competences [15]. It may be that the supervisor, for example, lacks the ability and preparation to give relevant and regular feedback [8].

The students put a lot of emphasis on aspects related to the mentor and the mentor-student relationship for experiencing good learning situations, and these aspects have also been documented in former studies [3, 4, 7]. However, the informants in the current study also acknowledged their own responsibility for achieving learning outcomes. This finding is quite interesting, and earlier research focusing on this aspect as a prerequisite for good learning experiences is sparse. The students' responsibility for their own learning in clinical studies is clearly described in the framework for nursing education [21]. In this respect, clarification of their current competences, and what individual learning goals they expect to achieve and how to achieve them, should be presented in the initial phase of the clinical studies. The assessment form and evaluation procedure which are currently used also require that the students continuously make up their mind and evaluate themselves concerning different types of competences. Self-assessment skills in nursing studies are described to be a necessity for competent performance and for developing autonomous and independent practitioners [22]. The informants further described that clarification of their own competence level and learning outcomes related to each practice placement facilitated for appropriate learning activities. Opportunities for further growth are more likely present when the nurse mentors are informed about, and comfortable with, the students' professional starting point, and it may be easier to find the balance between taking challenges and being reticent [7].

The aspect most often described by the informants to be of utmost importance for their development and learning in clinical studies was the quality of the relationship that they had with their supervisors. A relationship characterized by mutual respect, both as individuals and professionals, was highly empathized. Firstly, this respect included the students' recognition of the nurses' pedagogical and professional competences as well as their huge workload. Studies performed among nurse supervisors have reported that shortage of time and insufficient skills were perceived as challenging factors related to supervising students [3, 23]. In the same way, the students wanted the nurses to respect and regard their actual competence level and their individual needs for supervision and guidance as well as their need to take on challenges. Thus, having enough time for feedback and reflections, and having the opportunities to safely practice their skills, are particularly important [4, 11]. This means that the supervisor is attending and supporting when the student is practicing new skills. It also means that the student is challenged and is allowed to take responsibility and perform nursing procedures on their own. When they experience the supervisor's confidence in such situations, the students feel valued, seen, and respected [14].

The fact that they are continuously controlled and assessed in their clinical studies makes the students feel dependent and vulnerable [7]. Therefore, a relationship characterized by an open and inviting atmosphere, where both parties are encouraged to communicate positive as well as negative feedback, should be established. Such relationships can make a difference in how confident they are when it comes to seeking advice and assistance [13]. Terms such as friendly, supportive, welcoming, enthusiastic, and confident have been used to describe the characteristics of a good student-supervisor relationship [13]. Consequently, communication and feedback carried out in a respectful, friendly, and supportive way may result in good learning experiences and growth for the students, even in problematic situations.

5. Study Limitations

In qualitative studies it is not appropriate to make generalizations of the findings. In general, the purpose of qualitative studies is to explore the meaning of individuals' experiences or the nature of phenomena, and a transcribed interview text may be understood and interpreted in various ways. Therefore, the present interpretation should be viewed as one among many possibilities. However, the findings contribute to existing knowledge of what nursing students' perceive as important aspects for good learning experiences in their clinical studies. The interview text provided rich descriptions of the informants' experiences, and variations and similarities in these descriptions were recognized. The study sample was limited and consisted of students in the same class at one university. Despite these limitations, many of the experiences described by the students correspond to findings in other international and national studies.

6. Conclusions

The findings in this study showed that important conditions for nursing students' learning experiences and motivation in their clinical studies included individual, relational, and organizational aspects. Clinical studies constitute a major part of the bachelor program in nursing and, consequently, the quality of these studies is a crucial factor for the students to develop into competent professional nurses. To clarify the students' competence level and learning outcomes, as well as the students' and supervisors' mutual expectations, responsibility, and roles, seems to be decisive for the students' opportunities for personal and professional learning and growth. Feeling welcomed, included, and valued in the ward improves the students' motivation, self-confidence, and self-respect. In addition, the quality of the student-supervisor relationship and the supervisor's pedagogical and professional competences are highly emphasized.

Conflict of Interests

The authors declare that there is no conflict of interests.

References

[1] F. Sharif and S. Masoumi, "A qualitative study of nursing student experiences of clinical practice," *BMC Nursing*, vol. 4, article 6, 2005.

[2] P. A. Chesser-Smyth and T. Long, "Understanding the influences on self-confidence among first-year undergraduate nursing students in Ireland," *Journal of Advanced Nursing*, vol. 69, no. 1, pp. 145–157, 2013.

[3] Z. Wilkes, "The student-mentor relationship: a review of the literature," *Nursing Standard*, vol. 20, no. 37, pp. 42–47, 2006.

[4] C. Webb and P. Shakespeare, "Judgements about mentoring relationships in nurse education," *Nurse Education Today*, vol. 28, no. 5, pp. 563–571, 2008.

[5] C. Bradbury-Jones, S. Sambrook, and F. Irvine, "Empowerment and being valued: a phenomenological study of nursing students' experiences of clinical practice," *Nurse Education Today*, vol. 31, no. 4, pp. 368–372, 2011.

[6] M.-L. Kristofferzon, G. Mårtensson, A.-G. Mamhidir, and A. Löfmark, "Nursing students' perceptions of clinical supervision: the contributios of preceptors, head preceptors and clinical lectures," *Nurse Education Today*, vol. 33, no. 10, pp. 1252–1257, 2012.

[7] G. Haugan, E. Aigeltinger, and V. Sørlie, "The importance of the student nurse relationship to student nurses in clinical hospital praxis," *Sykepleien Forskning*, vol. 7, no. 2, pp. 152–159, 2012 (Norwegian).

[8] M. P. Clynes and S. E. C. Raftery, "Feedback: an essential element of student learning in clinical practice," *Nordic Nurse Education in Practice*, vol. 8, no. 6, pp. 405–411, 2008.

[9] A.-M. Skovgaard, "Dialogue and reflection between student nurses and their instructor in clinical practice," *Journal of Nursing Research*, vol. 24, no. 1, pp. 45–46, 2004.

[10] D. F. Polit and C. T. Beck, *Essentials of Nursing Research: Appraising Evidence for Nursing Practice*, Lippincott Williams & Wilkins, Philadelphia, Pa, USA, 7th edition, 2010.

[11] U. H. Graneheim and B. Lundman, "Qualitative content analysis in nursing research: concepts, procedures and measures to achieve trustworthiness," *Nurse Education Today*, vol. 24, no. 2, pp. 105–112, 2004.

[12] T. L. Beauchamp and J. F. Childress, *Principles of Biomedical Ethics*, Oxford University Press, New York, NY, USA, 6th edition, 2009.

[13] H. Courtney-Pratt, M. Fitzgerald, K. Ford, K. Marsden, and A. Marlow, "Quality clinical placements for undergraduate nursing students: a cross-sectional survey of undergraduates and supervising nurses," *Journal of Advanced Nursing*, vol. 68, no. 6, pp. 1380–1390, 2012.

[14] A. Löfmark and K. Wikblad, "Facilitating and obstructing factors for development of learning in clinical practice: a student perspective," *Journal of Advanced Nursing*, vol. 34, no. 1, pp. 43–50, 2001.

[15] N. B. D. Magobe, S. Beukes, and A. Müller, "Reasons for students' poor clinical competencies in the primary health care: clinical nursing, diagnosis treatment and care programme," *Journal of Interdisciplinary Health Sciences*, vol. 15, no. 1, pp. 181–186, 2010.

[16] A. James and Y. Chapman, "Preceptors and patients—the power of two: nursing student experiences on their first acute clinical placement," *Contemporary Nurse*, vol. 34, no. 1, pp. 34–47, 2009-2010.

[17] K. Haddeland and U. Söderhamn, "Nursing students' experiences of nurse-lead supervision in hospital practice. A phenomenological study," *Nordic Nursing Research*, vol. 3, no. 1, pp. 19–33, 2013 (Norwegian).

[18] M. Myall, T. Levett-Jones, and J. Lathlean, "Mentorship in contemporary practice: the experiences of nursing students and practice mentors," *Journal of Clinical Nursing*, vol. 17, no. 14, pp. 1834–1842, 2008.

[19] F. L. Luhanga, D. Billay, Q. Grundy, F. Myrick, and O. Yonge, "The one-to-one relationship: is it really key to an effective preceptorship experience? A review of the literature," *International Journal of Nursing Education Scholarship*, vol. 7, no. 1, article 21, 2010.

[20] C. L. Clarke, C. E. Gibb, and V. Ramprogus, "Clinical learning environments: an evaluation of an innovative role to support preregistration nursing placements," *Learning in Health and Social Care*, vol. 2, no. 2, pp. 105–115, 2003.

[21] Ministry of Education Research, *Norwegian Framework for Nursing Education*, 2008.

[22] A. Lofmark and I. Thorell-Ekstrand, "Evaluation by nurses and students of a new assessment form for clinical nursing education," *Scandinavian Journal of Caring Sciences*, vol. 14, no. 2, pp. 89–96, 2000.

[23] M. Bengtsson, J. Kvarnhäll, and P. Svedberg, "Swedish nurses' experiences of the process of supervising in clinical practice of nursing students," *Nordic Journal of Nursing Research*, vol. 31, no. 1, pp. 47–51, 2011 (Swedish).

13

Implementation Interventions Used in Nursing Homes and Hospitals: A Descriptive, Comparative Study between Austria, Germany, and The Netherlands

Helga E. Breimaier,[1] Ruud J. G. Halfens,[2] Doris Wilborn,[3] Esther Meesterberends,[2] Gunnar Haase Nielsen,[4] and Christa Lohrmann[1]

[1] *Institute of Nursing Science, Medical University of Graz, Billrothgaße 6, 8010 Graz, Austria*
[2] *Department of Health Services Research Focusing on Chronic Care and Ageing, Section of Nursing Science, Maastricht University, P.O. Box 616, 6200 MD Maastricht, The Netherlands*
[3] *Department of Nursing and Management, Faculty of Business & Social Sciences, Hamburg University of Applied Sciences, Alexanderstraße 1, 20099 Hamburg, Germany*
[4] *Department of Nursing and Health Sciences, Protestant University of Applied Sciences, Zweifalltorweg 12, 64293 Darmstadt, Germany*

Correspondence should be addressed to Helga E. Breimaier; helga.breimaier@medunigraz.at

Academic Editors: K. Clark, A. Green, B. Mandleco, K. G. Schepp, and D. Whitehead

Translating guidelines into nursing practice remains a considerable challenge. Until now, little attention has been paid to which interventions are used in practice to implement guidelines on changing clinical nursing practice. This cross-sectional study determined the current ranges and rates of implementation-related interventions in Austria, Germany, and The Netherlands and explored possible differences between these countries. An online questionnaire based on the conceptual framework of implementation interventions (professional, organizational, financial, and regulatory) from the Cochrane Effective Practice and Organization of Care (EPOC) data collection checklist was used to gather data from nursing homes and hospitals. Provision of written materials is the most frequently used professional implementation intervention (85%), whereas changes in the patient record system rank foremost among organisational interventions (78%). Financial incentives for nurses are rarely used. More interventions were used in Austria and Germany than in The Netherlands (20.3/20.2/17.3). Professional interventions are used more frequently in Germany and financial interventions more frequently in The Netherlands. Implementation efforts focus mainly on professional and organisational interventions. Nurse managers and other responsible personnel should direct their focus to a broader array of implementation interventions using the four different categories of EPOC's conceptual framework.

1. Introduction

Nurses are expected to deliver care that is regularly updated with research findings, and the volume of new scientific evidence for good clinical practice is growing quickly. This research-based knowledge should be used, for example, as a basis for decision making [1] and for providing evidence-based care to promote positive patient outcomes [2, 3]. Legal regulations commit governments to providing their citizens with healthcare based on the acknowledged state of scientific knowledge; for example, in Austria, there is the Health Care Quality Act (Section 3) [4]. Regulations also require nurses to update their knowledge and skills according to the latest scientific findings in nursing science. In Austria, this is governed by the Nursing Act (Section 4, paragraphs 1 and 2) [5]. However, numerous studies over the past decade have highlighted a failure to routinely translate research findings into daily practice [6–11]. A large gap between what is known from research and what happens in practice still exists [10, 12], and introducing change is far from straightforward [13]. As a consequence of this theory-practice gap, patients may suffer unnecessarily from inconveniences such as pain, pressure ulcers, and/or prolonged hospitalization [11, 14].

Much effort has been undertaken to implement new knowledge to change nursing practice. Clinical practice guidelines are seen as one means by which new knowledge can be instilled in practice [15] in order to change the process and the outcome of care provided by allied medical professionals [16]. However, knowledge distillation and the publication of research findings or guidelines do not ensure that practitioners will use them in their daily clinical practice [17, 18]. Translating research into healthcare decision making and practice remains a considerable challenge [19]. There are several reasons why research results are not implemented successfully in clinical practice, including, for example, characteristics of innovations [20], insufficient education/information, or inadequate organisational support [21]. Over the past decade, a growing number of articles have discussed interventions that implement new knowledge in healthcare [22–26]. This is especially true for medical but also, to an increasing extent, for nursing care. These articles show, among other things, why the effectiveness of implementation interventions varies in healthcare [27–30]. Alanen et al. revealed, for example, that the method of implementing a hypertension guideline in Finnish health centres varied widely. Health centres categorized as implementers used multiple strategies to promote the adoption of the guideline. Health centres categorised as disseminators did little to facilitate their adoption [31]. Earlier research disclosed that methods utilized to implement guidelines in primary healthcare were usually directive and passive [32]. According to Kortteisto et al., profession also has an effect on the intention to use clinical guidelines in patient care, and the authors recommended the use of different strategies when clinical guidelines are targeted at different professional groups [33].

There is a broad array of implementation interventions from which nurse managers, for example, may choose to implement new knowledge in their respective practical fields. The Cochrane Effective Practice and Organisation of Care Review Group compiled a checklist with a short description of each intervention, which was then grouped into four non-mutually exclusive categories: professional interventions (e.g., distribution of educational materials), organisational interventions (e.g., changes in medical records systems), financial interventions (e.g., fee-for-service), and regulatory interventions (e.g., changes in medical liability) [34, 35]. These implementation interventions are thought to facilitate the use of known knowledge and help to overcome barriers to its adoption in clinical settings [34]. In a systematic review, Medves et al. focussed on dissemination and implementation strategies of practice guidelines for healthcare teams and team-based practice. They identified 88 relevant studies that investigated 16 dissemination and implementation strategies. Four of these strategies are ranked as organisational interventions, one as patient-oriented, and one as structural interventions. Ten of these strategies were aimed at healthcare professionals and included the distribution of educational materials and educational meetings as the most common strategies [36]. In an explorative study, Meesterberends et al. found that interventions used in disseminating pressure-ulcer guidelines in nursing homes of six European countries differed in terms of number (2–4) and type. The most common implementation interventions were the use of the Internet and the presentation of the guideline at national or regional seminars or congresses [37]. According to the typology of EPOC, both interventions belong to the category of professional interventions [35]. However, the evidence supporting the use of the electronic retrieval of healthcare information (including the internet) by healthcare providers to improve practice and patient care was found to be insufficient [38]. Furthermore, attendance at seminars or congresses is a passive educational approach which is considered a less effective implementation intervention [39].

This indicates that interventions used are not in line with existing evidence regarding implementation and may be one of the reasons why innovations are not implemented sustainably. To resolve this inconsistency, the effectiveness of implementation interventions aimed at instilling new knowledge into nursing practice must be understood. To this end, this study sets out to discover which implementation strategies are actually used in nursing practice and whether the most frequently used implementation strategies are indeed effective ones. This can help nurse managers to find the best methods for implementing new knowledge and/or guidelines. To date, however, only little is known about which interventions are actively used to implement guidelines in nursing—be it in hospitals or in nursing homes.

To shed more light on this issue, an international research group from Austria, Germany and The Netherlands set itself the objective of (1) determining the current range and rates of the interventions used for implementation purposes regarding guidelines in nursing in these countries and (2) exploring whether there are any differences in the interventions employed between the three countries. For this purpose, four care problems were chosen on an exemplary basis—discharge management (in hospitals), urinary incontinence (in nursing homes), and malnutrition and pressure ulcers (in both settings)—as these are among the more common care problems in hospitals and nursing homes [40–42].

2. Methods

2.1. Design. Using a cross-sectional design, data were gathered from nursing homes and hospitals in Austria (A), Germany (D), and The Netherlands (NL).

2.2. Sample. Austrian, German, and Dutch hospitals and nursing homes were invited to participate in the study via email. In Austria, all nursing homes (692) and hospitals (268) nationwide were asked to participate. In Germany, for purposes of convenience, the survey was limited to the two federal states of Berlin and Hesse but included all nursing homes (Berlin: 228 and Hesse: 908) and hospitals (47 and 166, resp.). In The Netherlands, all 210 nursing homes and 70 hospitals which participated in the yearly National Prevalence Measurement of Care Problems (Landelijke Prevalentiemeting Zorgproblemen, LPZ) were invited to participate.

The ethical principles of good scientific practice according to the Declaration of Helsinki [43] were observed throughout the entire research process. In a cover letter, participating institutions were informed about the study. Anonymity and confidentiality were assured, and voluntary participation was guaranteed. Contact information for further questions was made available for all three institutions carrying out this project. Approval for filling out the questionnaire was given by the participating institutions. Consent was assumed on the basis of a returned and completed questionnaire.

2.3. Procedure and Data Collection. The management and nursing directors of nursing homes and hospitals received an email notification about the intention to investigate interventions used to implement guidelines in nursing practice. The contact details of the institutions in Austria were acquired through an extensive internet search and from lists of nursing homes published by the Federal Ministry of Labour, Social Affairs and Consumer Protection. Contact details in Germany were acquired from lists published by the Ministry of Health, by the Public Inspecting Authorities for Nursing Homes of Hesse, and by searching the internet. In The Netherlands, all participants of the National Prevalence Measurement of Care Problems (LPZ) [41] were contacted. Two weeks later, all managers and nursing directors received detailed information about the purpose of the proposed study, the researchers' intention to disseminate the results, the data collection procedure, the return of the questionnaire, and the time requirements (45 minutes) for completing the questionnaire. A link to the online questionnaire was attached. The email contact and collection of the completed questionnaires were carried out by an external organisation (Flycatcher, Internet Research, Maastricht). Two reminders were sent to all managers and nursing directors, and the deadline was extended twice to increase the response rate. After completing the data collection, the anonymized final data file was forwarded to authors 1, 2, and 3 for analysis. Thus, anonymity was ensured for all participants. The managers and nursing directors were asked to forward the questionnaire to the nurse responsible for implementing guidelines in their institution and to return it by June 2008.

2.3.1. Instrument. For comparison purposes, the modified typology of implementation interventions of the Cochrane Effective Practice and Organisation of Care (EPOC) Review Group [34, 35] was used for this study. The questionnaire included a total of four sets of questions based on the conceptual framework of four implementation interventions, namely, professional interventions, organisational interventions, financial interventions, and regulatory interventions [34, 35]. For each category of intervention, single interventions varying from bottom-up approaches (through participation) to top-down approaches (through instructions) were presented. Each intervention could be answered with *yes, no,* or *I do not know.* All questions were asked in relation to specific clinical domains. They were chosen on the basis of their prevalence in the three countries and the specific setting. In nursing homes, all questions relating to prevention of pressure ulcers, urinary incontinence, and malnutrition were asked. In hospitals, the clinical domain of *urinary incontinence* is less prevalent [44, 45] and was arbitrarily replaced by *discharge management*; its importance for hospitals has been pointed out previously [46–48]. The questionnaire consisted of 22 pages all together.

2.3.2. Translation. The intervention part of the English EPOC-Checklist [35] was translated into German by authors 3, 5, and 6. Based on this translation, a German version of the instrument, addressing implementation issues of particular concern to nursing, was developed. This version was revised for Austria in order to take into account the localized nuances of Austrian German. In The Netherlands, the intervention part of the English EPOC-Checklist [35] was translated into Dutch by authors 2 and 4. The Dutch version was then translated into German by a professional translator. Both German versions were cross-checked, and unclear items were discussed within the research group.

2.3.3. Content Validation. The questionnaire was developed by the researchers, and a content validation procedure was performed in all three countries. Three experts in the field (nursing and medicine) from each country were asked to indicate whether the included items were relevant to implementation issues in hospitals and nursing homes. Possible answers ranged from agree completely, partly agree/partly disagree, to disagree completely. The instrument was amended using the feedback from the content validation procedure. In this course, the existence of nursing guidelines and expert standards was highlighted in the questionnaire, and some items concerning financial interventions were modified or removed completely.

2.3.4. Pretest. After the process of content validation, an electronic web-based version of the questionnaire was developed. The questionnaire was piloted in three institutions per country to ensure that it was practical as well as easy to understand and read. The comments received were used to write the final electronic version of the questionnaire.

2.4. Analysis. Data were analyzed with SPSS 17.0. The percentage of each intervention was calculated by adding the answers of both the settings and the three care problems per intervention and dividing the result by the total number of institutions and then by three (care problems). The mean total number of each individual category of interventions and of the total interventions per setting and per care problem was calculated by adding the percentages of the respective individual items and dividing the result by 100. Next, the mean number of interventions of each category of intervention was calculated for each clinical domain and country. Differences between the three countries regarding the implementation interventions used were tested separately for each setting with one-way ANOVA. Due to the numerous tests, a P value of 0.01 was used for significance. The basis for the analysis was the net-response rates with $N_{\text{total}} = 333$.

3. Results

The response rates varied from 12.8% to 55.7%. In all countries, the response rate of hospitals was higher than nursing homes (between 8.3% and 28.6%). However, not all questionnaires were fully completed, so the net response of completed questionnaires (n = 333) was lower (8.7%–47.1%).

3.1. Implementation Interventions. In the three countries, various interventions were used during implementation, with a mean total of 19.6 interventions per setting per care problem. An overview of the interventions is shown in Table 1. The percentages presented are mean percentages calculated over the three care problems and over the institutions, which means that, for example, in Austria, professional internal written materials are used in 90% of the cases when implementing a guideline. The most frequently used implementation intervention is from the category of professional interventions, namely, providing written materials. On average this is used in 85% of cases. Other commonly used professional interventions (63%–66%) are internal consultations, internal audits and internal lectures. The organisational interventions used mostly (65%–78%) are changes in the patient record system, individual patient participation in treatment decisions, efforts to increase nurses' work satisfaction, regular use of assessment instruments, changes in structure and facilities of the institution, and management of patient complaints.

External electronic training and *the use of telemedicine* are the professional and organisational interventions which are least used (≤12%). Financial interventions for nurses are rarely used (10%), while an average of 1.3 regulatory interventions is used per setting per care problem.

3.2. Implementation Interventions per Country. When looking at the mean total of interventions used per country, it becomes apparent that settings in Austria and Germany used slightly more interventions than those in The Netherlands (resp., 20.3, 20.2, and 17.3; P = 0.007) (Table 1). This is also true for the mean total of professional (A: 10.6, D: 10.3, NL: 8.2; $P < 0.001$) and organisational (A: 8.5, D: 8.3, NL: 7.0; P = 0.004) interventions. Regulatory interventions are, however, used less in Austria (A: 1.0, D: 1.4, NL: 1.5; P = 0.001).

The most frequently used professional interventions with significant differences between the countries are *internal audits, internal lectures, regular team meetings about a clinical topic, local opinion leaders*, and *written/manual reminders* (Table 1). *Internal written materials, internal consultations* and *external lectures* are used less in The Netherlands. The least frequently used professional intervention with a significant difference is *external conferences*. With regard to organisational interventions, the results show differences between the *regular use of assessment instruments, efforts to improve nurses' work satisfaction, case management, changes in right to access documentation*, and *changes in number of staff*. Compared to Austria and Germany, *financial incentives* for nurses are used more frequently in The Netherlands. Within the regulatory interventions, *inspecting authorities* and *insurance-related regulations* differ significantly (Table 1).

The use of *internal written materials* ranks among the most frequently used professional interventions in all three countries, followed by *internal audits* and *internal lectures* in Germany, and *internal consultations, external conferences* as well as *internal audits* and *internal lectures* in Austria. In The Netherlands, the use of *internal written materials* is preceded by *regular team meetings about a clinical topic* and *manual reminders*. The three countries differ regarding the rank order of the most frequently used organisational interventions: in Austria these are *efforts to increase nurses' work satisfaction, changes in patient record systems* and *individual patient participation in treatment decisions*. In Germany the *regular use of assessment instruments* ranks first, whereas in The Netherlands *additional staff qualifications* is the third most frequent organisational intervention. The most often used regulatory intervention in Austria and The Netherlands is *inspecting authorities*, whereas in Germany *insurance-related regulations* is used most often (Table 1). An overview of the five most frequently used implementation interventions per country is provided in Table 2. In Austria and Germany, these are two professional and three organisational interventions. In The Netherlands, these are one regulatory, two professional, and two organisational interventions.

3.3. Implementation Interventions per Care Problem and Clinical Setting. These results are presented for each individual category of intervention.

3.3.1. Professional Interventions. The number of professional interventions used in nursing homes and hospitals does not differ between the countries regarding the care problems of *pressure ulcers* and *malnutrition* (Table 3). However, there are significant differences regarding the care problems of *incontinence* in nursing homes and *discharge management* in hospitals. In both cases, the number of professional interventions is less in The Netherlands. Regarding *incontinence*, an average of 7.4 professional interventions was used to implement guidelines in Dutch nursing homes compared to 10.9 in Austria and 10.1 in Germany (P = 0.001). In terms of *discharge management*, an average of 2.1 professional interventions was used to implement guidelines in hospitals in The Netherlands compared to 9.6 in Austria and 9.3 in Germany ($P < 0.001$).

3.3.2. Organisational Interventions. The evaluation of the organisational interventions yields a similar picture regarding differences between the settings and care problems in the three countries (Table 3). Regarding *incontinence*, an average of 6.3 organisational interventions were used to implement guidelines in Dutch nursing homes compared to 8.6 in Austria and 8.1 in Germany (P = 0.003). Regarding *discharge management*, an average of 3.2 organisational interventions was used to implement guidelines in hospitals in The Netherlands compared to 8.2 in Austria and 7.9 in Germany ($P < 0.001$).

3.3.3. Financial Intervention. Financial incentives for the implementation of guidelines regarding care problems are

Table 1: Percentage of implementation interventions used per setting per care problem in Austria, Germany and the Netherlands.

	Total%	Austria%	Germany%	The Netherlands%	*F*-values*	*P*
(1) Professional interventions (22 items)						
Internal written materials	85	90	90	67	22.584	<.001
Internal consultations	66	71	71	47	13.433	<.001
Internal audits	65	62	80	43	22.050	<.001
Internal lectures	63	62	73	45	13.896	<.001
Regular team meetings about a clinical topic	58	51	55	74	7.026	.001
External lectures	56	63	64	31	19.055	<.001
Local opinion leaders	55	70	58	21	33.755	<.001
Written/manual reminders	52	54	42	68	8.206	<.001
Patient- and relative-mediated interventions	50	56	51	36	6.109	.002
Internal electronic materials	49	56	47	39	3.388	.035
External conferences	49	69	47	19	36.794	<.001
Internal workshops	46	44	46	48	.184	.832
External consultations	43	51	41	33	5.137	.006
External audits	42	34	52	39	5.562	.004
Computerised reminders	42	51	42	28	6.082	.003
External workshops	39	45	39	31	3.423	.034
Supervision	36	35	33	44	1.605	.202
Internal training sessions	35	30	37	39	2.045	.131
External training sessions	28	34	23	25	3.022	.050
Other internal interventions	16	13	17	21	1.262	.284
External electronic training	12	13	14	7	1.121	.327
Other external interventions	7	3	8	12	4.264	.015
Mean total number of professional interventions	*9.7*	*10.6*	*10.3*	*8.2*	*10.430*	*<.001*
(2) Organisational interventions (19 items)						
Changes in patient record systems	78	78	82	69	3.781	.024
Individual patient participation in treatment decisions	74	77	75	65	2.889	.057
Efforts to improve nurses' work satisfaction	70	82	78	34	41.201	<.001
Regular use of assessment instruments	67	54	84	58	30.744	<.001
Changes in structure and facilities of institution	66	70	68	56	3.806	.023
Management of patient complaints	65	66	70	56	2.314	.101
Additional staff qualifications	58	58	56	62	.458	.633
Changes in size and type of services of the institution	56	60	59	42	5.161	.006
Multidisciplinary teams to support nursing	52	53	47	57	1.354	.260
Changes in professional responsibilities	49	55	50	39	3.626	.028
Case management	41	40	34	57	6.754	.001
Changing the right to access documentation	38	48	38	19	9.656	<.001
Changes in number of staff	26	36	24	13	7.924	<.001
Changes in composition of staff	16	19	13	14	1.176	.310
Participation of patient groups	14	18	12	9	2.304	.101
Use of telemedicine	11	15	8	11	1.449	.236
Other patient interventions	10	9	10	12	.144	.866
Other structural changes	9	6	7	17	5.713	.004
Other personal changes	9	6	10	12	1.251	.288
Mean total number of organisational interventions	*8.1*	*8.5*	*8.3*	*7.0*	*5.595*	*.004*
(3) Financial intervention (1 item)						
Availability of financial incentives for nurses	10	7	8	21	8.070	<.001
(4) Regulatory interventions (4 items)						
Inspecting authorities	46	37	42	69	12.872	<.001
Insurance companies	34	25	45	31	7.473	.001
Law	33	28	40	27	3.093	.047
Other regulatory interventions	12	7	13	19	3.708	.026
Mean total number of regulatory interventions	*1.3*	*1.0*	*1.4*	*1.5*	*6.975*	*.001*
Mean total number of interventions used	**19.6**	**20.3**	**20.2**	**17.3**	**5.024**	**.007**

*df = 2, 330.

TABLE 2: Overview of the five most used implementation interventions per country.

Austria	Germany	The Netherlands
Internal written materials (professional intervention)	Internal written materials (professional intervention)	Regular team meetings about a clinical topic (professional intervention)
Efforts to increase nurses' work satisfaction (organisational interventions)	Regular use of assessment instruments (organisational interventions)	Changes in patient record systems (organisational interventions)
Changes in patient record systems (organisational interventions)	Changes in patient record systems (organisational interventions)	Inspecting authorities (regulatory interventions)
Individual patient participation in treatment decisions (organisational interventions)	Internal audits (professional intervention)	Written/manual reminders (professional intervention)
Internal consultations (professional intervention)	Efforts to increase nurses' work satisfaction (organisational interventions)	Internal written materials (professional intervention)

TABLE 3: Mean number of professional, organisational, financial and regulatory implementation interventions.

	Professional interventions (n = 22)		Organisational interventions (n = 19)		Financial intervention (n = 1)		Regulatory interventions (n = 4)	
	Nursing homes	Hospitals	Nursing homes	Hospitals	Nursing homes	Hospitals	Nursing homes	Hospitals
Pressure ulcers								
Austria	11.0	12.1	9.0	9.5	6.5%	8.0%	1.2	.8
Germany	10.9	13.2	8.8	9.7	7.1%	20.0%	1.5	1.3
The Netherlands	11.6	11.6	9.0	9.6	28.2%	39.4%	1.9	1.6
F-values*	.412	1.231	.122	.046	8.122	6.568	5.438	4.493
P-values	.663	.296	.885	.995	<.001	.002	.005	.013
Malnutrition								
Austria	10.3	9.1	8.3	7.5	6.5%	6.0%	1.0	.6
Germany	10.3	7.3	8.4	5.6	3.0%	11.4%	1.6	.7
The Netherlands	8.3	7.5	7.2	6.6	12.8%	27.3%	1.8	1.1
F-values*	3.876	1.533	2.022	1.887	2.401	4.108	9.820	2.819
P-values	.022	.220	.135	.156	.093	.019	<.001	.064
Incontinence								
Austria	10.9	—	8.6	—	6.5%	—	1.1	—
Germany	10.1	—	8.1	—	5.1%	—	1.5	—
The Netherlands	7.4	—	6.3	—	17.9%	—	1.6	—
F-values*	9.042		6.022		3.421		3.347	
P-values	<.001	—	.003	—	.035	—	.037	—
Discharge management								
Austria	—	9.6	—	8.2	—	6.0%	—	1.0
Germany	—	9.3	—	7.9	—	20.0%	—	1.0
The Netherlands	—	2.1	—	3.2	—	3.0%	—	.6
F-values*		33.352		16.124		3.582		1.957
P-values	—	<.001	—	<.001	—	.031	—	.146
Mean								
Austria	10.7	10.3	8.6	8.4	6.1%	6.7%	1.1	0.8
Germany	10.4	10.0	8.4	7.8	5.1%	17.1%	1.5	1.0
The Netherlands	9.1	7.1	7.5	6.4	19.7%	23.2%	1.8	1.1
F-values*	2.697	7.832	1.898	3.258	5.576	3.288	6.202	1.045
P-values	.070	.001	.152	.042	.004	0.041	.002	.355

*df (nursing homes) = 2, 212; df (hospitals) = 2, 115.

available in only a few organizations (Table 3). In Dutch nursing homes they are used in total significantly more often (19.7%) than in Austrian (6.1%) and German (5.1%; P = 0.004) ones. This also holds true for the care problem of *pressure ulcers* (28.2%/6.5%/7.1%; $P < 0.001$). In hospitals, financial interventions are used less in Austria (6.7%) compared to Germany (17.0%) and The Netherlands (23.3%; $P = 0.004$) with the exception of *discharge management* ($P = 0.041$).

3.3.4. Regulatory Interventions. The mean number of regulatory interventions is significantly lower in Austrian nursing homes (1.1) than in German (1.5) and Dutch ones (1.8; P = 0.002) (Table 3). The same is true for the individual care problem of *pressure ulcers* (1.2/1.5/1.9; $P < 0.005$) and *malnutrition* (1.0/1.6/1.8; $P < 0.001$). There is no significant difference between hospitals in the three countries, neither in total nor for the individual care problems.

4. Discussion

Until now, "studies on the implementation of evidence based practice in nursing care make a very small contribution to the overall evidence on effective implementation" [49, p. 1163]. This study sought to gain an insight into ranges and rates of interventions used to implement nursing guidelines in Austria, Germany, and The Netherlands.

4.1. Ranges and Rates of Implementation Interventions. The results describing implementation interventions revealed that, on average, a broad array of implementation interventions was used. The most frequent ones were found within professional and organisational strategies. Financial and regulatory interventions were rarely used. This is in line with findings from the literature [37, 50] and, although indirectly, comparable with findings of a systematic review about the effectiveness of the dissemination and implementation interventions of practice guidelines for (multidisciplinary) healthcare teams. In this review, Medves et al. revealed that of the 16 interventions (classified according to the EPOC taxonomy), ten were professional and five were organisational/structural interventions [36]. Robertson and Jochelson conclude from their review that there is less research into organisational-level interventions than those targeted at individuals [51].

Among the five most frequently used interventions, the distribution of *written materials* as a professional intervention ranks first. This may be due to the advantage that printed educational materials can be distributed relatively cheaply and easily to a large number of professionals. Furthermore, its dissemination aims at improving the awareness, knowledge, attitudes, skills, and professional practice of nurses as well as patient outcomes [52]. This intervention is also among the five most frequently used interventions of a study investigating described implementation strategies in published abstracts [50], and it is the most commonly investigated one [36]. Although the majority of reviewed studies reported significant findings, it was not possible to attribute this intervention to the described effect. Grimshaw et al. concluded from their review that the distribution of written materials is a less effective method and that the addition of educational materials to other interventions did not seem to increase effectiveness [27]. This is supported by Farmer et al., who found a slightly beneficial effect on process outcomes but not on patient outcomes [52].

Four organisational interventions are ranked next: *changes in the patient record system, individual patient participation in treatment decisions, efforts to increase nurses' work satisfaction, and regular use of assessment instruments.* These measures do not force nurses to actively react to recommendations of an implemented guideline. Nonetheless, these measures seem to be a necessary basis which makes their use possible, in that, for example, it should be possible to record recommended care once it is carried out. Work satisfaction, which is associated with autonomy, good collaboration between nurses and physicians along with reduced job stress [53], was found to be an important individual characteristic of research utilization [54]. Out of these four most often used organisational interventions, *changes in the patient record system* was the only one included in Medves et al.'s work [36]. No conclusions could be drawn as to their effectiveness. In a former systematic review, however, Urquhart et al. found some limited evidence of effects on practice attributable to changes in nursing record systems [55]. A systematic review of reviews about organisational interventions found limited evidence in organisational interventions. None of the interventions produced consistent effects [56].

Additional frequently used interventions directed to professionals include *internal consultations, internal audits* and *internal lectures.* In these internally directed interventions, nursing managers may see a possible advantage in tailoring the specific content to the necessities of the respective setting in which they are delivered and/or a cost effective intervention possibility to introduce change. Often, audits are found to be investigated together with feedback as an implementation intervention. In general, their effect is consistently described as small to moderate for health practitioners [27, 28, 51, 57–60], yet not mandatory [61], and their effect could be increased where baseline adherence to recommended practice is low and when feedback is delivered more intensively [28]. An investigation by Dulko et al. in acute nursing care also showed their effectiveness [25].

Internal lectures are part of educational interventions which are usually regarded to be of limited [62] or no effect when used as a single intervention [39, 51, 57]. Simpson and Doig unexpectedly found that in-servicing (didactic lectures) was ranked highly, that is, as an effective practice change intervention, by participants [63]. In general, it can be said that educational meetings which include courses, conferences, lectures, workshops, seminars, and symposia can have a small effect on improving professional practice and healthcare outcomes [27, 39]; however, interactive educational strategies such as small-scale interactive meetings and workshops appear to be more successful in changing practice [51] and were consistently reported as effective [57, 64]. Yet, workshops, on average, were offered in less than half of the participating settings. Studies which reveal the effects of different educational implementation interventions showed only modest or moderate effects on processes or outcomes of care [27, 29, 39].

In general, financial and regulatory interventions were rarely used. Financial interventions, especially *financial incentives*, are seldom used to implement innovations in hospitals and nursing homes. The industrial sector, on the other hand, makes widespread use of financial incentives to encourage employees to achieve certain goals in their individual fields of responsibility. In the healthcare sector, however, this seems to be a rare measure to foster and implement quality improvement policies—at least in nursing. Actually, the use of financial incentives seems almost impossible considering that a separate budget for innovation implementation, which might be used for providing financial incentives, is very rare in the healthcare sector [16, 37]. Nevertheless, the effect of financial incentives was found to be inconclusive and provided no evidence that the magnitude of the incentive influenced compliance [57]. Flodgren et al. concluded that financial incentives may be effective in changing healthcare professional practice but not in improving patient outcomes [65]. Based on sparse observational studies found regarding regulatory interventions, Robertson and Jochelson summarized that regulation is associated with improvements in healthcare quality [51].

4.2. Comparison between the Three Countries. A count of the amount of implementation interventions shows that more interventions were used in Austria and Germany than in The Netherlands. However, when evaluating implementation interventions, limiting the perspective to mere numbers is not necessarily useful. Studies have revealed no relationship between the number of component interventions and the effects of multifaceted interventions on improvements in care [27]. It is still not clear how many and which combination of strategies are required to be successful [36].

For this reason, the authors of this study have focused their evaluation on the most common implementation interventions. In Austria and Germany, the five implementation interventions used most frequently are part of professional and organisational interventions with a ratio of 2 : 3. In The Netherlands they are part of professional, organizational, and regulatory interventions with a ratio of 3 : 1 : 1. The configuration of the used categories of implementation interventions shows a broader approach of implementation interventions in Dutch nursing homes and hospitals than in Germany and Austria. Moreover, in The Netherlands, interventions are also used which seem to focus on the ward-level, such *as regular team meetings about a clinical topic* and *written/manual reminders*, in addition to interventions applied on an institutional level. This might address nurses more directly and force them to react in a short time frame. According to Prior et al., the use of reminders consistently resulted in significant practical improvements, and computer-delivered reminders had a slightly greater effect than manual- or paper-based reminders [57]. Furthermore, in all but one of the five most used interventions per country, there was a significant difference between the countries. This exception is *individual patient participation in treatment decisions*, although ranked differently in the top-five list. Robertson and Jochelson found some evidence that providing educational materials to patients can help in the implementation of guidelines [51]. *Inspecting authorities* was among the five most used interventions in Dutch settings and is significantly more applied there than in Austrian and German settings. Inspection in its function of external oversight refers to surveillance and enforcement to ensure minimum standards are met [51]. The differences between the countries regarding these top-five interventions might be due to a higher awareness of the relevance of the process and steps of implementation in Dutch hospitals and nursing homes than in German and Austrian settings because of the longer history of nursing science in The Netherlands. Furthermore, The Netherlands started to develop national guidelines, for example, for pressure-ulcer prevention and treatment, as early as 1985 [66], whereas, in Germany, this process was started in 1999 with the development of *expert standards* (a type of guideline) [67], and education as the recommended implementation intervention [68]. In Austria, there exists no equivalent institution on a national level which is responsible for the development of national guidelines for relevant care problems in nursing. The difference regarding *inspecting authorities* might be due to the fact that, in The Netherlands, the Health Care Inspectorate regularly controls whether healthcare institutions meet their standards. Dutch healthcare settings are obliged to collect data about the so-called "norms of safe care", for example, in the form of the annual prevalence survey, which was launched in 1998 [69].

4.3. Implementation Interventions per Care Problem. With regard to the amount of used professional and organisational interventions, no differences were found for *pressure ulcers* and *malnutrition* in the three countries. A possible explanation may be that these problems occur to a similar extent and that the amount of intervention reflects the magnitude of the care problems. This applies to malnutrition where prevalence rates are similarly high in nursing homes and hospitals: 25.7%/25.1% (A), 20.2%/22.8% (NL), and 23.0% in German nursing homes. In contrast, the prevalence rates of pressure ulcers are found to be highest in Dutch hospitals (10.2%) and lowest in German nursing homes (4.0%) [45]. In the field of incontinence care in nursing homes and discharge management in hospitals, there was a remarkably lower amount of professional and organisational implementation interventions in The Netherlands. It might be that these topics are regarded as less essential in Dutch nursing care. *Pressure ulcers*, *malnutrition*, and *incontinence* seem to be equally important areas in nursing care in Austria and Germany, and this might be due to their epidemiological relevance. Furthermore, since 2008 it has been mandatory for German nursing homes to implement what are known as *expert standards* [70], a kind of guideline focusing, among other things, on these care problems. Therefore, the high number of implementation interventions used in relation to those problems seems reasonable. Financial and regulatory interventions do not seem to play an important role regarding specific care problems, although they are used more frequently in The Netherlands relating to *pressure ulcers*.

Finally one should consider that the majority of the cited literature did not focus on the nursing profession but on healthcare professionals and medical doctors. Yet, interventions to implement guidelines should be tailored to different groups of stakeholders [15]. For this reason we should know the effectiveness of the used interventions.

4.4. Limitations. The results of this study might be limited due to low response rates—especially from nursing homes, which made comparison between hospitals and nursing homes difficult. Although low response rates are rather common nowadays [71, 72], several aspects could have had a negative influence, such as the use of a web-based questionnaire. Even though the questionnaire was developed in a very user-friendly way and tested for applicability, it could have been a problem for some respondents to fill in a web-based questionnaire. Also, the persons contacted might have considered the completion time for this task to be too long. Proposed participants were, however, notified beforehand of the forthcoming study. One further reason for low response rates may be that the questionnaire was distributed by a Dutch company, thus influencing possible participants from Austria and Germany. Furthermore, a high percentage of questionnaires was not fully completed; that is, the respondents stopped after the first few questions. In those cases, we decided to only use completely filled-out questionnaires.

Another limitation might lie in the fact that neither the characteristics of the person who filled out the questionnaire nor their role in the nursing team of each respective institution was identified. It is, therefore, possible that nurses in different positions with a variety of views about and responsibilities regarding implementation interventions filled in the questionnaire and this may, in turn, have influenced the results.

5. Conclusions

This study suggests that the most widely used implementation interventions to translate guidelines into nursing practice focus on professionals and organisations. There are only a few marked differences between the three countries, a fact which may be attributed to different familiarity with the field of nursing science and a different significance of problems in nursing care. After investigating the effectiveness of the most frequently used single interventions in the literature, it can be concluded that these are either of little or modest to moderate effect or that their effectiveness still lacks evidence. Furthermore, one should consider that the majority of the cited literature did not focus on the nursing profession.

Nurses responsible for implementing nursing guidelines in practice should not focus mainly on a few implementation interventions with modest or even unknown effectiveness. On the contrary, at the beginning of an implementation process it might be worth considering what exactly has to be achieved and, based on this, selecting appropriate implementation strategies from all four different implementation categories. Yet to date, it is unknown how many implementation interventions, in which combination and from which EPOC-framework category [34, 35], would be effective in implementing a guideline into nursing practice. More research is necessary to explore whether a wide variety of implementation interventions is more effective than focussing on professional and organisational interventions alone.

Acknowledgments

Upon request, a list of all nursing homes in Hesse was kindly made available by the Public Inspecting Authorities for Nursing Homes (Heimaufsicht) of the Regional Administrative Authority of the Federal State of Hesse in Gießen (Regierungspräsidium in Gießen). The Regional Administrative Authority in Gießen also very kindly supported the survey in Hesse by conveying greetings to all nursing homes as part of the introduction to the electronic questionnaire encouraging nursing homes to participate in the study.

References

[1] D. J. McCloskey, "Nurses' perceptions of research utilization in a corporate health care system," *Journal of Nursing Scholarship*, vol. 40, no. 1, pp. 39–45, 2008.

[2] P. Hart, L. A. Eaton, M. Buckner et al., "Effectiveness of a computer-based educational program on nurses' knowledge, attitude, and skill level related to evidence-based practice," *Worldviews on Evidence-Based Nursing*, vol. 5, no. 2, pp. 75–84, 2008.

[3] M. Kirshbaum, "Translation to practice: a randomised, controlled study of an evidence-based booklet for breast-care nurses in the United Kingdom," *Worldviews on Evidence-Based Nursing*, vol. 5, no. 2, pp. 60–74, 2008.

[4] "Federal Act on the Quality of Health Services (Health-Care Quality Act—Gesundheitsqualitätsgesetz—GQG)," Excerpt from the 2005 Health Reform Act, Fed. Law Gaz. I no. 179/2004, 2004, http://www.bmg.gv.at/cms/home/attachments/3/4/1/CH1063/CMS1043931577060/health_care_quality_act.pdf.

[5] G. Flemmich and W. Nöstlinger, Eds., *GesUndheits-Und Krankenpflegegesetz*, Gesetze und Kommentare NR 180, Verlag des Österreichischen Gewerkschaftsbundes GmbH, Vienna, Austria, 2004.

[6] R. Grol, "Successes and failures in the implementation of evidence-based guidelines for clinical practice," *Medical Care*, vol. 39, no. 8, pp. II46–II54, 2001.

[7] R. Grol and J. Grimshaw, "From best evidence to best practice: effective implementation of change in patients' care," *The Lancet*, vol. 362, no. 9391, pp. 1225–1230, 2003.

[8] J. Grimshaw, M. Eccles, and J. Tetroe, "Implementing clinical guidelines: current evidence and future implications," *The Journal of Continuing Education in the Health Professions*, vol. 24, supplement 1, pp. S31–S37, 2004.

[9] D. S. Thompson, C. A. Estabrooks, S. Scott-Findlay, K. Moore, and L. Wallin, "Interventions aimed at increasing research use in nursing: a systematic review," *Implementation Science*, vol. 2, article 1, 2007.

[10] T. van Achterberg, L. Schoonhoven, and R. Grol, "Nursing implementation science: how evidence-based nursing requires evidence-based implementation," *Journal of Nursing Scholarship*, vol. 40, no. 4, pp. 302–310, 2008.

[11] E. Meesterberends, R. J. G. Halfens, C. Lohrmann, J. M. G. A. Schols, and R. de Wit, "Evaluation of the dissemination and implementation of pressure ulcer guidelines in Dutch nursing homes," *Journal of Evaluation in Clinical Practice*, vol. 17, no. 4, pp. 705–712, 2011.

[12] M. L. Koehn and K. Lehman, "Nurses' perceptions of evidence-based nursing practice," *Journal of Advanced Nursing*, vol. 62, no. 2, pp. 209–215, 2008.

[13] K. Gerrish, "Evidence-based practice," in *The Research Process in Nursing*, K. Gerrish and A. Lacey, Eds., pp. 491–505, Blackwell Publishing, Oxford, UK, 5th edition, 2007.

[14] L. Wallin, "Knowledge translation and implementation research in nursing," *International Journal of Nursing Studies*, vol. 46, no. 4, pp. 576–587, 2009.

[15] J. Ploeg, B. Davies, N. Edwards, W. Gifford, and P. E. Miller, "Factors influencing best-practice guideline implementation: lessons learned from administrators, nursing staff, and project leaders," *Worldviews on Evidence-Based Nursing*, vol. 4, no. 4, pp. 210–219, 2007.

[16] L. H. Thomas, N. A. Cullum, E. McColl, N. Rousseau, J. Soutter, and N. Steen, "Guidelines in professions allied to medicine," *Cochrane Database of Systematic Reviews*, no. 2, article CD000349, 2000.

[17] S. Campbell, H. Hancock, and H. Lloyd, "Implementing evidence-based practice," in *The Research Process in Nursing*, K. Gerrish and A. Lacey, Eds., pp. 506–520, Blackwell Publishing, Oxford, UK, 5th edition, 2007.

[18] S. E. Straus, J. Tetroe, and I. Graham, "Defining knowledge translation," *The Canadian Medical Association Journal*, vol. 181, no. 3-4, pp. 165–168, 2009.

[19] K. Seers, K. Cox, N. J. Crichton et al., "FIRE (Facilitating Implementation of Research Evidence): a study protocol," *Implementation Science*, vol. 7, article 25, 2012.

[20] R. Grol and M. Wensing, "Characteristics of successful innovations," in *Improving Patient Care. The Implementation of Change in Clinical Practice*, R. Grol, M. Wensing, and M. Eccles, Eds., pp. 60–70, Elsevier, Edinburgh, UK, 2005.

[21] H. E. Breimaier, R. J. G. Halfens, and C. Lohrmann, "Nurses' wishes, knowledge, attitudes and perceived barriers on implementing research findings into practice among graduate nurses in Austria," *Journal of Clinical Nursing*, vol. 20, no. 11-12, pp. 1744–1756, 2011.

[22] M. Eccles, E. McColl, N. Steen et al., "Effect of computerised evidence based guidelines on management of asthma and angina in adults in primary care: cluster randomised controlled trial," *The British Medical Journal*, vol. 325, no. 7370, pp. 941–944, 2002.

[23] J. Rashotte, M. Thomas, D. Grégoire, and S. Ledoux, "Implementation of a two-part unit-based multiple intervention: moving evidence-based practice into action," *The Canadian Journal of Nursing Research*, vol. 40, no. 2, pp. 94–114, 2008.

[24] M. Dobbins, P. Robeson, D. Ciliska et al., "A description of a knowledge broker role implemented as part of a randomized controlled trial evaluating three knowledge translation strategies," *Implementation Science*, vol. 4, article 23, 2009.

[25] D. Dulko, E. Hertz, J. Julien, S. Beck, and K. Mooney, "Implementation of cancer pain guidelines by acute care nurse practitioners using an audit and feedback strategy," *Journal of the American Academy of Nurse Practitioners*, vol. 22, no. 1, pp. 45–55, 2010.

[26] E. Fineout-Overholt, K. M. Williamson, B. Kent, and A. M. Hutchinson, "Teaching EBP: strategies for achieving sustainable organizational change toward evidence-based practice," *Worldviews on Evidence-Based Nursing*, vol. 7, no. 1, pp. 51–53, 2010.

[27] J. M. Grimshaw, R. E. Thomas, G. MacLennan et al., "Effectiveness and efficiency of guideline dissemination and implementation strategies," *Health Technology Assessment*, vol. 8, no. 6, iii–iv, pp. 1–72, 2004.

[28] G. Jamtvedt, J. M. Young, D. T. Kristoffersen, M. A. O'Brien, and A. D. Oxman, "Audit and feedback: effects on professional practice and health care outcomes," *Cochrane Dtabase of Systematic Reviews*, vol. 2, article CD000259, 2006.

[29] M. A. O'Brien, S. Rogers, G. Jamtvedt et al., "Educational outreach visits: effects on professional practice and health care outcomes," *Cochrane Database of Systematic Reviews*, vol. 4, article CD000409, 2007.

[30] K. G. Shojania, A. Jennings, A. Mayhew, C. R. Ramsay, M. P. Eccles, and J. Grimshaw, "The effects of on-screen, point of care computer reminders on processes and outcomes of care," *Cochrane Database of Systematic Reviews*, vol. 3, article CD001096, 2009.

[31] S. I. Alanen, R. Johannala-Kemppainen, J. J. Ijäs et al., "Evaluation of current care effectiveness: a survey of hypertension guideline implementation in Finnish health centres," *Scandinavian Journal of Primary Health Care*, vol. 25, no. 4, pp. 232–236, 2007.

[32] S. Miilunpalo, E. Toropainen, and P. Moisio, "Implementation of guidelines in primary health care: a challenge for the municipal health centres in Finland," *Scandinavian Journal of Primary Health Care*, vol. 19, no. 4, pp. 227–231, 2001.

[33] T. Kortteisto, M. Kaila, J. Komulainen, T. Mäntyranta, and P. Rissanen, "Healthcare professionals' intentions to use clinical guidelines: a survey using the theory of planned behaviour," *Implementation Science*, vol. 5, article 51, 2010.

[34] T. Thorsen and M. Mäkelä, "A framework for guidelines implementation studies," in *Changing Professional Practice. Theory and Practice of Clinical Guidelines Implementation*, T. Thorsen and M. Mäkelä, Eds., pp. 23–53, Danish Institute for Health Services Research, Copenhagen, Denmark, 1999.

[35] Cochrane Effective Practice and Organisation of Care Review Group (EPOC), "Data collection checklist," 2002, http://epoc.cochrane.org/sites/epoc.cochrane.org/files/uploads/datacollectionchecklist.pdf.

[36] J. Medves, C. Godfrey, C. Turner et al., "Systematic review of practice guideline dissemination and implementation strategies for healthcare teams and team-based practice," *International Journal of Evidence-Based Healthcare*, vol. 8, no. 2, pp. 79–89, 2010.

[37] E. Meesterberends, R. Halfens, C. Lohrmann, and R. de Wit, "Pressure ulcer guideline development and dissemination in Europe," *Journal of Clinical Nursing*, vol. 19, no. 11-12, pp. 1495–1503, 2010.

[38] J. L. McGowan, R. Grad, P. Pluye et al., "Electronic retrieval of health information by healthcare providers to improve practice and patient care," *Cochrane Database of Systematic Reviews*, vol. 3, article CD004749, 2009.

[39] L. Forsetlund, A. Bjørndal, A. Rashidian et al., "Continuing education meetings and workshops: effects on professional practice and health care outcomes," *Cochrane Database of Systematic Reviews*, vol. 2, CD003030, 2009.

[40] T. Dassen, Ed., *Bundesweite Erhebung Zu Pflegeproblemen 2009*, Studie aus Pflegeheimen und Krankenhäusern, Charité-Universitätsmedizin Berlin, Centrum 1 Human- und Gesundheitswissenschaften, Institut für Medizin-, Pflegepädagogik und Pflegewissenschaft, Berlin, Germany, 2009.

[41] R. J. G. Halfens, J. M. M. Meijers, J. C. L. Neyens, and J. M. G. A. Schols, "Rapportage resultaten. Landelijke Prevalentiemeting Zorgproblemen 2009," Report of the National Prevalence Measurement, Universiteit Maastricht, Onderzoeksinstituut Caphri,

Department of Health Care and Nursing Science, Maastricht, The Netherlands, 2009.

[42] C. Lohrmann, Ed., *Prävalenzerhebung 07. April 2009*, Medizinische Universität Graz, Institut für Pflegewissenschaft, Graz, Austria, 2009.

[43] WMA, (World Medical Association), "Declaration of Helsinki—Ethical principles for Medical Research involving Human Subjects," 2008, http://www.wma.net/en/30publications/10policies/b3/.

[44] G. Schmitz, "Inkontinenz," in *Pflegeprobleme in Deutschland. Ergebnisse Von 10 Jahren Forschung in Pflegeheimen Und Kliniken 2001–2010*, T. Dassen, Ed., pp. 51–57, Charité-Universitätsmedizin Berlin, Berlin, Germany, 2010.

[45] R. J. G. Halfens, J. M. G. A. Schols, S. Bartholomeyczik et al., International Prevalence Measurement of Care Problems (LPZ): 2009-2010. At a glance, Datawyse, Maastricht, 2011.

[46] S. Bartholomeyczik, "Reparaturbetrieb Krankenhaus. DRGs und ihre Auswirkungen aus Sicht der Pflege," Langfassung des Artikels aus Dr. med. Mabuse Nr. 166, März/April 2007, http://www.mabuse-verlag.de/chameleon/outbox/public/4/166_Bartholomeyczik.pdf.

[47] B. Braun, P. Buhr, and R. Müller, "Pflegearbeit im Krankenhaus. Ergebnisse einer wiederholten Pflegekräftebefragung und einer Längsschnittanalyse von GEK-Routinedaten," GEK-Edition, Schriftenreihe zur Gesundheitsanalyse, Band 60, Asgard-Verlag, St. Augustin, Germany, 2008, http://www.barmer-gek.de/barmer/web/Portale/Presseportal/Subportal/Infothek/Studien-und-Reports/GEK-Schriftenreihe-Gesundheitsanalyse/Berufsleben-Gesundheit/PDF-Pflegekraefte-60,property=Data.pdf.

[48] Deutsches Netzwerk für Qualitätsentwicklung in der Pflege (DNQP), Ed., *Expertenstandard Entlassungsmanagement in Der Pflege*, Aktualisierung, University of Applied Sciences Osnabrück, Osnabrück, Germany, 2009, http://www.dnqp.de/ExpertenstandardEntlassungsmanagement_Atk.pdf.

[49] T. van Achterberg and A. E. Sales, "Implementation Science for nursing: evidence needed! Call for papers for a special issue," *International Journal of Nursing Studies*, vol. 48, no. 10, pp. 1163–1164, 2011.

[50] D. Mazza, P. Bairstow, H. Buchan et al., "Refining a taxonomy for guideline implementation: results of an exercise in abstract classification," vol. 8, article 32, 2013.

[51] R. Robertson and K. Jochelson, *Interventions That Change Clinician Behaviour: Mapping the Literature*, NICE, London, UK, 2006, http://www.nice.org.uk/media/AF1/42/HowToGuideKingsFundLiteratureReview.pdf.

[52] A. P. Farmer, F. Légaré, L. Turcot et al., "Printed educational materials: effects on professional practice and health care outcomes," *Cochrane Database of Systematic Reviews*, vol. 3, article CD004398, 2008.

[53] G. A. Zangaro and K. L. Soeken, "A meta-analysis of studies of nurses' job satisfaction," *Research in Nursing and Health*, vol. 30, no. 4, pp. 445–458, 2007.

[54] J. E. Squires, C. A. Estabrooks, P. Gustavsson, and L. Wallin, "Individual determinants of research utilization by nurses: a systematic review update," *Implementation Science*, vol. 6, article 1, 2011.

[55] C. Urquhart, R. Currell, M. J. Grant, and N. R. Hardiker, "Nursing record systems: effects on nursing practice and healthcare outcomes," *Cochrane Database of Systematic Reviews*, vol. 1, article CD002099, 2009.

[56] M. Wensing, H. Wollersheim, and R. Grol, "Organizational interventions to implement improvements in patient care: a structured review of reviews," *Implementation Science*, vol. 1, 1, article 2, 2006.

[57] M. Prior, M. Guerin, and K. Grimmer-Somers, "The effectiveness of clinical guideline implementation strategies—a synthesis of systematic review findings," *Journal of Evaluation in Clinical Practice*, vol. 14, no. 5, pp. 888–897, 2008.

[58] B. Gardner, C. Whittington, J. McAteer, M. P. Eccles, and S. Michie, "Using theory to synthesise evidence from behaviour change interventions: the example of audit and feedback," *Social Science and Medicine*, vol. 70, no. 10, pp. 1618–1625, 2010.

[59] A. Boaz, J. Baeza, A. Fraser, and The European Implementation Science Collaborative Group (EIS), "Effective implementation of research into practice: an overview of systematic reviews of the health literature," *BMC Research Notes*, vol. 4, article 212, 2011.

[60] T. Sinuff, N. E. Cahill, R. Dhaliwal, M. Wang, A. G. Day, and D. K. Heyland, "The value of 'audit and feedback reports' in improving nutritional therapy in the intensive care unit: a multicentre observational study," American Society for Parenteral and Enteral Nutrition ASPEN, s.a., http://www.nutritioncare.org/Index.aspx?id=4568.

[61] P. Sudsawad, *Knowledge Translation: Introduction To Models, Strategies, and Measures*, Southwest Educational Development Laboratory, National Center for the Dissemination of Disability Research, Austin, TX, USA, 2007, http://www.ncddr.org/kt/products/ktintro/ktintro.pdf.

[62] N. Opiyo and M. English, "In-service training for health professionals to improve care of the seriously ill newborn or child in low and middle-income countries," *Cochrane Database of Systematic Reviews*, vol. 4, article CD007071, 2010.

[63] F. Simpson and G. S. Doig, "The relative effectiveness of practice change interventions in overcoming common barriers to change: a survey of 14 hospitals with experience implementing evidence-based guidelines," *Journal of Evaluation in Clinical Practice*, vol. 13, no. 5, pp. 709–715, 2007.

[64] S. C. Kim, C. E. Brown, W. Fields, and J. F. Stichler, "Evidence-based practice-focused interactive teaching strategy: a controlled study," *Journal of Advanced Nursing*, vol. 65, no. 6, pp. 1218–1227, 2009.

[65] G. Flodgren, M. P. Eccles, S. Shepperd, A. Scott, E. Parmelli, and F. R. Beyer, "An overview of reviews evaluating the effectiveness of financial incentives in changing healthcare professional behaviours and patient outcomes," *Cochrane Database of Systematic Reviews*, vol. 7, article CD009255, 2011.

[66] I. C. Buss, R. J. G. Halfens, H. H. Abu-Saad, and G. Kok, "Pressure ulcer prevention in nursing homes: views and beliefs of enrolled nurses and other health care workers," *Journal of Clinical Nursing*, vol. 13, no. 6, pp. 668–676, 2004.

[67] Deutsches Netzwerk für Qualitätsentwicklung in der Pflege (DNQP), "Expertenstandards in der Pflege: Zur Entwicklung wissenschaftsbasierter Expertenstandards," s.a., http://www.dnqp.de/Projekte.htm.

[68] Deutsches Netzwerk für Qualitätsentwicklung in der Pflege (DNQP), Ed., *Methodisches Vorgehen Zur Entwicklung, Einführung Und Aktualisierung Von Expertenstandards in Der Pflege*, University of Applied Sciences, Osnabrück, Germany, 2011.

[69] "LPZ—Résumé," CAPHRI School for Public Health and Primary Care, Maastricht University, s.a., http://www.lpz-um.eu/eng/home.

[70] "Bundesgesetzblatt, Gesetz zur strukturellen Weiterentwicklung der Pflegeversicherung (Pflege-Weiterentwicklungsgesetz) vom 28. Mai 2008," Bundesgesetzblatt Jahrgang, Teil I Nr. 20, ausgegeben zu Bonn am 30, 113a, 3, 2008, http://www.mdk-qualitaetsberichte.de/files/080528-pfwg-mit-aenderungen.pdf.

[71] M. B. Hamilton, "Online survey response rates and times. Background and Guidance for Industry," 2009, http://www.supersurvey_white_paper_response_rates.pdf.

[72] D. F. Polit and C. T. Beck, *Nursing Research. Generating and Assessing Evidence For Nursing Practice*, Wolters Kluwer Health, Lippincott Williams and Wilkins, Philadelphia, Pa, USA, 9th edition, 2012.

A Statewide Case Management, Surveillance, and Outcome Evaluation System for Children with Special Health Care Needs

Karen A. Monsen,[1] Scott A. Elsbernd,[2] Linda Barnhart,[3] Jacquie Stock,[3] Carla E. Prock,[4] Wendy S. Looman,[1] and Maria Nardella[3]

[1] *University of Minnesota, Minneapolis, MN 55455, USA*
[2] *Children's Hospitals and Clinics of Minnesota, Minneapolis-Saint Paul, MN 55404, USA*
[3] *Children with Special Health Care Needs Program, Washington State Department of Health, Olympia, WA 98504, USA*
[4] *Benton-Franklin Health District, Kennewick, WA 98336, USA*

Correspondence should be addressed to Scott A. Elsbernd; scottelsbernd@gmail.com

Academic Editors: L.-Y. Chien and A. Green

Objectives. To evaluate the feasibility of implementing a statewide children with special health care needs (CSHCN) program evaluation, case management, and surveillance system using a standardized instrument and protocol that operationalized the United States Health and Human Services CSHCN National Performance Measures. *Methods.* Public health nurses in local public health agencies in Washington State jointly developed and implemented the standardized system. The instrument was the Omaha System. Descriptive statistics were used for the analysis of standardized data. *Results.* From the sample of CSHCN visit reports ($n = 127$), 314 problems and 853 interventions were documented. The most common problem identified was growth and development followed by health care supervision, communication with community resources, caretaking/parenting, income, neglect, and abuse. The most common intervention category was surveillance (60%), followed by case management (24%) and teaching, guidance, and counseling (16%). On average, there were 2.7 interventions per problem and 6.7 interventions per visit. *Conclusions.* This study demonstrates the feasibility of an approach for statewide CSHCN program evaluation, case management, and surveillance system. Knowledge, behavior, and status ratings suggest that there are critical unmet needs in the Washington State CSHCN population for six major problems.

1. Introduction

Children with special health care needs (CSHCN) are at increased risk for poor health outcomes [1]. The CSHCN population is growing, the need for services is increasing, and the capacity to provide CSHCN services is decreasing due to public sector financial constraints [2]. It is critical to demonstrate the needs of this vulnerable population and evaluate the effectiveness and value of CSHCN programs [2, 3]. Public health nurses (PHNs) in Washington State serving CSHCN sought to describe CSHCN client needs and evaluate CSHCN programs using a standardized terminology, the Omaha System [4]. They selected the Omaha System because many of the local Washington State public health jurisdictions used electronic health records and the Omaha System for clinical documentation. Standardized terminologies have potential to advance the development of practice standards and assessment guidelines and overall quality improvement policies and procedures [5–7]. This work builds on previous efforts to describe care and evaluate outcomes in other states and programs [8].

The Maternal Child Health Bureau (MCHB) defines CSHCN as "those who have or are at increased risk for a chronic physical, developmental, behavioral, or emotional condition and who also require health and related services of a type or amount beyond that required by children generally" [1]. The MCHB has advanced a national agenda for achieving and measuring the success of CSHCN programs. The purpose of this agenda is "to provide and promote family-centered, community-based, coordinated care for CSHCN and to facilitate the development of community-based systems of services for such children and their families" [1]. Since the 1980s, this agenda has guided state and federal programs through the identification of six key indicators of progress. These indicators describe the necessity for the early identification of problems in order to provide an opportunity for intervention, as well as the organization of services in order to provide accessible and appropriate interventions [1].

Identifying health care problems experienced by CSHCN and their families provides information about the larger service system, while a successful system of services results in high levels of child and family health and well-being [9]. Partnering across jurisdictions to define, measure, and monitor a system of care for CSHCN at the state level may lead to the promotion of best practice [10]. Uniform data, specifically, state-level data from the National Surveys of CSHCN, is a key in driving system of care improvements and facilitating state and local program planning efforts [11, 12]. However, little research exists describing the role or benefits of a standardized process for PHN agencies to assess and document nursing activities related to CSHCN programs [13].

Programs that address the unique needs of CSCHN have long been a component of the public health system [2]. Public health nursing contributes a unique service for this population and the health system by assessing health status and access to other health services, assuring that families receive the services they need, and providing findings to policy makers [2]. CSHCN often require long-term services for complex needs, consuming a disproportionate share of health care dollars spent on children. Therefore, they are especially vulnerable to health care issues such as access, quality, and cost containment (denial of care). In Washington State, the CSHCN program goal is to "assure children and youth with special health care needs achieve the healthiest life possible by promoting access to integrated, family-centered, culturally competent, and community-based programs and services" [14].

The adoption of electronic health records and public health information systems varies across jurisdictions in the United States [12]. Many local public health jurisdictions in Washington State implemented commercial and agency-developed public health information systems over the past several years [11]. However, some local public health jurisdictions continue to use paper systems for all data tracking and documentation. The diversity of these documentation methods presents a challenge in uniform statewide data collection. The PHNs developed a solution to this challenge, through the use of a common standardized terminology in all paper or computerized platforms (the Omaha System) [4, 15]. The resulting uniform data could then be combined across all jurisdictions, regardless of how the data were collected.

The objective of this study was to evaluate the feasibility of implementing a state-wide case management, surveillance, and program evaluation system for CSHCN program using a standardized Omaha System protocol and visit report. This paper reports preliminary data from the first four months after the implementation of the standardized data collection protocol.

2. Materials and Methods

The University of Minnesota Institutional Review Board and State of Washington Institutional Review Board approvals were obtained for this study. All local public health agencies in Washington State were invited to a statewide training on the data collection system (September 2010) and to participate in the data collection starting November 2010. The data collection period for this study ended in February 2011. Visit reports were submitted to State of Washington Department of Health CSHCN officials for program evaluations by 25 of the 35 local agencies during this time period. The Department of Health entered the deidentified data into a spreadsheet and provided the spreadsheet to the research team for analysis [15].

2.1. Instrument: The Omaha System. The Omaha System [4] was selected by Washington State CSHCN directors for this statewide program evaluation, because it is a standardized interface terminology used widely for computerized documentation in community care settings [4]. It is recognized by the American Nurses Association and other informatics organizations [16]. The Omaha System does not include medical diagnoses or tests. Instead, it provides a comprehensive, holistic architecture for describing, documenting, and evaluating health care by enabling practitioners to collect relevant clinical data and identify client strengths and needs. A previous study compared Omaha System KBS ratings for high risk families including families of CSHCN served in PHN home visiting programs by four local public health agencies in another state (Minnesota) [8]. The Omaha System consists of three components: the Problem Classification Scheme, the Intervention Scheme, and the Problem Rating Scale for Outcomes [4].

The Problem Classification Scheme is used to identify and classify health-related issues and includes 42 problems. Problems are uniquely identified by distinctive definitions and signs and symptoms (s/sx). The Intervention Scheme is used for addressing the problems which are described using the four-level Intervention Scheme. The four terms of the Intervention scheme are: problem from the Problem Classification Scheme, category (action term), target (defined term that further specifies the intervention), and care description (undefined, customizable term) [4].

The Problem Rating Scale for Outcomes is used to measure client knowledge, behavior, and status (KBS) related to each client problem. KBS ratings are documented using a Likert-type ordinal scale from 1 (lowest) to 5 (highest). The knowledge scale measures what the client understands and knows. The behavior scale measures the appropriateness of client actions. The status scale describes the level of severity of client sign and symptoms [4]. The definitions of KBS ratings are provided in Table 1.

2.2. Development of the Evaluation Protocol. The State of Washington Department of Health together with PHNs serving CSHCN sought to develop a uniform CSHCN evaluation protocol including the development of practice standards and assessment guidelines. The purpose of their project was to

Table 1: Definitions of knowledge, behavior, and status ratings [4].

	Knowledge—behavior—status rating key		
5	Superior knowledge	Consistently appropriate behavior	No signs/symptoms
4	Adequate knowledge	Usually appropriate behavior	Minimal no signs/symptoms
3	Basic knowledge	Inconsistently appropriate behavior	Moderate signs/symptoms
2	Minimal knowledge	Rarely appropriate behavior	Severe signs/symptoms
1	No knowledge	Not appropriate behavior	Extreme signs/symptoms

generate data for overall quality improvement and outcomes reporting. They created the evaluation protocol in response to three important trends: (1) the need to respond to federal maternal-child health national performance measures, (2) the fact that many of the public health agencies had the electronic capacity to collect standardized data, and (3) many of the agencies were using the Omaha System for other maternal-child health programs [15]. Title V technical assistance funds supported consultation for this project from a nationally known expert in the use of the Omaha System for program evaluation. PHNs serving CSHCN in Washington State created a logic model for program evaluation based on HHS Title V National Performance Measures (NPM) for addressing CSHCN National Performance Measures (Table 2) [1]. During a ten-month period, PHNs in local public health agencies jointly developed and implemented a standardized visit report operationalizing the National Performance Measures using the Omaha System. Over a series of four meetings, they selected eight problems for the standardized visit report: income, residence, communication with community resources, caretaking/parenting, abuse, neglect, growth and development, and health care supervision. The visit report was available in electronic and paper form (see example in Figure 1). It is available online [17]. Data quality for new Omaha System users was supported by peer training, and by the use of the KBS Rating Guide Supplement, also available online [17].

2.3. Sample. There were CSHCN visit reports (n = 127). The client demographics were excluded from analysis because of Washington State data deidentification protocols. The only known characteristics of the sample were that the CSHCN who received PHN visits qualified for services through the HHS Title V CSHCN definitions and criteria.

2.4. Variables. Omaha System variables were problems; s/sx; intervention categories and targets; and knowledge, behavior, and status ratings for client problems. For dependent clients such as CSHCN, the knowledge rating reflects the caregiver's knowledge while behavior and status ratings reflect the child's behavior and status.

2.5. Analysis. The Omaha System Partnership for Knowledge Discovery and Health Care Quality [18] provided in-kind data management and analysis for the project. Descriptive statistics were used to quantify the number of clients and s/sx by problem for all problems with 10 or more instances in the data.

3. Results

From the visit reports (n = 127), 314 problems and 853 interventions were documented. The most common problem identified was growth and development followed by health care supervision, communication with community resources, caretaking/parenting, income, neglect, and abuse. The most common intervention category was surveillance (60%), followed by case management (24%) and teaching, guidance, and counseling (16%). On average, there were 2.7 interventions per problem and 6.7 interventions per visit. The mean KBS ratings for each problem are reported in Figure 2.

3.1. Growth and Development. For the growth and development problem (n = 80), the most common s/sx were abnormal results of developmental screening tests (40%), inadequate achievement/maintenance of developmental tasks (40%), age-inappropriate behavior (30%), and abnormal weight/height/head circumference in relation to growth/age standards (23%).

3.2. Health Care Supervision. For the health care supervision problem (n = 57), the most common s/sx were inability to coordinate multiple appointments/treatment plans (23%), inadequate source of health care (21%), inadequate treatment plan (21%) fails to obtain routine/preventative health care (18%), inconsistent source of health care (11%), fails to return as requested by health care provider (9%), and fails to seek care for symptoms requiring evaluation/treatment (7%).

Table 2: Proposed outcomes of the project based on national performance measures for children with special health care needs [1] as operationalized by the Omaha System Problem Classification Scheme [4].

NPM: children are screened early and continuously for special health care needs (Growth and development)*
Developmental screening results are within normal limits or referrals are made
NPM: child has a medical home (Health care supervision)*
Caregiver knows when and how to seek emergency, chronic, and acute illness and preventive care
Caregiver follows prescribed/recommended treatment plan and preventive care
Consistently uses medical home and health care resources appropriately
Child receives appropriate timely health care in a medical home
NPM: community resources are organized so families can use them easily (Communication with community resources)*
Caregiver is aware of community resources as needed and knows how to access them
Caregiver uses resources/services consistently
Caregiver uses resources/services appropriately
NPM: families have adequate private and/or public insurance to pay for the services they need (Income)*
Caregiver knows how to navigate resources
Caregiver completes financial paperwork accurately and on time for medical care
Health care expenses are covered or paid for
NPM: families are decision makers in their child's care and are satisfied with the services they receive (Caretaking/parenting)*
Caregiver knows how to contact CSHCN program as needed.

NPM: National Performance Measure.
*(Omaha System problems corresponding to each NPM noted in parentheses).

3.3. Communication with Community Resources. For the communication with community resources problem (n = 57), the most common s/sx were unfamiliar with options/procedures for obtaining services (58%), language, cultural, educational, transportation barriers (38%), difficulty understanding roles/regulations of service providers (36%), inability to communicate concerns to provider (24%), dissatisfaction with services (20%), limited access to care/services/goods (14%), and inability to use/have inadequate communication devices/equipment (2%).

3.4. Caretaking/Parenting. For the Caretaking/parenting problem (n = 48), the most common s/sx were difficulty providing physical care/safety (33%), difficulty providing cognitive learning experiences and activities (33%), difficulty providing preventative and therapeutic health care (31%), expectations incongruent with the stage of growth and development (19%), difficulty providing emotional nurturance (17%), dissatisfaction/difficulty with responsibilities (15%), difficulty interpreting or responding to verbal/nonverbal communication (15%), and neglectful or abusive (4.2%).

3.5. Income. The most common s/sx of the income problem (n = 45) were low/no income (78%), ability to buy only necessities (33%), uninsured medical expenses (18%), difficulty buying necessities (18%), and difficulty with money management (11%).

3.6. Residence. For the residence problem (n = 18), the most common s/sx were cluttered living space (44%), structural barriers (11%), homelessness (11%), structurally unsound (6%), inadequate heating/cooling (6%), steep, unsafe stairs, (6%) inadequate/obstructed exits and entries (6%), presence of lead based paints (6%), and unsafe equipment/wiring (6%).

3.7. Neglect. For the neglect problem (n = 12), the most common s/sx were of the signs and symptoms documented in the neglect problem included *inadequate/delayed medical care* (25%), included *lacks necessary supervision* (17%), while *lacks adequate physical care* (8%), *lacks emotional support* (8%).

3.8. Abuse. Of the 127 visit reports, four abuse problems were recorded, which is less than the threshold of 10 cases established a priori. Therefore, the frequency of s/sx and mean KBS ratings were not reported for the abuse problem.

4. Discussion

The Washington State CSHCN program developed and implemented a state-wide case management, surveillance, and program evaluation system using the Omaha System, demonstrating the feasibility of this approach. Preliminary data suggest serious needs in the CSHCN population that should be further investigated, especially related to health care access for CSHCN and services needed to address developmental issues. The findings of this study were reported to the CSCHN program in April 2011 [15]. The PHNs suggested the very low KBS ratings for the growth and development problem may reflect the fact that funding reductions have severely limited PHN services in local health jurisdictions. As a result, the CSHCN program policy shifted to focus on a small subset of the most seriously affected children.

4.1. Characteristics and Needs of CSHCN and Families. Omaha System s/sx data provide insight into the characteristics and needs of CSHCN and families. In this study, the s/sx and very low KBS ratings for the health care supervision and communication with community resources problems suggest that there are serious gaps in the sources of health care and treatment plans for CSHCN and that families have difficulty accessing care due to barriers in the system. The s/sx also suggest that very few families are unwilling to access care or use resources. These findings relate to the NPM: "Community

CV/OV☐ HV☐ TV☐			Initial ☐ Interim☐ Final☐	
K 1 2 3 4 5	B 1 2 3 4 5		Growth and development Ratings 1 2 3 4 5	Not applicable or unable to address today (circle one)
Signs and symptoms	Category	Target	Client specific information	Notes
☐ Abnormal results of developmental screening tests ☐ Abnormal weight/height/head circumference in relation to growth/age standards ☐ Age-in appropriate behavior ☐ Inadequate achievement/ maintenance of developmental tasks ☐ Other	S	Bonding/attachment	Parent/child interaction	
	S	Growth/devel.care	Developmental tasks for age, developmental test ratings	
	S	Rest/sleep	Forage/condition, consistent patterns	
	S	S/S physical	Physical growth/variations	
	S	S/S physical	Voiding ands tooling	
	S	S/Smental/emotional	Behavior concerns	
	CM	S/S mental/emotional	Intervention programs for behavioral health	
	CM	S/S physical	HC provider, WIC, lactation consultant, and community support group	
	CM	Growth/devel.care	Education/developmental resources	
K 1 2 3 4 5	B 1 2 3 4 5		Abuse Ratings 1 2 3 4 5	Not applicable or unable to address today (circle one)
☐ Harsh/excessive discipline ☐ Attacked verbally ☐ Welts/bruises/burns/questionable injuries ☐ Fearful/hyper vigilant behavior ☐ Violent environment ☐ Consistent negative messages ☐ Assaulted sexually ☐ Other	S	S/S mental/emotional	Behavioral extremes	
	S	S/S physical	Unexplained injuries, evidence of abuse	
	CM	Legal system	Child protective services and lawen forcement	

S: surveillance, CM: case management, K: knowledge, B: behavior, S: status.

FIGURE 1: Children with special health care needs visit report example [17].

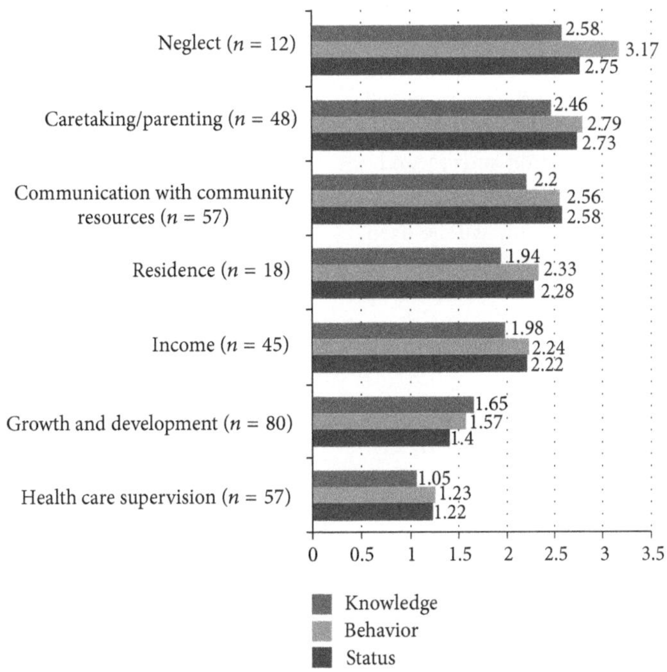

FIGURE 2: Baseline knowledge, behavior, and status scores for problems of children with special health care needs ($n = 127$).

resources are organized so families can use them easily," "Child has a medical home," and "Families are decision-makers in their child's care and are satisfied with the services they receive."

The s/sx of the caretaking/parenting problem most often related to providing adequate physical care, cognitive learning experiences, and health care. Very few families had s/sx related to parental dissatisfaction or emotional issues. The s/sx of the income problem most often related to income shortages, while few families had budgeting difficulties. These findings relate to the NPM: "Families have adequate public and/or private insurance to pay for the services they need."

The s/sx of the residence problem most often related to excessive household clutter, while few homes had structural deficits and few families were homeless. The most common s/sx of the neglect problem were related to medical neglect and child supervision. Very few CSHCN did not receive appropriate physical care or emotional nurturance. Overall, these results describe the stressful circumstances that families of CSHCN in this study experienced on a daily basis. Consistent with the goal of the CSHCN program, PHNs have traditionally worked with families to promote access to services (program website). The use of the CSHCN visit reports will generate large data sets that will enable further evaluation of the effectiveness of PHN interventions for these problems. Previous studies have described intervention tailoring and effectiveness for high risk families [19–21]. Further research is needed to identify approaches most successful in supporting families of CSHCN, so that resources can be used efficiently and effectively, and the NPM goals for CSHCN and their families can be achieved.

4.2. Use of the Omaha System for Uniform Data Collection. The use of the Omaha System enabled the aggregation of standardized CSHCN data for program evaluation. Assessments and intervention data from 25 of 35 local health jurisdictions were included in this study. The 127 visit reports were submitted to the Department of Health on the paper visit report forms. Data from electronic documentation of CSHCN assessments and interventions were not included in this study but will be available in the future. The interoperability of electronic systems continues to be a challenge. It is essential for state and local health jurisdictions, software vendors, and policy makers to work together to achieve the goals of standardized, interoperable systems to support uniform data collection for program evaluation and research.

4.3. Policy Significance. The results of this study will be used by the Washington State CSHCN program to focus nursing activities on the problems most likely to be encountered by PHNs serving the CSHCN population. Additionally, these results will be used to further refine the program evaluation process.

National, state, and local officials have a responsibility to develop, support, and maintain CSHCN programs [1, 22]. Public funding for CSHCN programs in Washington State has been greatly reduced since the inception of this CSHCN program evaluation initiative and continues to be in jeopardy [14, 23]. The data obtained in this study suggest that serious needs are likely to be unmet in the current economic climate due to funding shortfalls and related reductions in CSHCN program staffing.

4.4. Limitations. With all research using large observational data sets, limitations of the data include observer bias and fidelity to documentation procedures. While the sample of 127 clients from 25 local health jurisdictions demonstrates the feasibility of the approach, bias toward submitting forms for clients with the greatest need may exist. This limitation is supported by the PHN interpretation of the findings reported in Section 5.0. Therefore, alternative explanations for the findings must be considered. In this study, many of the local health jurisdictions started to use the Omaha System for the CSHCN at the beginning of the data collection period. Documentation quality was supported by peer training and the use of KBS rating guide supplements. However, no evaluation of documentation quality was included in the program evaluation protocols. Further research is needed to create quality assurance measures that can be implemented as an integral part of program evaluation.

5. Conclusions

This study demonstrates the feasibility of a structured approach to case management, surveillance, and program evaluation for CSHCN using a standardized terminology. The use of the Omaha System facilitated uniform data collection of client assessments and services across 25 of 35 local health jurisdictions in the first four months of the evaluation. Preliminary findings suggest that critical needs existed among CSHCN in Washington State. In the future, larger data sets will be used to evaluate the quality of PHN services, inform public policy, and improve the health CSHCN and their families.

Acknowledgments

The authors are clinical experts in the area of CSHCN and/or informatics specialists with expertise in the use of the Omaha System in education and research. All authors declare no conflict of interests in the preparation of this paper. The content is solely the responsibility of the authors and does not necessarily represent the official views of the authors' employers. One author (K. Monsen) provided consultation to the Washington State CSHCN program, supported by an MCH Bureau Title V Technical Assistance Grant. The authors would like to acknowledge the funding support for this project from the MCH Title V Technical Assistance Grant to the Washington State CSHCN Program and to thank the public health nurses, the families of children with special health care needs, and the Omaha System Partnership for Knowledge Discovery and Health Care Quality.

References

[1] United States Department of Health and Human Services, Health Resources and Services Administration: Maternal and Child Health Bureau, Children with Special Health Care Needs MCHB agenda, 2012, http://mchb.hrsa.gov/AZ/azdescriptions.html.

[2] B. B. Strickland, P. C. Van Dyck, M. D. Kogan et al., "Assessing and ensuring a comprehensive system of services for children with special health care needs: a public health approach," *American Journal of Public Health*, vol. 101, no. 2, pp. 224–231, 2011.

[3] S. L. Parish, P. T. Shattuck, and R. A. Rose, "Financial burden of raising CSHCN: association with state policy choices," *Pediatrics*, vol. 124, supplement 4, pp. S435–S442, 2009.

[4] K. S. Martin, *The Omaha System: A Key to Practice, Documentation, and Information Management*, Health Connections Press, Omaha, Neb, USA, 2nd edition, 2005.

[5] K. A. Monsen, C. Neely, G. Oftedahl, M. J. Kerr, M. Cella, and O. Farri, "Translating Institute for Clinical Systems Improvement standards into practice through the electronic health record using the Omaha System," *Journal of Biomedical Informatics*, vol. 45, pp. 719–725, 2012.

[6] K. A. Monsen, D. J. Foster, T. Gomez, J. K. Poulsen, J. Mast, B. L. Westra et al., "Evidence-based standardized care plans for use internationally to improve home care practice and population health," *Applied Clinical Informatics*, vol. 2, pp. 373–384, 2011.

[7] B. L. Westra, C. W. Delaney, D. Konicek, and G. Keenan, "Nursing standards to support the electronic health record," *Nursing Outlook*, vol. 56, no. 5, pp. 258–266.el, 2008.

[8] K. A. Monsen, J. A. Fulkerson, A. B. Lytton, L. L. Taft, L. D. Schwichtenberg, and K. S. Martin, "Comparing maternal child health problems and outcomes across public health nursing agencies," *Maternal and Child Health Journal*, vol. 14, no. 3, pp. 412–421, 2010.

[9] S. J. Blumberg and A. C. Carle, "The well-being of the health care environment for CSHCN and their families: a latent variable approach," *Pediatrics*, vol. 124, supplement 4, pp. S361–S367, 2009.

[10] R. N. Roberts, D. D. Behl, and A. L. Akers, "Building a system of care for children with special healthcare needs," *Infants and Young Children*, vol. 17, no. 3, pp. 213–222, 2004.

[11] S. De Fries, V. Sharp, M. Nardella, and R. Peters, "A data driven process in Washington State to improve systems of care for Children With Special Health Care Needs: The National Survey of CSHCN," *Maternal and Child Health Journal*, vol. 9, supplement 2, pp. S117–S120, 2005.

[12] Institute of Medicine, *For the Publica Health: The Role of Meaaurement in Action and Accountability*, National Academies Press, Washington, DC, USA, 2011.

[13] K. A. Monsen, B. Bekemeier, R. P. Newhouse, and F. D. Scutchfield, "Development of a public health nursing data infrastructure," *Public Health Nursing*, vol. 29, pp. 343–351, 2012.

[14] Children with special health care needs program, 2012, http://www.doh.wa.gov/YouandYourFamily/InfantsChildrenandTeens/HealthandSafety/ChildrenwithSpecialHealthCareNeeds.aspx.

[15] S. Elsbernd, L. Barnhart, J. Stock, K. A. Monsen, and C. Prock, "Washington State public health nurse use of the Omaha system in serving children with special health care needs," in *Proceedings of the Omaha System International Conference*, Eagan, Minn, USA, 2011.

[16] ANA recognized terminologies and data element sets, 2012, http://www.nursingworld.org/npii/terminologies.htm.

[17] Minnesota Omaha System Users Group, 2012, http://omahasystemmn.org.

[18] Omaha System Partnership for Knowledge Discovery and Health Care Quality, 2012, http://omahasystempartnership.org/.

[19] K. A. Monsen, D. M. Radosevich, M. J. Kerr, and J. A. Fulkerson, "Public health nurses tailor interventions for families at risk," *Public Health Nursing*, vol. 28, no. 2, pp. 119–128, 2011.

[20] K. A. Monsen, A. Chatterjee, and B. L. Westra, "Relationships between client characteristics, nursing interventions, and client outcomes in family home visiting" . In Review.

[21] K. A. Monsen, D. B. McNaughton, K. Savik, and O. Farri, "Problem stabilization: a metric for problem improvement in home visiting clients," *Applied Clinical Informatics*, vol. 2, pp. 437–446, 2011.

[22] S. J. Blumberg and M. D. Bramlett, "Comparing states on outcomes for children with special health care needs," *Maternal and Child Health Journal*, vol. 9, supplement 2, pp. S121–S128, 2005.

[23] Local health department budget cuts in the news, 2012, http://www.naccho.org/press/coverage/budgetcuts/index.cfm.

15

The Factors Affecting the Refusal of Reporting on Medication Errors from the Nurses' Viewpoints: A Case Study in a Hospital in Iran

Mohammadkarim Bahadori,[1] Ramin Ravangard,[2] Amin Aghili,[3] Jamil Sadeghifar,[3] Mahdi Gharsi Manshadi,[3] and Javad Smaeilnejad[1]

[1] *Health Management Research Centre, Baqiyatallah University of Medical Sciences, Tehran, Iran*
[2] *School of Management and Medical Information Sciences, Shiraz University of Medical Sciences, Shiraz, Iran*
[3] *Students' Scientific Research Center, School of Management and Medical Information, Tehran University of Medical Sciences, Tehran, Iran*

Correspondence should be addressed to Jamil Sadeghifar; jamil.sadeghifar@gmail.com

Academic Editors: R. Constantino and B. Roberts

Objective. Medication errors are the most common types of medical errors which considerably endanger the patient safety. This survey aimed to study the factors influencing not reporting on medication errors from the nurses' viewpoints in Abbasi Hospital of Miandoab, Iran. *Methods.* This was a cross-sectional, descriptive and analytical study conducted in 2012 in which all nurses ($n = 100$) working in different inpatient units were studied using a consensus method. Required data were collected using a questionnaire. Collected data were analyzed through some statistical tests including Independent t-test, ANOVA, and chi-square. Results. According to the results, the most important reasons for not reporting on medication errors were related to the managerial factors (3.56 ± 0.996), factors related to the process of reporting (3.32 ± 0.797), and fear of the consequences of reporting (3.01 ± 1.039), respectively. Also, there was a significant relationship between employment status and fear of the Consequences of reporting on medication errors ($P < 0.008$). *Conclusion.* This study results showed that managerial factors had the greatest role in the refusal of reporting on medication errors. Therefore, for example, establishing a mechanism to improve quality rather than focus only on finding the culprits and blaming them can result in improving the patient safety.

1. Introduction

One of the most fundamental components of health care quality is the patient safety [1]. The patient safety is a priority for every health care system which follows the ensuring and improving of the quality of health care [2] and also is one of the main concerns of all health care systems [3, 4]. The principle of "no harm" in the Hippocratic Oath is a confirmation of this issue [5]. The patient safety is known as to avoid injuries to the patients or occurring unexpected adverse events of health care processes [6].

Adverse events and medical errors are the main factors endangering the patient safety which are the most important problems of all health care systems, and all of these systems try to reduce their resulted injuries [5]. Statistics show that from 2.9% to 16.6% of hospital inpatients suffer from treatment-related adverse events [7, 8]. On the other hand, the rate of medical errors throughout the world is so high that is accounted for one of the five major causes of deaths [9].

One of the most common types of medical errors is medication error which because of their high prevalence and potential risks to patients, the rate of medication errors is considered as an indicator to determine the level of the patient safety in hospitals [3, 9, 10]. Medication error has been defined as the preventable misuse of the drugs [11, 12].

In the patient safety management issues, from the 1990s onwards, determining the factors influencing the occurrence of errors as well as the barriers to reports on occurred errors has been focused instead of only detection and prevention of errors [13]. The occurrence of medication errors among nurses is more than that among other health care professionals [14]. The results of studies have shown that among approximately 44000 to 98000 annual deaths due to medical errors, 7000 deaths have been related to the medication errors [9]. Reporting on the medication errors can cause maintaining the safety of patients as well as providing a valuable database of information to prevent medication errors in the future [15].

Several studies have been conducted on determining the barriers to report on medication errors. Tol and colleagues in their study on a group of nurses conducted at a teaching hospital concluded that the managerial factors were the most important barriers to report on medication errors [16]. The results of Wakefield and colleagues' study on 1300 nurses showed that using medication errors for reprimanding nurses by their supervisors was one of the factors affecting the refusal of reporting on medication errors [17]. Based on the results of a study conducted in Japan, the main cause of occurring medication errors among newly graduated nurses was related to the wrong administration of intravenous drugs which, in turn, was due to their little knowledge of pharmacology [18].

The researchers of the present study in their searches found that most of the researches had been focused only on identifying the causes of medication errors and few researches had conducted to determine the factors influencing the refusal of reporting on medication errors or barriers to reporting on these errors. Because determining the factors influencing not reporting on the medication errors can result in taking appropriate managerial and individual measures to increase the rate of reporting on medication errors and finally decrease the occurrence of these errors, the present survey aimed to study the factors influencing not reporting on medication errors from the nurses' viewpoints in Abbasi Hospital of Iran.

2. Methods

This was a cross-sectional, descriptive analytical study conducted in 2012 in which all nurses ($n = 100$) working in different inpatient units of Abbasi Hospital in Miandoab, an Iranian hospital affiliated to Urmia University of Medical Sciences, were studied using a consensus method.

Required data were collected using a questionnaire consisting of two sections: the first section included nurses' demographic characteristics such as age, sex, marital status, education level, employment status, types of work shifts, experience, and their service unit. The second section, also, included 19 questions in 3 domains: fear of the consequences of reporting (with 11 items), managerial factors (with 5 items), and factors related to the process of reporting (with 3 items). The five-point Likert scale was used to determine the factors affecting the refusal of reporting on medication errors, whereby 1 refers to strongly disagree and 5 as strongly agree. Though the validity and reliability of this questionnaire had been confirmed in Tol and colleagues' study [16], in the present study, the reliability of this questionnaire was approved again ($\alpha = 0.82$). For collecting data, one of the researchers attended the mentioned hospital in three work shifts—morning, evening, and night—and distributed the questionnaire among studied nurses after obtaining oral consent from them for participating in this study and explaining the objectives of the study and assuring the confidentiality of collected data.

Finally, collected data were analyzed using SPSS 19.0 through some statistical tests including independent t-test, ANOVA, and chi-square. $P < 0.05$ was considered statistically significant.

3. Results

The response rate was 83%. The results showed that among 83 nurses who participated in this study, most of them ($n = 65$, 78.3%) were female, 71% were married ($n = 59$), 55.5% were in the 25–35 age group ($n = 46$), 86.8% had a bachelor's degree ($n = 72$), 49.4% were employed officially ($n = 41$), 38.6% had lower than 5 years job experience ($n = 32$), 88% were working in rotating work shifts ($n = 73$), and 39.7% were working in the Intensive Care Units ($n = 33$) (Table 1).

The mean self-reported scores of studied domains for not reporting on medication errors were as follows.

Fear of the consequences of reporting (3.01 ± 1.039), managerial factors (3.56 ± 0.99), and factors related to the process of reporting (3.32 ± 0.79). Therefore, managerial factors were the most important reason for not reporting on the medication errors.

The results showed that the highest mean score in the managerial factors domain was related to "the heads' focus only on finding the culprits and blaming them, regardless of other factors involved in the occurrence of errors" (3.674 ± 1.21). The highest mean scores in the domain of fear of the consequences of reporting was related to "fear of judicial affairs following reporting on medication errors" (3.68 ± 1.21), and in the domain of factors related to the process of reporting was associated with "lack of a clear definition of medication errors" (3.144 ± 1.29).

The frequency, mean, and standard deviation of nurses' responses to the questions related to each studied domains (fear of the consequences of reporting, managerial factors, and factors related to the process of reporting) and their items have been shown in Table 2 based on their importance in occurring medication errors from the nurses' viewpoints.

Also, the results showed that there were not any significant relationships between some nurses' demographic characteristics (such as marital status, types of work shifts, age, education level, employment status, and service units) and the studied domains of not reporting on medication errors (including fear of the consequences of reporting, managerial factors, and factors related to the process of reporting) (P-value > 0.05). However, there was a significant relationship between employment status and fear of the consequences of reporting on medication errors ($P < 0.008$).

4. Discussion

Identification and reduction of medication errors requires a system to be designed for finding the root causes of occurring

TABLE 1: The demographic characteristics of studied nurses.

Variables	Frequency (%)
Age (year)	
Less than 25	10 (12%)
25–35	46 (55.5%)
35–45	15 (18.1%)
More than 45	6 (7.2%)
Missing	6 (7.2%)
Sex	
Male	17 (20.5%)
Female	65 (78.3%)
Missing	1 (1.2%)
Marital status	
Single	23 (27.8%)
Married	59 (71%)
Missing	1 (1.2%)
Education level	
Diploma	7 (8.4%)
Associate degree	4 (4.8%)
Bachelor's degree	72 (86.8%)
Employment status	
Official employee	41 (49.4%)
Contractual employee	29 (34.9%)
Other	12 (14.5%)
Missing	1 (1.2%)
Types of work shift	
Fixed shifts	10 (12%)
Rotating shifts	73 (88%)
Job experience (year)	
Less than 5	32 (38.6%)
5–10	27 (32.5%)
More than 10	17 (20.5%)
Missing	7 (8.4%)
Service unit	
General Care Units	23 (27.8 %)
Intensive Care Units	33 (39.7%)
Missing	27 (32.5%)

them. Based on such a system, first the occurred errors should be reported, and then, the major causes of occurring them should be found in an intimate and scientific situation. In this regard, the present survey aimed to study the factors influencing not reporting on medication errors from the nurses' viewpoints in Abbasi Hospital, Miandoab.

The study results showed that managerial factor was the most one causing not reporting on medication errors, and other factors including factors related to the process of reporting and fear of the consequences of reporting had the next priorities for not reporting on medication errors from the viewpoint of nurses. Tol and colleagues in a similar study conducted among the nurses of Baharloo hospital in Tehran also found the same results [16]. The similarity of these two studies in using the same methods and population studies (viz., the nurses of public hospitals) is a reason for those similar results. Kouhestani and Baghcheghi in their study on the nursing students reported the fear of the consequences of reporting errors as the most important factors of not reporting on medication errors by them [19]. The different population study of mentioned studies (viz., nursing student and nurses) can be a reason for their different results. In another study carried out by Osborne and colleagues the most important reasons for not reporting on medication errors were fear of being blamed, fear of being labeled as incompetent nurses and inadequacy, fear of their future professional career, fear of judicial issues, and adverse reactions of their heads and colleagues [20].

According to the results of the present study, among the studied managerial variables, "the heads' focus only on finding the culprits and blaming them, regardless of other factors involved in the occurrence of errors," had the greatest impact on not reporting on medication errors from the viewpoints of nurses. The results of the Tol and colleagues' study [16] as well as Hosseinzadeh and colleagues' study [21] confirm the present study results.

In the current study, unlike other researches in this field [3, 15, 17, 22], the factor of fear of the consequences of reporting had approximately the same mean score as the factor of managerial. Among the studied variables in the factor of fear of the consequences of reporting, "fear of judicial issues following reporting on medication errors" was introduced as the most important variable influencing not reporting on medication errors.

One of the new trends that are emerging today and should be paid particular attention is patients' litigation against possible and unwanted medical errors and malpractices throughout the diagnosis and treatment processes [23]. Kouhestani and Baghcheghi in their study had reported "fear of the impact of reporting of errors on the students' evaluation scores and their educational outcomes" as the most important variable in the factor of fear of the consequences of reporting which does not confirm the present study results. The difference between the population studies of these two studies can be a reason for the results differences [19]. However, the results of Tol and colleagues' study confirm this result of the present study [16].

Among the studied variables related to the process of reporting, "lack of a clear definition of medication errors" was the most important variable influencing not reporting on medication errors from the studied nurses' viewpoints. Hosseinzadeh and colleagues showed similar results in their study [21]; however, the results of Tol and colleagues' study [16] as well as Kouhestani and Baghcheghi's study [19], which had introduced "not paying attention to the reporting on some medication errors" as the most important reason for not reporting on medication errors, do not confirm the present study results in the mentioned domain.

Nurses are the second group protecting against medication errors because they play an important role in the distribution, preparation, and administration of medication orders [24].

Nurses' proper and appropriate function of reporting on medication errors will prevent doing possible harm to the patients and also is considered as a source of valuable

TABLE 2: The frequency (%), mean, and standard deviation of nurses' responses to the variables based on their importance in occurring medication errors from their viewpoints.

Factors	Variables	Strongly agree *F* (%)	Agree *F* (%)	Scale neutral *F* (%)	Disagree *F* (%)	Strongly disagree *F* (%)	Mean ± SD *F* (%)	Mean ± SD total
Fear of the consequences of reporting	Fear of the impact of reporting of errors on the personnel's annual evaluation	13 (15.9%)	19 (23.2%)	8 (9.8%)	30 (36.6%)	12 (14.6%)	3.11 ± 1.35	3.01 ± 1.039
	Fear of the impact of reporting of errors on their salary and benefits	10 (12.2%)	25 (30.5%)	11 (13.4%)	28 (34.1%)	8 (9.8%)	2.99 ± 1.24	
	Fear of being blamed by nursing heads	6 (7.2%)	16 (19.3%)	7 (8.4%)	34 (41%)	20 (24.1%)	3.55 ± 1.25	
	Fear of being blamed by doctors	9 (11%)	18 (22%)	7 (8.5%)	33 (40.2%)	15 (18.3%)	3.33 ± 1.30	
	Fear of being blamed by colleagues	16 (9.8%)	31 (38.3%)	13 (16%)	16 (19.8%)	5 (6.2%)	3.54 ± 1.19	
	Fear of producing side effects in patients	11 (13.8%)	14 (17.5%)	2 (2.5%)	29 (36.3%)	24 (30%)	3.51 ± 1.43	
	Fear of being labeled as incompetent nurses and inadequacy	14 (17.1%)	17 (20.7%)	8 (8.9%)	32 (39%)	11 (13.4%)	3.11 ± 1.35	
	Fear of colleagues' behavior	13 (15.9%)	27 (32.9%)	14 (17.1%)	19 (23.2%)	9 (11%)	2.8 ± 1.27	
	Fear of expressing a negative attitude towards the nurse(s) making errors by the patient and his/her family	5 (6.2%)	17 (21%)	7 (8.6%)	39 (48.1%)	13 (16%)	3.47 ± 1.17	
	Fear of judicial issues following reporting on medication errors	6 (7.4%)	11 (13.6%)	7 (8.6%)	36 (44.4%)	21 (25.9%)	3.68 ± 1.21	
	Fear of informing colleagues working in other units and other facilities about one's medication error	4 (4.9%)	19 (23.5%)	8 (9.9%)	34 (42%)	16 (19.8%)	3.48 ± 1.19	
Managerial factors	Lack of receiving positive feedback from the nursing heads following to report on medication errors	4 (4.8%)	17 (20.5%)	10 (12%)	28 (33.7%)	24 (28.9%)	3.61 ± 1.24	3.56 ± 0.99
	False beliefs in nursing heads and managers	5 (6%)	19 (22.9%)	12 (14.5%)	27 (32.5%)	20 (24.1%)	3.46 ± 1.25	
	The heads' focus only on finding the culprits and blaming them, regardless of other factors involved in the occurrence of errors	5 (6%)	12 (14.5%)	12 (14.5%)	30 (36.1%)	24 (28.9%)	3.67 ± 1.21	
	Disproportionate reactions of the heads to the error seriousness	4 (4.8%)	20 (24.1%)	2 (2.4%)	35 (42.2%)	22 (26.5%)	3.24 ± 1.61	
	Disproportionate reactions of the heads to the error importance	3 (3.7%)	22 (27.2%)	9 (11.1)	25 (30.9)	22 (27.2%)	3.50 ± 1.25	
Factors related to the process of reporting	Not paying attention to the reporting on some medication errors	21 (25.6)	14 (17.1%)	11 (13.4%)	28 (34.1%)	8 (9.8%)	2.85 ± 1.39	3.32 ± 0.79
	Lack of a clear definition of medication errors	8 (9.6%)	25 (30.1%)	11 (13.3%)	25 (30.1%)	14 (16.9%)	3.14 ± 1.28	
	To forget reporting on the medication errors	13 (15.7%)	20 (24.1%)	11 (13.3%)	28 (33.7%)	11 (13.3%)	3.05 ± 1.32	

information to avoid occurring similar errors in the future and finally can dramatically provide safety for patients [15]. In other words, it can be said that as a rule, making errors is inevitable; however, reporting them and following their subsequent harm can prevent recurrence of those errors for the other patients [25].

The present study had some limitations such as studying only on one hospital and a small sample as well as its limitation of results generalizability. Therefore, it is suggested that similar studies should be carried out on other public and also private hospitals using large samples and population studies, and then those results should be compared with the present study results. Also, future studies should be conducted using interventional designs to identify the major causes of occurring medication errors, other reasons for not reporting them, and strategies to prevent or reduce their occurrence.

5. Conclusion

The current study results showed that managerial factors had the greatest role in the refusal of reporting on medication errors. Therefore, designing a system for reporting on medication errors properly and accurately, training nurses in the quality of reporting on medication errors, and above all, establishing a mechanism to improve quality rather than focus only on finding the culprits and blaming them can result in more reporting on medication errors, reducing their occurrence, and, finally, improving patient safety.

Acknowledgment

The authors would like to thank the hospital's heads and nursing staff of Abbasi Hospital for their kind cooperation with the researchers in collecting and analyzing the data.

References

[1] World Alliance for Patient Safety Forward Programme, "2008," Geneva, Switzerland, 2004, http://www.who.int/patient-safety/en.

[2] R. Westat, J. Sorra, T. Famolaro, M. P. S. N. Dyer, K. Khanna, and D. Nelson, *Hospital Survey on Patient Safety Culture: 2010 User Comparative Database Report*, 2010.

[3] K. M. Stratton, M. A. Blegen, G. Pepper, and T. Vaughn, "Reporting of medication errors by pediatric nurses," *Journal of Pediatric Nursing*, vol. 19, no. 6, pp. 385–392, 2004.

[4] E. L. Allan and K. N. Barker, "Fundamentals of medication error research," *American Journal of Hospital Pharmacy*, vol. 47, no. 3, pp. 555–571, 1990.

[5] S. Bodur and E. Filiz, "Validity and reliability of Turkish version of "hospital survey on patient safety culture" and perception of patient safety in public hospitals in Turkey," *BMC Health Services Research*, vol. 10, article 28, 2010.

[6] P. Aspden, *Patient Safety: Achieving a New Standard For Care*, National Academy Press, Washington, DC, USA, 2004.

[7] T. A. Brennan, L. L. Leape, N. M. Laird et al., "Incidence of adverse events and negligence in hospitalized patients: results of the Harvard Medical Practice Study I," *Quality & Safety in Health Care*, vol. 13, no. 2, pp. 145–151, 2004.

[8] M. Zegers, M. C. De Bruijne, C. Wagner et al., "Adverse events and potentially preventable deaths in Dutch hospitals: results of a retrospective patient record review study," *Quality and Safety in Health Care*, vol. 18, no. 4, pp. 297–302, 2009.

[9] A. Milstein, R. S. Galvin, S. F. Delbanco et al., "Improving the safety of health care: the leapfrog initiative," *Effective Clinical Practice*, vol. 3, no. 6, pp. 313–316, 2000.

[10] D. W. Bates, D. J. Cullen, N. Laird et al., "Incidence of adverse drug events and potential adverse drug events," *Journal of the American Medical Association*, vol. 274, no. 1, pp. 29–34, 1995.

[11] R. A. Hansen, S. B. Greene, C. E. Williams et al., "Types of medication errors in north carolina nursing homes: a target for quality improvement," *American Journal Geriatric Pharmacotherapy*, vol. 4, no. 1, pp. 52–61, 2006.

[12] C. U. Lehmann, K. G. Conner, and J. M. Cox, "Preventing provider errors: online total parenteral nutrition calculator," *Pediatrics*, vol. 113, no. 4 I, pp. 748–753, 2004.

[13] D. J. Anderson and C. S. Webster, "A systems approach to the reduction of medication error on the hospital ward," *Journal of Advanced Nursing*, vol. 35, no. 1, pp. 34–41, 2001.

[14] M. T. Mrayyan, K. Shishani, and I. Al-Faouri, "Rate, causes and reporting of medication errors in Jordan: nurses' perspectives," *Journal of Nursing Management*, vol. 15, no. 6, pp. 659–670, 2007.

[15] H. Y. Chiang and G. A. Pepper, "Barriers to nurses' reporting of medication administration errors in Taiwan," *Journal of Nursing Scholarship*, vol. 38, no. 4, pp. 392–399, 2006.

[16] A. Tol, A. Pourreza, G. Sharifirad, B. Mohebbi, and Z. Gazi, "The causes of not reporting medication errors from the viewpoints of nursing in baharlo hospital," *Journal of Hospital*, vol. 9, no. 1-2, pp. 19–24, 2011.

[17] D. S. Wakefield, B. J. Wakefield, T. Uden-Holman, T. Borders, M. Blegen, and T. Vaughn, "Understanding why medication administration errors may not be reported," *American Journal of Medical Quality*, vol. 14, no. 2, pp. 81–88, 1999.

[18] H. Kawamura, "The approaches to factors which cause medication error–from the analyses of many near-miss cases related to intravenous medication which nurses experienced," *Japanese Journal of Cancer and Chemotherapy*, vol. 28, no. 3, pp. 304–309, 2001.

[19] H. Kouhestani and N. Baghcheghi, "Refusal in reporting medication errors from the viewpoints of nursing students in arak university of medical sciences," *Iranian Journal of Medical Education*, vol. 8, no. 2, pp. 285–292, 2009.

[20] J. Osborne, K. Blais, and J. S. Hayes, "Nurses' perceptions: when is it a medication error?" *Journal of Nursing Administration*, vol. 29, no. 4, pp. 33–38, 1999.

[21] M. Hosseinzadeh, P. E. Aghajari, and N. Mahdavi, "Reasons of nurses' medication errors and persepectives of nurses on barriers of error reporting," *Hayat*, vol. 18, no. 2, pp. 66–75, 2012.

[22] M. A. Blegen, T. Vaughn, G. Pepper et al., "Patient and staff safety: voluntary reporting," *American Journal of Medical Quality*, vol. 19, no. 2, pp. 67–74, 2004.

[23] A. Shahraky and M. Hamule, *Principal of Nursing Documentation*, Salemi Population, 2008.

[24] R. G. Hughes and E. Ortiz, "Medication errors: why they happen, and how they can be prevented," *The American Journal of Nursing*, vol. 105, no. supplement 3, pp. 14–24, 2005.

[25] B. L. Marquis and C. J. Huston, *Leadership Roles and Management Functions in Nursing: Theory and Application*, Lippincott Williams & Wilkins, 2008.

Young Registered Nurses' Intention to Leave the Profession and Professional Turnover in Early Career: A Qualitative Case Study

Mervi Flinkman,[1] Ulpukka Isopahkala-Bouret,[2] and Sanna Salanterä[1,3]

[1] *Department of Nursing Science, University of Turku, 20014 Turku, Finland*
[2] *Faculty of Behavioural Sciences, University of Helsinki, P.O. Box 9, 00014 Helsinki, Finland*
[3] *Hospital District of Southwest Finland, Bureau of Administration, Turku University Hospital, P.O. Box 52, 20521 Turku, Finland*

Correspondence should be addressed to Mervi Flinkman; mervi.flinkman@utu.fi

Academic Editors: S. Keeney and J. Scholes

In a time of global nursing shortages an alarming number of young registered nurses have expressed a willingness to leave the profession. In this qualitative case study we investigate in depth why young nurses leave nursing profession and reeducate themselves for a new career. The study is based on longitudinal interviews of three young registered nurses in Finland. These nurses were first interviewed between December 2006 and May 2007, when they were 29–32 years old and having an intention to leave the profession. The second interview took place four years later, from January 2011 to March 2011 when all of them had made the transition to a new career. Data were analyzed in two stages. In the first stage, comprehensive career story narratives were formed on the basis of the interviews. In the second stage, emerging themes in these stories were compared, contrasted, and interpreted in the context of the overall career histories. Nursing as a second career choice and demanding work content as well as poor practice environment and the inability to identify with the stereotypical images of nurses were main themes that emerged from these career stories. The results of this interpretative qualitative study reflect a shift toward insights into understanding professional turnover as a complex and long-lasting process.

1. Introduction

Nurses are the largest group of professionals within the global health care system, with a total of 19.3 million nursing and midwifery personnel in the world [1]. The current and growing shortage of registered nurses (RNs) in health care systems is thus a global concern [2, 3]. In fact, the European Commission has estimated that there will be a shortage of 590,000 nurses by the year 2020 [4]. In the United States, employment of RNs is expected to grow faster than the expected average for all occupations [5]. Most countries within the Organization for Economic Cooperation and Development (OECD) have reported a nursing shortage [6], which is predicted to get worse because the current nursing population is aging [7]. This shortage of RNs influences the delivery of health care and negatively affects patient outcomes; an insufficient nurse staffing level is associated with negative patient outcomes [8, 9] and decreased nurse job satisfaction [10].

At the same time of this global nursing shortage, many nurses are considering leaving their job, profession or are out of the nursing workforce. According to Flinkman et al. [11] literature review, nurses' intention to leave the profession varied from 4% up to 54% across the studies internationally. In a NEXT (nurses early exit) study, conducted in ten European countries (N = 30,330), 13% of nurses had thought about leaving the profession frequently [12]. According to an RN4CAST (nurse forecasting in Europe) study (N = 33,659 nurses/Europe; 27,509 nurses/United States), the proportion of nurses planning to leave their current job ranged from 49% (Finland, Greece) to 14% (United States) [13]. In European sample of this study, every tenth (9%) of nurses was having intention to leave the profession [14]. Furthermore, in Salminen [15] study, nearly half (37%, N = 343) of young RNs (under 35 years) working in hospitals have reported frequent intention to leave the profession in Finland. In Sweden, 10–20% of new graduates have considered leaving the profession [16]. In the United States, it was reported that the percentage of RNs intending to leave nursing within 3 years was low, at 3%. Yet, of the total licensed RN population in 2008, it was estimated that more than 15% (n = 466,564) were not actually employed within nursing [17].

Turnover intention appears to be a multistage process consisting of psychological, cognitive, and behavioral components [18] and has been found to predict the actual decision to leave the profession [12, 19, 20]. According to a study by Hasselhorn et al. [12], the majority of leavers began the process with serious consideration in the final year preceding leaving, and the actual decision to leave was then made within the 6 months prior to determination. In Carless and Arnup's [21] study, one year prior to changing careers, actual career changers were actively looking for a new career and had a high intention to leave their current job. Furthermore, another study revealed that nurses left nursing within 6 months of their decision to leave [22]. The final decision to leave the profession is likely to be the result of an individual reflection process [21, 23] with multiple underlying causes [11, 12].

From the society's and healthcare's points of view, professional turnover is a more significant form of work transitions than organizational turnover [24, 25]. Those RNs, who are leaving the profession, are reducing the total number of nurses in the manpower, which has an impact on the present nursing shortage [2] and is leading to a permanent loss of productivity [18]. Nurses leaving the profession take their tacit knowledge, experience, and contribution from the organizations and also from the nursing workforce [11]. The financial investments used on nurse's education, orientation, and continuing education are lost. Moreover, nurse turnover is also costly to organizations: first, because it results in the direct and indirect costs of filling the positions, and second, because of the loss of organizational productivity and knowledge [26].

The youngest generation of nurses are the most willing to leave the job and the nursing profession [12, 15, 16, 27, 28]. Kovner and Djukic [29] have reported that in the United States more RN graduates left their first nursing job (26%) than nursing profession (2%) during the first two years in career. According to NEXT study [12], in most European countries the intent to leave the profession was highest in the age groups between 25 and 35 years of age. In Robinson et al. [30] study, diploma-qualified nurses' movement into other activities was highest around the age of 28 and declined thereafter. According to Barron and West [31] study, rate of leaving the nursing profession for a better job was highest at the age of 32. However, conflicting findings also exist. According to an RN4CAST-study, older nurses were having higher intention to leave the profession than younger nurses [14].

Several factors are related to young RNs' intentions to leave the profession, including an imbalance of effort and reward, high psychological demands, and higher job strain, which all influence young nurses' intention to resign from their nursing careers [32]. According to a Swedish study of Rudman et al. [16], graduates of a younger age are more vulnerable to early career burnout, which is associated with the intention to leave the profession. In a study by Flinkman et al. [33], both the survey questionnaire and the open-ended questions showed that young nurses' intentions to leave the profession were connected with the highly demanding work, burnout and dissatisfaction with salary levels.

Experiences of resent graduates have been widely examined in the nursing research [34–36]. However, less research is available concerning graduate nurses' intention to leave the profession. In a study by Scott et al. [37], graduates (mean age 29) who did not like being a nurse reported a higher desire to leave the profession. In a study by Lavoie-Tremblay et al. [38], those young graduates (24 or younger) who reported having poor work environment, were more likely to state they would leave the profession.

Most of the earlier turnover research is concerned with nurses leaving the job or the organization [27]; less research is conducted on what motivates nurses to leave their profession [11, 25]. This is understandable, because nurse turnover is expensive and organizations are usually more concerned with their own nursing manpower than workforce in a whole [11]. Studies concerning nurses' turnover and their intent to leave the profession have been mainly executed using quantitative methods and survey questionnaires [11, 27, 39], revealing the need to explore this phenomenon using qualitative methods and to produce studies with more in-depth understanding. Accordingly, qualitative research and research from generational perspective has been recommended in order to get a more comprehensive picture of turnover [27, 40].

Knowing that young nurses' transition from a student to nursing career is a demanding and stressful process and thus could lead to nurse turnover from the profession [37, 38], it is important to explore views and perceptions regarding early career experiences from the young nurses point of view. Therefore, the aim of this study was to gain a deeper understanding of young nurses' career transition processes, as experienced by young registered nurse, aged between 29 and 32 years. Young registered nurse (RN) in this study refers to a person who has completed Bachelor of Health Care degree in the University of Applied Sciences and whose intention to leave the profession has started before the age of 30 years.

2. Material and Methods

2.1. Design. This inquiry has been designed as a longitudinal qualitative case study using interpretive narrative method. A "case" is being defined as a longitudinal career story interpreted by a young registered nurse.

2.2. Theoretical Framework. This is a qualitative case study [41], in which an interpretative narrative approach [42, 43] is adopted. Qualitative case study has been defined as a research methodology grounded in an interpretive, constructivist paradigm [41]. Case studies often contain narratives that approach the complexities and contradictions of real life [44] and can be used for exploring, describing, and understanding a phenomenon in its context [44, 45]. An intensive investigation of cases can provide contextual knowledge of real-life phenomena that would be unobtainable with a population-based approach [45]. Case-centred research can add knowledge of how people experience career transitions and construct new career identities [46].

According to Sharp [47] case-centred approaches are an excellent and relevant way of doing nursing research, because nursing practice is centred on cases (patients and in broader sense organizations and social context). Even though "nurses have not fully embraced case study as a comprehensive approach for research" [45, page 103], case studies can be seen as an option for many nursing studies, because it allows to use various sources of evidence and it has a potential to uncover multiple realities [48].

Both the interview material and data analysis method in this study can be defined as narrative. The underlying assumption of narrative inquiry is the idea that individuals make sense of their world by telling stories [49]. Narrative approach does not assume objectivity, but rather it privileges positionality, pluralism, relativism, and subjectivity [50, 51]. There is an underlying assumption in a narrative approach that "there is neither a single, absolute truth in human reality nor one correct reading or interpretation of a text" [50, page 2]. Narrative turn is a part of a paradigmatic shift from realism toward constructivism in science, which then further refers to fundamental changes in beliefs concerning reality and knowledge [52].

Events in a narrative are selected, organized, connected, and evaluated in accordance with the audience to which the narrative is told (e.g., the interviewer) [53]. Interpretation is inevitable because stories are representations, and a researcher does not have direct access to another's experiences [51]. Stories are usually composed and received in context, telling much about the society, culture, and the social reality the teller is living in [54]. Stories are a way for a person to make sense of disruptive events in their lives or when there has been a breach between the ideal and real, self and society [51].

Cochran [55] suggests that narrative study is a paradigm in career research, because the topic of the career is not ultimately focused on the distinct parts of the story but instead on how the different elements of a professional history are interrelated and brought together. Transitions from one profession to another involve always narrative reflection [56]. By narrating their professional history and transitions, people try to find a meaningful connection between their past and new careers [46]. A successful transition to a new workplace or occupation could be considered as completed once a person is able to resolve the conflicts and contradictions in his or her career narrative [57].

2.3. Recruitment Procedure and the Participants. The selection of participants was purposeful [53], as we were seeking "key informants" or "critical cases" that were knowledgeable about the phenomenon of interest [44]. In the year 2006, we invited young nurses to write the narrative stories of their nursing careers and why they had an intention to leave nursing. We advertised in *Tehy*—the magazine of the Union of Health and Social Care Professionals—and in an open discussion forum for nurses via the Internet (http://www.hoitajat.net). To be eligible for the study, we required the participants to

(i) be a registered nurse,

(ii) have work experience in nursing,

(iii) have an intention to leave a nursing profession that had started before the age of 30,

(iv) have a willingness to articulate, and reflect upon, their experiences in their nursing career.

We requested that they add their contact information if they wanted participate the interviews concerning the intention of leaving the nursing profession.

Three young female registered nurses were willing to tell their story to the interviewer and met the inclusion criteria. We decided to accomplish longitudinal career story interviews with these three nurses in order to get an in-depth understanding of the phenomenon of interest. We considered that three young nurses was a sufficient number, because in case study method sample sizes are nonrepresentative [47] and narrative interview data usually accumulate with a large quantity of rich data [51]. The participants were 29–32 years old during the course of the first interview. The nurses were living in different parts of Finland, one in a large city and the remaining two in smaller cities. They all had degrees of Bachelor of Health Care. Nursing education in Finland is arranged in universities of applied sciences, and study consists of 210 credit points.

2.4. Conducting the Interviews. Young nurses were interviewed twice. The first author conducted all of the interviews: a female researcher who was at the time in her 30s, a registered nurse, and a PhD student in nursing science. The process of gathering the initial data was conducted between December 2006 and May 2007. In the beginning of the first interview the interviewees were asked to draw—on A3-sized paper—their pathway as a nurse and put into this drawing the significant events in, and experiences of, their nursing career. Narratives of personal experiences or life stories are often told in response to open-ended questions, which do not limit or specify the type and the form of the narrative [58]. In the first interview, an open question was posed: *"I would like you to tell me, freely and with your own words, your story as a nurse. You can start your story at any point of your life that you have felt to be significant for you becoming a nurse. You can end your story at any point in your life that you want."* After this open-ended question, the interviewer acted as an active listener and avoided interrupting the participant's narrative.

When the complete story had been obtained, some detailed relevant questions were presented to encourage further elaboration on the narrative (e.g., "*could you tell more about why you applied to nursing school?*"). Further questioning helps participants to recall details, turning points, and other meaningful events in their narrative story [53]. In the last phase of the interview, the interviewer asked the participant whether she wanted to say anything else; the interviews ended when the participant did not want to add anything further.

The second interviews took place four years later, between January and March 2011, when all of these young nurses had made the transition to a new career. In the beginning of the second interview, the participants were asked to continue their earlier career-pathway drawing and were asked to continue their story of being a nurse from any point in their life that they chose.

The lengths of the interviews varied from 113 minutes (longest first interview) to 25 minutes (shortest second interview). One nurse chose to be interviewed at her workplace, and the other participants were interviewed in their homes. Interviews were recorded on a digital recorder and were transcribed verbatim by the first author, because analysis and interpretation of such data depends on the adequacy of a carefully prepared manuscript [59].

2.5. Data Analysis. Narrative data guided the data analysis method we chose for this inquiry. Data were analyzed in two stages. Firstly, we followed the holistic-content method developed by Lieblich et al. [50], where the life story of a person is taken as a whole; researchers studying life histories and case studies also use this approach. After the first readings of the data, the first author formed three career story narratives on the basis of the interviews, career-pathway drawings and written stories. In these narratives, the first author selected and organized the separate events from the nurses' careers into complete narratives with a chronological order. Polkinghorne [42] describes this kind of method as narrative analysis, where the researcher configures a new narrative on the basis of the narrative material. These career stories were then reviewed and discussed with the coauthors.

We found in the preliminary readings that while these narratives were unique, certain main themes also appeared to be reflected both within and between these stories. A thematic approach to narratives is useful when trying to find common thematic elements across research participants and the events they report [53]. As Sandelowski and Leeman [60, page 1407] conclude, "The identification of themes is foundational to qualitative research of all kinds". The first author followed these particular themes throughout the stories and compared, contrasted, and interpreted these themes in the context of the overall career histories. These emerging interpretations and themes were discussed, reviewed, and refined with the coauthors. The results of the analysis are reported in accordance with these themes. By presenting cases and themes simultaneously it was possible to reach a more holistic and multidimensional perspective to these stories.

2.6. Trustworthiness. To evaluate the validity of narrative studies, Riessman [43] argues that it is trustworthiness, rather than truth, which should be evaluated in narrative studies. We established the trustworthiness for this study in four ways. First, our data analysis is described in detail, and direct citations from the narratives are provided in relation to each story to reveal the basis from which the analysis was conducted. According to Polkinghorne [61, page 6], "Readers should be able to follow the presented evidence and argument enough to make their own judgment as to the relative validity of the claim." Second, we used data triangulation (narrative interviews, career-pathway drawings, and written stories) to enhance the trustworthiness of the analysis. Third, the narrative stories and themes were reviewed in research seminars in a doctoral school of nursing science and in a narrative summer school to ensure that the chosen themes resonated with the narrative stories. Fourth, the accuracy was reviewed by sending the final paper draft to the participants, to allow them to verify the authenticity of the data and ensure that they agreed with the interpretations. As the original transcripts were in Finnish, the citations used in this paper have been translated into English by a professional translator in order to reproduce the citations as accurately as possible and maintain the authenticity of the participant's responses.

2.7. Ethical Considerations. We followed the ethical guidelines described by the Finnish Advisory Board on Research Integrity [62]. The participants gave their oral and written informed consent to participation. We informed them that they had the right to withdraw at any stage, and that the collected data would be treated with confidentiality. We removed the following details from the career stories: places of residence, names of the health care organization, names of family members, and names of colleagues. We also changed some minor details in these career stories, which we considered to be insignificant, in order to protect participants' identity. Furthermore, we used pseudonyms to protect participant anonymity. Because nurses participated voluntarily and in their leisure time, no additional ethical committee approval was needed.

3. Results and Discussion

3.1. Starting the Stories: Introducing the Career Story Narrators. At the time of the first interview, Anna (a pseudonym) was a young woman at a crossroad in her nursing career. She showed a strong intention for a career change, yet at the same time she was tired and distressed because she was not sure how such a career change would be possible. Anna was very analytical and told her story in an animated way. Her narrative was detailed, complex, and often included cynical humor and sarcasm; she also often vocalized direct quotations from other people's speech to make parts of her narrative more dramatic. Anna used a great amount of time in the first interview analyzing what she wanted for her future career and what she might be capable of doing if she were to leave nursing work. She had talked about this career change with her relatives and friends and had thought deeply about the advantages and disadvantages of leaving the nursing profession.

Betty (a pseudonym) already had a new university education at the time of her first interview. She told her story in a good-humored way, often laughing. During her story, Betty mentioned frequently that her nursing job had mostly been "nice" and the patients were also mostly "nice". There were some more dramatic stories—for example, an unsuccessful resuscitation of a small baby—but mainly her nursing career story was positive and optimistic. She had, however, stayed in her nursing career for quite a short time.

Cecilia (a pseudonym) was very calm and analytical when telling her story. Her narratives were well structured, and she used a flowing narrative style to tell her stories. Cecilia had mainly enjoyed nursing work and taking care of patients. She had a strong sense of treating other people in a fair and just way. During her time at the nursing school confidential tasks were already being given to Cecilia, and teachers were saying that she would become a good teacher. She had already begun to be interested in management when she was in the nursing school and was willing to develop herself professionally from the beginning of her nursing career.

3.2. Theme One: Nursing as a Second Career Choice. When Anna was in both grammar school and high school, she had no intention of becoming a nurse. She considered many careers, for example, a veterinarian or journalist, but was not sure, or at least confident, of what she wanted to do in her forthcoming career. After high school she applied to university to read nonnursing discipline but was not accepted. She was at that time in practical training in a hospital and liked the work, despite the fact that it was not exactly the work she was considering as a career choice. Not knowing what else to do, she however applied to a nursing school and was accepted. Anna related that she did not know anything about nursing when she was applying to nursing school, but she was confident that she was never going to work as a bedside nurse. In the admission test she achieved a very high overall score but a low motivation score. In her retrospective analysis she reflected that the test had probably quite accurately measured the reality of the situation: she was not especially eager to get into the nursing school. At that time her mother and friends had said that a career in nursing might not be right for Anna's personality.

> *Well, it was some sort of drifting, that I had never any kind of calling. And then I thought that I really did not know where to apply, so then it was the nursing school, because perhaps nursing was something kind of similar to psychology, although I did not really want to admit to myself that it wasn't really like that.*

Betty was also not interested in a nursing career when she was in high school. After high school Betty applied to university but, disappointingly for her, was not accepted. She was doing voluntary work during a "gap" year and through this became interested in nursing work. She decided to apply for a nursing education because she thought that nursing could be a stepping stone for working in developing countries or in becoming a physician. At the very beginning of her nursing studies she had already started to hesitate: was she choosing the right career? In the beginning of her story she recalled

> *I do not even know how to say why I ended up becoming a nurse, but I feel that I have sort of drifted or something.*

Cecilia too believed that she became a nurse through serendipity, and a nursing career had not been a childhood dream for her either. After high school Cecilia decided to move abroad and to start university studies there. Before leaving, Cecilia was working for a few months in a hospital and started to consider what it would be like to be a nurse. Coincidentally she noticed an advertisement for the nursing studies in a newspaper, decided to apply, and was accepted. One of her relatives had worked in a hospital when Cecilia was a small child. She thought that there was a certain attraction to nursing work, although at the same time the hospital was quite a frightening place, with white working clothes and with peculiar smells. She recalled

> *But a nursing career was never a dream job for me. It's not as if I had thought that I would like to work in a hospital. Maybe this has been more like destiny that I have gone there.*

Even though these young nurses did not have nursing as a first career option, they all graduated from nursing school with good grades. They also all received positive feedback from the school and from clinical practices, and their memories from the nursing school were mainly positive in their narratives.

3.3. Theme Two: Demanding Work Content and Poor Practice Environment. Since the beginning of her nursing career, Anna had been working in a ward where many patient were alcoholic, drug abusers, or elderly patients with no hope of recovery. She said that she did not like the routine tasks related to patient hygiene and housekeeping within the ward. Anna did not like working close to the patients; she highlighted nursing tasks that were menial, unpleasant, and intimate. Perhaps because of the work-related burnout, she recalled

> *I'm just so irritated by our patients to be honest. When we think of the picture that the so-called "normal" people have of a hospital, that there nurses take care of car-crash patients and make them healthy and heal them and all kinds of things. And the reality is some are intoxicated, some alcoholic, and then there are old people with many diseases whose nursing feels more like torturing them.*

Betty also had to take on a great deal of responsibility as a graduate nurse: in some wards she was the only RN during a shift, as all the others were nursing aids. There was insufficient staffing level, and patient care was demanding. When she was employed in her last summer job as a nurse she thought that the nurses where she was working had an increased workload, and that they were extremely busy. She was no longer enjoying nursing work, and she felt that being productive was seen as more important than taking good care of the patients. She told a story about one nightshift when the workload was almost overwhelming

> *That hospital, it was a place like, it was really something like eight people in the same room and*

some of those people were screaming all night long. That's also when I thought that this is not making any sense! And there's two of us nurses and over forty patients on the wards. That was totally insane.

Cecilia liked nursing work related to the patients and their care and enjoyed both the atmosphere of the workplace and her coworkers. The nursing job was demanding but also rewarding. At the same time as relating how much she liked her job, Cecilia also verbalized feelings of guilt and of being burdened because she thought that she was unable to provide the level of care that she considered adequate. She told a story of her last summer in the hospital when there were many inexperienced doctors on the ward. She had subsequently thought that she had to supervise and look after those doctors. She recalls

We had had some really difficult patient cases and that summer for some reason there happened to be some really, really inexperienced doctors at the beginning of their careers, candidates of medical science, and all the time you had to be kind of mentoring their actions. It felt like you had to watch out all the time, and that besides your own work you kind of had to also take care of how everything else runs there.

There was a strong hierarchy in the hospitals, and the lowest in the hierarchy were nursing students—in some workplaces they were not even permitted to go into the coffee room—yet graduate nurses and new nurses in the ward were also low down. Betty noticed during her nursing education that medical students were even lower in the hierarchy than nursing students; after this realisation she decided against pursuing a medical career. Strong hierarchy was a disappointment for these young nurses; however, they felt that they could not change the situation.

During her interviews, Cecilia often recounted her experiences of poor management in the hospital. For example, she had supervised students, often using her own leisure time to do so, but these efforts were not compensated; furthermore, she had lacked feedback about what she was good at, and what she needed to do in order to develop. She had wanted to participate in further education, but as a temporary worker she was not offered this possibility. Cecilia felt that managers in the hospital did not actually understand how demanding the nurses' work was, and that they had very unrealistic proposals about how to develop patient care. She also confronted ethical problems in the ward; she felt that nurses in the ward were not able to provide humane and proper care. She recalled

And then, like I told you, my husband came to pick me up from work and then I started to cry that I cannot take this anymore, this is terrible, I cannot. I cannot, I feel like nobody takes good care of these patients.

Anna felt that nursing would not provide her with intellectual challenges after a few years of work, and that nurses had no career development possibilities. Similarly, Betty had sought career development opportunities but was not able to see the potential for pursuing them in her nursing career; she had hoped that nurses would have some kind of career ladder, to allow for such progress. Thus, this lack of professional development was a common concern, as expressed by Betty

I find it kind of terrible to think that you graduate as a nurse and then you will be a nurse for the rest of your life. That maybe you move from one ward to another ward or from place to place but the work is always the same everywhere.

All of these nurses were dissatisfied with their salaries. Anna thought that even a much higher salary would not compensate for work that was otherwise unsatisfactory. Betty said that the salary was too low when compared to the responsibilities of nursing work; she was getting a better salary in her new job outside nursing, even though there she was not able to "kill anyone." She also thought that higher salaries would improve the image of nursing.

Anna, Betty, and Cecilia all did shift work during their nursing career. Combining private life with shift work was demanding for them, because they found planning their lives around it challenging. Recovering from night shifts was also difficult, because it was hard to be awake at nights and sleep during the day. Betty, furthermore, said that if she did not get enough sleep, she was prone to suffer from migraines.

All of these nurses were working under fixed-term contracts at the beginning of their career, because during the economic depression, graduate nurses were mainly offered only fixed-term employments. Anna felt that the charge-nurse in the ward was using fixed-term contracts as a way to exert power. This power relation changed when there started to be a shortage of nurses in the ward, which provided Anna with a bargaining opportunity. After telling the ward sister that she was looking for a new job, she was offered longer fixed-term contracts. Anna finally secured a permanent work contract after a few years. She thought that getting a permanent job was a good thing for gaining control over one's own life, although at the same time she also thought that she was then somewhat "trapped."

There were these fixed-term contracts which could be from two weeks to three months or then for six months. They couldn't give me their word that there would be longer periods which made me feel really insecure when I thought about my future.

Betty did not work in nursing for long and only with temporary work contracts. While studying for a new career she worked for short periods in numerous hospitals. In some places there was no proper orientation for the job, and there was no support for a recently graduated, inexperienced nurse. Cecilia also started with temporary work contracts, working in many different hospitals. She had the possibility to apply for a permanent contract but never did so; she did not want a permanent job because she was sure that she was not going to work for the next forty years as a nurse.

3.4. Theme Three: The Inability to Identify with the Stereotypical Images of Nurses. Within the narratives, all these young nurses described what kind of people nurses are: nurturing, altruistic, and willing to serve. They did not, however, place themselves within these expected images of nurses. In their stories, these young nurses narrate nursing as a profession, not as a vocational calling. They construct themselves as talented and ambitious and striving for career advancement. Throughout Anna' story, she described herself as intellectual, creative, and systematic, but that she was not able to use any of these qualities in nursing. She thought that many other nurses were hoping to change career but found it impossible because of the demands of their families. Her boyfriend concurred, as he had said that she was too bright and talented for a nursing work

> *My husband used to tell me "well with that mind, with those talents, with that brain, it is obvious you're not going to enjoy it there", that he has always been saying to me that you're in the wrong profession.*

Betty also related that she had not been a nurturer when she was a child. When Betty applied to the nursing school, her parents said that she was too ambitious for a nursing career, and that she would not stay in nursing for long. However, Betty was a strong-minded woman and decided at that time to continue, despite her parents' worries. After graduation, Cecilia worked on a ward taking care of elderly patients. She was afraid that she was going to be "stuck" in that ward, where she was not capable of using her knowledge and talents as a nurse. Cecilia also produced stereotypical images of nurses in her stories: she described that nurses had a role within the hospital of the physicians' handmaids. She thought that nurses had a lower professional status in the hospital than physicians and that a nurse's role was not autonomous.

> *Nurses are physicians' handmaids in the hospital. So developing your own thinking skills, development, was kind of incomplete.*

Anna also said that people did not know what the nursing profession requires. She also thought that the average person did not know how demanding the nursing job is or how many skills nursing work requires, and that she did not like the stereotypical picture of nurses given in the media and on television

> *I'm disgusted by the word "Nursey" who's just the typical sort of little blond scrubber that just fools around with the doctors and giggles and puts her cool hand to the feverish patient's forehead wearing a short skirt with her bottom up.*

3.5. Life in a New Career: The End of the Story? In her search for a new career Anna tried to discover one that would better suit her personality as an intellectual, creative, and systematic person. Her decision for changing careers had started as a "sinking" feeling, although the interviews did not reveal a single instance where this intention would have started. This transition process had lasted for many years and was difficult for Anna; indeed a number of times during the interview she remembered that she had often cried and had occasionally felt very tired. However, she presented herself as an active actor who had the power to change a situation that was not satisfactory to her. After the first interview Anna applied to university for a nonnursing discipline, and was accepted. She graduated, and she found a new workplace outside nursing, and also resigned from her permanent nursing job. Anna was the only one of these three nurses who thought that she would never work as a registered nurse again. As Anna shared

> *I guess it was pretty much the whole thing and many people have asked me why because this is such a dramatic career change. That it is a bunch of various things.*

According to Betty's story, how she ended up in a different career was as serendipitous as her initial choice to become a nurse. A friend had given her an extra application form for the entrance exam to study nonnursing discipline in the university; after sending in the application she decided to prepare carefully for the exam, studied hard, and was accepted. She managed her financial problems while studying by working as a nurse and by living frugally, which required both self-discipline and sacrificing her own comfort. After graduating from a university, she received a demanding work outside the nursing field. At the time of the second interview Betty had some thoughts of continuing her education in university to doctoral level and also doing some nursing work occasionally under temporary contracts. In Finland reregistration is not required, so Betty would have the possibility to return to nursing.

> *At the moment I cannot even imagine what I would be if I had not gone through the nursing school. Although I've thought many times that me being a nurse has been a total waste, that I've been squandering the resources of society or something like that. I think that I would be missing something if I would've not done that. It has given me a lot.*

During the transition process many changes were happening in Cecilia's private life. Her family was very supportive of her career change, because they saw that she was not satisfied with nursing. Cecilia applied to the university to study nonnursing discipline and was accepted. She graduated, and because she was having a university degree, she got a new demanding job in human resource management in a large organization. She enjoyed her new work, even though it was demanding and the workdays were long.

> *I do not know if it has been a bad choice, "cause it has made many things possible, but the choice that I've clearly made intentionally has been to leave" cause I've been thinking that it is possible to do things better. But maybe the path that has leaded me away from nursing to here, where I am now, could've been more direct.*

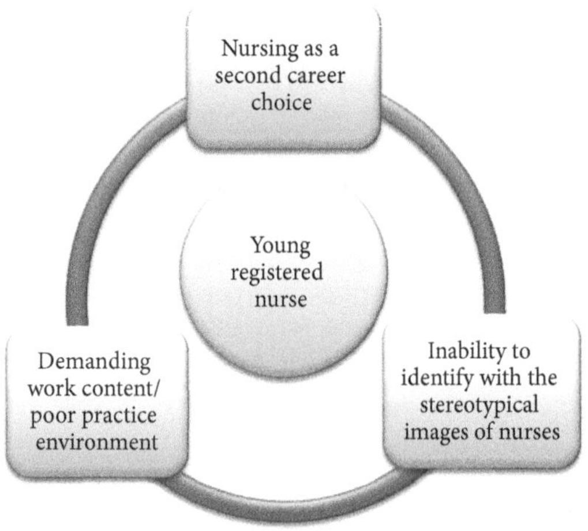

FIGURE 1: Framework enlightening themes associated with young registered nurse career transition.

3.6. Discussion. In this inquiry, we used a qualitative case-study approach to form an in-depth investigation into the reasons why young registered nurses may leave nursing profession. This study produced three rich, detailed accounts of career transition from a perspective of a young generation. The results of this exploratory qualitative study reflect a shift toward insights into understanding professional turnover as a complex and long-lasting process. These transition processes cannot be simply captured with questionnaires. This could be one reason why earlier quantitative studies do not provide a clear picture of the reasons why nurses leave nursing.

All of these career stories are unique but also have similarities (see Figure 1). Firstly, no single incident triggered the decision to leave nursing. None of these young nurses had nursing as a childhood dream; it was more serendipitous that they had ended up as nurses. The work content of nursing was demanding, and the practice environment was not ideal in terms of nurse-patient ratios, rush, shift hours, working contracts, salary, and general appreciation. Furthermore, these young women felt that they did not fit to the stereotypical picture and image of nurses. And finally, nursing was not able to provide the career development possibilities and intellectual challenges that these women were able to gain by applying to university studies and by starting a new career. Although these nurses narrated their career changes as having happened serendipitously, they also constructed themselves as active and competent actors. Throughout their career transition process, these nurses had the possibility to make financial and personal sacrifices for a new education, and they were supported by their families.

Findings of this inquiry support the work of others; for example, in Takase's [18] literature review turnover intention was described as a multistage process, with a range of factors considered as the antecedents. Additionally, according to Cheung's [63] qualitative interview study of former nurses the decision to leave the profession was a difficult one for nurses, and represents a complex psychological process. The case studies here present three phases of a career transition: nurses reassessed their work; they began the transition process (e.g., by getting a new education); and finally there was a socialization phase for the new job. Trice and Morand [64] described similar phases based on the literature: separation from the old role, transition, and then integration into the new role. As typical for voluntary career transitions these nurses had both time and the possibility to consider options for new education and for a new career [65]. There was no single particular experience or crisis that made these nurses leave the profession. This is contrary to the findings of Cheung [63] and Morrell [66] studies, and where also a single, jarring event or shock initiated nurse's thoughts of quitting.

As seen in this inquiry, the long-lasting process of career transition can actually start even before young nurses enter the nursing education. None of these nurses who shared their stories held nursing as a childhood dream; they described their career choices as a "second career choice," or that they had "drifted" into nursing, rather than as a purposefully selected occupation. After being a while in a nursing career all of these nurses applied to their primary educational choice, to study at the university. This finding resonates with previous research. Nursing career chosen as a "default choice" [22] or not having nursing as a childhood career dream [67] has been associated with a shorter tenure in nursing. Also a study conducted in Sweden gave similar results; of graduates (N = 672) who were negative or uncertain about their career choice (26%), a majority had considered leaving the profession [68]. In an earlier study by Santamäki et al. [69], approximately one-third of Finnish nurses (35%, N = 3,352) reported that they had chosen nursing coincidentally, or as a second-best alternative. By investigating nurses' longitudinal career stories there is an opportunity to gain understanding of the complex dynamics of why nurses choose their career [70] and how leaving considerations and behaviors evolve over time [40]. However, future research is needed into whether the motives for choosing nursing career affect the length of the career in nursing.

According to these young nurses stories, the work content of nursing was demanding, and the nursing practice environment was not ideal in terms of nurse-patient ratios, rush, shift hours, and general appreciation. Nurses felt tired because they could not provide as adequate nursing care as they were willing. Nurses' narratives bought up ethical dilemmas associated with not being able to provide humane and proper care. Not being able to do one's best and not being able to influence working conditions were in contradiction with the talent and ambitions of these young women. Similar themes came up in McGillis Hall and Kiesners [71] study, where nurses related narratives about guilt and over commitment when the working environment prevented them from providing complete and high-quality care. We believe that narrative stories can provide "a window into people's beliefs and experience" [72, page 209] and can provide richer understanding of how young nurses experienced the reality of nursing and how these lived experiences affected their career decisions.

Young nurses reproduced cultural images and stereotypes of a nurse's role and behaviour. They described what kind of people nurses are supposed to be: nurturing, altruistic, and willing to serve. Similar traditional stereotypes of "good women" have been presented on media and in public when nursing has been presented as a "virtue script" [73]. Nursing, as paradigmatically women's work, has been historically devalued [74]. Nursing profession has been associated with femininity [75] and powerlessness [76, 77], and stereotypical public images—such as angels with pretty faces and empty heads, physicians' handmaids, or naughty nurses—still exist in Western countries [77]. These young nurses did not, however, place themselves within these expected stereotypic images of nurses. This could be one reason why these nurses left profession—talented and bright women did not fit the stereotypes of nurses as nurturing and serving and of being lower in the hospital hierarchy.

As seen in this inquiry, public stereotypes can have negative impact on nurses' self-esteem [78] and could lead nurses to leave their profession [79]. Although there is considerable amount of research concerning stereotypes and images of nurses [77, 80], a search of the literature revealed only few earlier studies where the low status of the profession was connected to nurse turnover [78, 81]. More quantitative and also qualitative research is needed on how public stereotypes and image of nursing possibly affect young nurse's turnover. Stories can reveal deeply hidden assumptions that influence the actions of people [72]; through stories we can better understand how nurses explain and make sense of the stereotypes and images associated with the profession. By investigating in-depth stories there is a possibility to gain deeper understanding of the historical, sociocultural, and gendered perceptions which partly could lead younger generation of nurses to leave their profession.

In these stories, young nurses described themselves as talented and determined to go ahead in their career, attributes not historically attached to nurses [77, 80]. For example, in the UK [82, page 305], media tend to view "ambition in nurses as being an undesirable characteristic." Nursing profession was not able to provide the career development possibilities and intellectual challenges that these women were able to gain by applying to university studies and by starting a new career. Similar findings have been discussed in other studies. For example, in a study by Salminen [15], RNs who judged that they had the potential to carry out more challenging tasks had a higher intention to leave the profession. Additionally, Hasselhorn et al. [12] found that former nurses had indicated "too low demands" of nursing work as one reason to leave the profession, and former nurses in a Swedish study by Fochsen et al. [81] stated that a lack of professional opportunities and restricted professional autonomy were central reasons for leaving.

Most of this earlier literature was focused on turnover from the perspectives of organizations or professions, with the researchers viewing it as a preventable or negative result [11, 27]. However, as seen in this inquiry, turnover can also be beneficial for an individual nurse [12, 23]. Changing workplace, and even career, can provide nurses with the opportunity to move to positions better suited to their motives, ambitions, skills, and career goals. According to Hasselhorn et al. [12], a proportion of nurses with an intention to leave the profession are young, highly qualified, and seeking a new challenge. In light of this study, we think that it would be beneficial to health care systems to retain this group of nurses within the profession by opening up to them new possibilities and challenges within nursing. On the contrary, nurses who display a low level of work ability might benefit from leaving the nursing profession. In-depth investigations of career stories could give a broader perspective to the research of nurse's turnover, by focusing on career transition from a perspective of an individual nurse and by enlightening how a single nurse can benefit from a change of career.

What kind of new knowledge of nurses' professional turnover can we expect to get based on qualitative case-study approach? The purpose of this inquiry was not to seek universal explanations of why young nurses leave nursing profession. The results are not meant to be generalized to a certain population [44] as case study research commonly needs to be generalized theoretically [47, 53]. It is clear that no one methodology by itself will be able to address nurse turnover as a multifaceted phenomenon effectively. There is still a need to statistically measure and model variables connected with turnover [40]; also interventions to reduce turnover intention need to be developed and tested [18]. The advantage of large sample sized research is the breath and the empirical generalizability of the evidence [47]. However, as Flyvbjerg [44] remains, the disadvantage of this kind of knowledge is one of depth; therefore, qualitative case studies are needed as well.

The findings of this study are significant for three reasons. First, nurses were given an opportunity to tell their own story of why they had initially intended to leave, and why they eventually left, nursing. The voices of nurses who have intended to leave nursing have rarely been studied from their own perspective. Second, in contrast to the majority of previous studies that have mainly focused on turnover intentions and not actual turnover, a unique feature of this study is its longitudinal nature, which allows the reader to follow nurses through the process of their career transition. Third, nurses here provided stories of negative images and stereotypes in relation to their intention to leave nursing; in earlier studies of professional turnover, nurses' own negative stereotypes and images have not been significant factors in causing an intention to leave. Furthermore, it provides unique real-life contextual knowledge of young nurses' experiences of leaving a nursing career. This knowledge can be used as a basis for further studies and in discussions concerning nurses' intentions to leave nursing from a generational perspective. More in-depth research is needed in order to better understand why nurses leave, and even more significantly, what could motive the younger generation of nurses to stay in nursing. In addition, there is also a need for longitudinal research that tracks nurses throughout the career change processes.

3.7. Limitations. The findings should be viewed in light of the study's limitations. The findings reported in this study may be limited due to the sampling methods which were used. It is possible that the nurses who volunteered, and thus were prepared to tell their career stories, were different from other nurses who had also considered leaving the profession. These nurses were interested in the subject under investigation, they had all thought about the motives for why they had an intention to leave and were willing to narrate their experiences. All of the nurses who participated were open to the experience, sociable, and talkative. These are all also characteristics that are associated with persons who are more likely to change their career [21].

All of these nurses had the personal and financial opportunities to gain a new education at university, something that is not possible for all nurses with an intention to leave. Furthermore, the participants were all aware of the interviewer's occupation as a registered nurse; thus it is possible that this knowledge may have influenced the way in which they recounted their career stories. They were also aware that the topic of the research was the intention to leave nursing; this in turn might have brought up more negative issues from their career, in order to justify their reasons for leaving it.

4. Conclusions

The use of the qualitative case study method made it possible to examine nurses' career turnover as an ongoing and multidimensional process, in which several causes consequently impacted on the final decision to leave the nursing profession. We demonstrated that narrative career interviews are a feasible way of collecting data regarding career transition processes. We also claim that in-depth narrative stories can provide unique real-life contextual knowledge of nurses' experiences when living through these kinds of career transitions. We conclude that the qualitative case-study approach is a potential and novel way of doing turnover research in nursing science. Given the complex nature of nurse turnover, such a qualitative, in-depth approach is essential, alongside with quantitative studies, for a sound development of the nurse turnover research.

Acknowledgments

The authors are deeply grateful to all nurses who participated in the interviews and shared their experiences. University of Turku, the Finnish Association of Nursing Research, and the Finnish Foundation of Nursing Education provided financial support for this research.

References

[1] World Health Organization, *World Health Statistics 2011*, WHO, 2011, http://www.who.int/whosis/whostat/2011/en/index.html.

[2] J. Buchan and L. H. Aiken, "Solving nursing shortages: a common priority," *Journal of Clinical Nursing*, vol. 17, no. 24, pp. 3262–3268, 2008.

[3] S. P. Juraschek, X. Zhang, V. K. Ranganathan, and V. W. Lin, "United States Registered Nurse Workforce Report Card and Shortage Forecast," *American Journal of Medical Quality*, vol. 27, no. 3, pp. 241–249, 2012.

[4] W. Sermeus and L. Bruyneel, "Investing in Europe's health workforce of tomorrow: scope for innovation and collaboration," Summary Report of the Three Policy Dialogues, 2010, http://www.healthworkforce4europe.eu/downloads/Report_PD_Leuven_FINAL.pdf.

[5] Bureau of Labor Statistics, U.S. Department of Labor, *Occupational Outlook Handbook*, 2011, http://www.bls.gov/ooh/healthcare/registered-nurses.htm.

[6] S. Simoens, M. Villeneuve, and J. Hurst, "Tackling nurse shortages in OECD countries," OECD Health Working Papers 19, 2005, http://www.oecd.org/health/health-systems/34571365.pdf.

[7] World Health Organization, "Working together for health," The World Health Report, WHO, 2006, http://www.who.int/whr/2006/whr06_en.pdf.

[8] J. Needleman, P. Buerhaus, V. S. Pankratz, C. L. Leibson, S. R. Stevens, and M. Harris, "Nurse staffing and inpatient hospital mortality," *The New England Journal of Medicine*, vol. 364, no. 11, pp. 1037–1045, 2011.

[9] X. W. Zhu, L. M. You, J. Zheng et al., "Nurse staffing levels make a difference on patient outcomes: a multisite study in Chinese hospitals," *Journal of Nursing Scholarship*, vol. 44, no. 3, pp. 266–273, 2012.

[10] A. M. Rafferty, S. P. Clarke, J. Coles et al., "Outcomes of variation in hospital nurse staffing in English hospitals: cross-sectional analysis of survey data and discharge records," *International Journal of Nursing Studies*, vol. 44, no. 2, pp. 175–182, 2007.

[11] M. Flinkman, H. Leino-Kilpi, and S. Salanterä, "Nurses' intention to leave the profession: integrative review," *Journal of Advanced Nursing*, vol. 66, no. 7, pp. 1422–1434, 2010.

[12] H.-M. Hasselhorn, B. H. Müller, and P. Tackenberg, "Nursing in Europe: intention to leave the nursing profession," in *NEXT Scientific Report*, H. M. Hasselhorn, B. H. Mueller, and P. Tackenberg, Eds., pp. 17–24, 2005, http://www.next.uni-wuppertal.de/EN/index.php?articles-and-reports.

[13] L. H. Aiken, W. Sermeus, K. Van den Heede et al., "Patient safety, satisfaction, and quality of hospital care: cross sectional surveys of nurses and patients in 12 countries in Europe and the United States," *British Medical Journal*, vol. 344, no. 7851, Article ID e1717, 2012.

[14] M. M. Heinen, T. van Achterberg, R. Schwendimann et al., "Nurses' intention to leave their profession: a cross sectional observational study in 10 European countries," *International Journal of Nursing Studies*, vol. 50, no. 2, pp. 174–184, 2013.

[15] H. Salminen, "Turning the tide: registered nurses' job withdrawal intentions in a Finnish university hospital," *SA Journal of Human Resource Management*, vol. 10, no. 2, pp. 1–11, 2012.

[16] A. Rudman, M. Omne-Pontén, L. Wallin, and P. J. Gustavsson, "Monitoring the newly qualified nurses in Sweden: The Longitudinal Analysis of Nursing Education (LANE) Study," *Human Resources for Health*, vol. 8, article 10, 2010.

[17] HRSA, U.S. Department of Health and Human Services, *Registered Nurse Population. Findings From the 2008 National Sample Survey of Registered Nurses*, 2010, http://bhpr.hrsa.gov/healthworkforce/rnsurveys/rnsurveyfinal.pdf.

[18] M. Takase, "A concept analysis of turnover intention: implications for nursing management," *Collegian*, vol. 17, no. 1, pp. 3–12, 2010.

[19] M. Krausz, M. Koslowsky, N. Shalom, and N. Elyakim, "Predictors of intentions to leave the ward, the hospital, and the nursing profession: a longitudinal study," *Journal of Organizational Behavior*, vol. 16, no. 3, pp. 277–288, 1995.

[20] I. M. Lane, R. C. Mathews, and P. H. Presholdt, "Determinants of nurses' intentions to leave their profession," *Journal of Organizational Behavior*, vol. 9, no. 4, pp. 367–372, 1998.

[21] S. A. Carless and J. L. Arnup, "A longitudinal study of the determinants and outcomes of career change," *Journal of Vocational Behavior*, vol. 78, no. 1, pp. 80–91, 2011.

[22] C. Duffield, L. O'Brien Pallas, and L. M. Aitken, "Nurses who work outside nursing," *Journal of Advanced Nursing*, vol. 47, no. 6, pp. 664–671, 2004.

[23] M. Laine, B. I. J. M. van der Heijden, G. Wickstrom, H.-M. Hasselhorn, and P. Tackenberg, "Job insecurity and intent to leave the nursing profession in Europe," *International Journal of Human Resource Management*, vol. 20, no. 2, pp. 420–438, 2009.

[24] K. D. Carson, P. P. Carson, and A. G. Bedeian, "Development and construct validation of a career entrenchment measure," *Journal of Occupational and Organizational Psychology*, vol. 68, no. 4, pp. 273–368, 1995.

[25] M. Simon, B. H. Müller, and H. M. Hasselhorn, "Leaving the organization or the profession—a multilevel analysis of nurses' intentions," *Journal of Advanced Nursing*, vol. 66, no. 3, pp. 616–626, 2010.

[26] Y. Li and C. B. Jones, "A literature review of nursing turnover costs," *Journal of Nursing Management*, vol. 21, no. 3, pp. 405–418, 2013.

[27] L. J. Hayes, L. O'Brien-Pallas, C. Duffield et al., "Nurse turnover: a literature review—an update," *International Journal of Nursing Studies*, vol. 49, no. 7, pp. 887–905, 2012.

[28] J. Blythe, A. Baumann, I. U. Zeytinoglu et al., "Nursing generations in the contemporary workplace," *Public Personnel Management*, vol. 37, no. 2, pp. 137–159, 2008.

[29] C. T. Kovner and M. Djukic, "The nursing career process from application through the first 2 years of employment," *Journal of Professional Nursing*, vol. 25, no. 4, pp. 197–203, 2009.

[30] S. Robinson, T. Murrells, and P. Griffiths, "Investigating the dynamics of nurse migration in early career: a longitudinal questionnaire survey of variation in regional retention of diploma qualifiers in England," *International Journal of Nursing Studies*, vol. 45, no. 7, pp. 1064–1080, 2008.

[31] D. Barron and E. West, "Leaving nursing: an event-history analysis of nurses' careers," *Journal of Health Services Research & Policy*, vol. 10, no. 3, pp. 150–157, 2005.

[32] M. Lavoie-Tremblay, L. O'Brien-Pallas, C. Gélinas, N. Desforges, and C. Marchionni, "Addressing the turnover issue among new nurses from a generational viewpoint," *Journal of Nursing Management*, vol. 16, no. 6, pp. 724–733, 2008.

[33] M. Flinkman, M. Laine, H. Leino-Kilpi, H.-M. Hasselhorn, and S. Salanterä, "Explaining young registered Finnish nurses' intention to leave the profession: a questionnaire survey," *International Journal of Nursing Studies*, vol. 45, no. 5, pp. 727–739, 2008.

[34] J. E. B. Duchscher, "Transition shock: the initial stage of role adaptation for newly graduated registered nurses," *Journal of Advanced Nursing*, vol. 65, no. 5, pp. 1103–1113, 2009.

[35] L. B. Zinsmeister and D. Schafer, "The exploration of the lived experience of the graduate nurse making the transition to registered nurse during the first year of practice," *Journal for Nurses in Staff Development*, vol. 25, no. 1, pp. 28–34, 2009.

[36] Y. T. Teoh, L. H. Pua, and M. F. Chan, "Lost in transition—a review of qualitative literature of newly qualified Registered Nurses' experiences in their transition to practice journey," *Nurse Education Today*, vol. 33, no. 2, pp. 143–147, 2013.

[37] E. S. Scott, M. Keehner Engelke, and M. Swanson, "New graduate nurse transitioning: necessary or nice?" *Applied Nursing Research*, vol. 21, no. 2, pp. 75–83, 2008.

[38] M. Lavoie-Tremblay, E. Leclerc, C. Marchionni, and U. Drevniok, "The needs and expectations of generation Y nurses in the workplace," *Journal for Nurses in Staff Development*, vol. 26, no. 1, pp. 2–8, 2010.

[39] Z. C. Chan, W. S. Tam, M. K. Lung, W. Y. Wong, and C. W. Chau, "A systematic literature review of nurse shortage and the intention to leave," *Journal of Nursing Management*, vol. 21, no. 4, pp. 605–613, 2013.

[40] B. C. Holtom, T. R. Mitchell, T. W. Lee, and M. B. Eberly, "Turnover and retention research: a glance at the past, a closer review of the present, and a venture into the future," *The Academy of Management Annals*, vol. 2, no. 1, pp. 231–274, 2008.

[41] S. Anthony and S. Jack, "Qualitative case study methodology in nursing research: an integrative review," *Journal of Advanced Nursing*, vol. 65, no. 6, pp. 1171–1181, 2009.

[42] D. E. Polkinghorne, "Narrative configuration in qualitative analysis," *Qualitative Studies in Education*, vol. 8, no. 1, pp. 5–23, 1995.

[43] C. K. Riessman, *Narrative Analysis*, vol. 30 of *Qualitative Research Methods*, Sage, Thousand Oaks, Calif, USA, 1993.

[44] B. Flyvbjerg, "Five misunderstandings about case-study research," *Qualitative Inquiry*, vol. 12, no. 2, pp. 219–245, 2006.

[45] L. Luck, D. Jackson, and K. Usher, "Case study: a bridge across the paradigms," *Nursing Inquiry*, vol. 13, no. 2, pp. 103–109, 2006.

[46] K. LaPointe, "Narrating career, positioning identity: career identity as a narrative practice," *Journal of Vocational Behavior*, vol. 77, no. 1, pp. 1–9, 2010.

[47] K. Sharp, "The case for case studies in nursing research: the problem of generalization," *Journal of Advanced Nursing*, vol. 27, no. 4, pp. 785–789, 1998.

[48] C. Jones and C. Lyons, "Case study: design? Method? Or comprehensive strategy?" *Nurse researcher*, vol. 11, no. 3, pp. 70–76, 2004.

[49] J. Bruner, "Life as narrative," *Social Research*, vol. 54, no. 1, pp. 11–32, 1987.

[50] A. Lieblich, R. Tuval-Mashiach, and T. Zilber, *Narrative Research: Reading, Analysis, and Interpretation*, vol. 47, Sage, Thousand Oaks, Calif, USA, 1998.

[51] C. K. Riessman, "Narrative analysis," in *The Qualitative Researcher's Companion*, A. M. Huberman and B. M. Miles, Eds., pp. 217–270, Sage, Thousand Oaks, Calif, USA, 2002.

[52] H. Heikkinen, "Whatever is narrative research?" in *Narrative Research: Voices of Teachers and Philosophers*, R. Huttunen, H. Heikkinen, and L. Syrjälä, Eds., pp. 13–28, Jyväskylä, Finland, SoPhi, 2002.

[53] C. K. Riessman, *Narrative Methods for the Human Sciences*, Sage, Thousand Oaks, Calif, USA, 2008.

[54] J. F. Gubrium and J. A. Holstein, *Analyzing Narrative Reality*, Sage, Thousand Oaks, Calif, USA, 2009.

[55] L. R. Cochran, "Narrative as a paradigm for career research," in *Methodological Approaches to the Study of Career*, R. A. Young and W. A. Borger, Eds., pp. 71–86, Praeger, New York, NY, USA, 1990.

[56] U. Isopahkala-Bouret, *Joy and struggle for renewal: a narrative inquiry into expertise in job transitions [Ph.D. thesis]*, Helsinki University Press, Helsinki, Finland, 2005, http://ethesis.helsinki.fi/julkaisut/kay/kasva/vk/isopahkala-bouret/joyandst.pdf.

[57] H. Ibarra, "Career transition and change," Insead Faculty & Research, Working paper series 2004/97/OB, 2004, http://www.insead.edu/facultyresearch/research/doc.cfm?did=1477.

[58] A. De Fina, "Narratives in interview—the case of accounts for an interactional approach to narrative genres," *Narrative Inquiry*, vol. 19, no. 2, pp. 233–258, 2009.

[59] E. Mischler, *Research Interviewing: Context and Narrative*, Harvard University Press, Cambridge, Mass, USA, 1986.

[60] M. Sandelowski and J. Leeman, "Writing usable qualitative health research findings," *Qualitative Health Research*, vol. 22, no. 10, pp. 1404–1413, 2012.

[61] D. E. Polkinghorne, "Validity issues in narrative research," *Qualitative Inquiry*, vol. 13, no. 4, pp. 471–486, 2007.

[62] The Finnish Advisory Board on Research Integrity (TENK), "Responsible conduct of research and procedures for handling allegations of misconduct in Finland," 2012, http://www.tenk.fi/sites/tenk.fi/files/HTK_ohje_2012.pdf.

[63] J. Cheung, "The decision process of leaving nursing," *Australian Health Review*, vol. 28, no. 3, pp. 340–348, 2004.

[64] H. M. Trice and D. A. Morand, "Rites of passage in work careers," in *Handbook of Career Theory*, M. B. Arthur, D. T. Hall, and B. S. Laurence, Eds., pp. 397–416, Cambridge University Press, New York, NY, United States, 1989.

[65] N. A. Fouad and J. Bynner, "Work transitions," *American Psychologist*, vol. 63, no. 4, pp. 241–251, 2008.

[66] K. Morrell, "Towards a typology of nursing turnover: the role of shocks in nurses' decisions to leave," *Journal of Advanced Nursing*, vol. 49, no. 3, pp. 315–322, 2005.

[67] K. Louise Barriball and A. E. While, "The similarities and differences between nurses with different career choice profiles: findings of an interview survey," *Journal of Advanced Nursing*, vol. 23, no. 2, pp. 380–388, 1996.

[68] B. Enberg, H. Stenlund, G. Sundelin, and A. Öhman, "Work satisfaction, career preferences and unpaid household work among recently graduated health-care professionals—a gender perspective," *Scandinavian Journal of Caring Sciences*, vol. 21, no. 2, pp. 169–177, 2007.

[69] K. Santamäki, T. Kankaanranta, L. Henriksson, and P. Rissanen, "Sairaanhoitaja 2005. Perusraportti. Työraportteja 83/2009," Tampereen yliopisto, yhteiskuntatieteen yksikkö, Työelämän tutkimuskeskus, Finnish, 2009, http://tampub.uta.fi/handle/10024/65551.

[70] S. Price, "Future directions for career choice research in nursing: a discussion paper," *International Journal of Nursing Studies*, vol. 46, no. 2, pp. 268–276, 2009.

[71] L. McGillis Hall and D. Kiesners, "A narrative approach to understanding the nursing work environment in Canada," *Social Science & Medicine*, vol. 61, no. 12, pp. 2482–2491, 2005.

[72] J. S. Bell, "Narrative inquiry: more than just telling stories," *TESOL Quarterly*, vol. 36, no. 2, pp. 207–213, 2002.

[73] S. Gordon and S. Nelson, "An end to angels," *American Journal of Nursing*, vol. 105, no. 5, pp. 62–69, 2005.

[74] K. Fletcher, "Image: changing how women nurses think about themselves. Literature review," *Journal of Advanced Nursing*, vol. 58, no. 3, pp. 207–215, 2007.

[75] J. A. Seago, J. Spetz, A. Alvarado, D. Keane, and K. Grumbach, "The nursing shortage: is it really about image?" *Journal of Healthcare Management*, vol. 51, no. 2, pp. 96–108, 2006.

[76] K. White, "Nursing as vocation," *Nursing Ethics*, vol. 9, no. 3, pp. 279–290, 2002.

[77] P. Darbyshire and S. Gordon, "Exploring popular images and representations of nurses and nursing," in *Professional Nursing: Concepts, Issues, and Challenges*, J. Daly, S. Speedy, D. Jackson, V. Lambert, and C. Lambert, Eds., pp. 69–93, Springer, New York, NY, USA, 2005.

[78] M. Takase, P. Maude, and E. Manias, "Impact of the perceived public image of nursing on nurses' work behaviour," *Journal of Advanced Nursing*, vol. 53, no. 3, pp. 333–343, 2006.

[79] H. Janiszewski Goodin, "The nursing shortage in the United States of America: an integrative review of the literature," *Journal of Advanced Nursing*, vol. 43, no. 4, pp. 335–343, 2003.

[80] J. M. Bridges, "Literature review on the images of the nurse and nursing in the media," *Journal of Advanced Nursing*, vol. 15, no. 7, pp. 850–854, 1990.

[81] G. Fochsen, K. Sjögren, M. Josephson, and M. Lagerström, "Factors contributing to the decision to leave nursing care: a study among Swedish nursing personnel," *Journal of Nursing Management*, vol. 13, no. 4, pp. 338–344, 2005.

[82] K. Gillett, "A critical discourse analysis of British national newspaper representations of the academic level of nurse education: too clever for our own good?" *Nursing Inquiry*, vol. 19, no. 4, pp. 297–307, 2012.

17

A Comparative Analysis of Cultural Competence in Beginning and Graduating Nursing Students

Helen Reyes, Lance Hadley, and Deborah Davenport

Department of Nursing, West Texas A&M University, P.O. Box 60969, Canyon, TX 79016, USA

Correspondence should be addressed to Helen Reyes; hreyes@wtamu.edu

Academic Editors: P. N. Clarke, A. Green, and B. Mandleco

The ethnic proportions of the population in the United States are rapidly changing, with the nation's minority population at approximately 101 million. This is also true for the West Texas region, where locally in a city with 183,000 residents, 43 different languages are spoken suggesting that cultural education needs to be included in nursing program curricula. Therefore, a study was conducted during a period of curriculum revision to determine if the current nursing curriculum at a public university offers enough education and experience for graduating nurses to care for such a diverse population by comparing their perceptions of cultural competence with beginning sophomore nursing students' perceptions. Participants were asked to complete the Cultural Competence Assessment (CCA) tool in order to evaluate perceptions of cultural competence. Upon analysis of the data, perceptions of cultural competence among graduating nursing students were significantly higher ($P = .002$) than the perceptions of cultural competence among beginning nursing students. These results support that nursing students perceive that they have become culturally competent during their nursing education, leading to implications of the need for continued education relating to this concept, beginning with the first course and continuing throughout the nursing curriculum.

1. Introduction

Cultural diversity is an issue that faces all health-care workers today. The immigrant population in the United States is increasing, which suggests that education is needed in transcultural nursing to allow nurses to provide culturally competent care. The nation's minority population has reached approximately 101 million, and it is estimated that one in three United States residents is a person belonging to a minority group [1–3]. It is expected by the year 2050 that the Black, Hispanic, and Asian ethnic group percentages within the population will rise dramatically, and the Caucasian population will drop significantly [4], with the USCB (2013) projecting that the United States will become a majority-minority nation, no single group making up the majority, by 2043. Yet, according to the Department of Health and Human Services (DHHS) Office of Minority Health [5], it is estimated that only 10% of registered nurses in the United States claim minority group status. The lack of diversity in the nursing profession mandates a need for cultural competence education in order to provide culturally competent care to an ethnically diverse patient population that is increasing [6, 7].

Currently, there are no education requirements from the Texas Board of Nursing for transcultural nursing [8]. Cultural competence education concepts remain an option for professional nursing education programs. The American Association of Colleges of Nursing (AACN) believes that diversity and equality of opportunity are core values of all educational systems, and one goal is to create a community of culturally competent scholars, including faculty, students, staff, and practitioners [9]. Decreasing inequities in the health-care system will require culturally competent nurses and other health care providers to meet the needs of disenfranchised groups [10]. The Joint Commission on Accreditation of Health-care Organizations [11] emphasizes the importance of cultural competence in terms of safety and outcomes and believes that it is now essential for nurses to examine their practices related to cultural elements.

The challenge is growing for professional nurses to care for a culturally diverse population. The American Nurses

Association (ANA) believes that nurses and health care providers have a responsibility to provide an environment that recognizes differences and is free from discrimination, including discrimination based on racial and ethnic differences [12]. It is difficult to remain aware of the myriad of cultural groups that reside in the United States. However, healthcare professionals should be aware of the dominant cultures within their local area. For example, there are approximately 43 different languages spoken in a city with a population of 183,021 people, which is located in the southwestern United States. Increasing awareness of these different groups will allow nurses to gain additional insight regarding the care of these individuals.

According to the ANA, nurses should provide care with respect for human dignity as well as considering the uniqueness of the individual client [12]. Unrealized or unacknowledged biases may prevent nurses from providing optimal quality care. Acknowledging the practices of diverse cultures will allow professional nurses to provide a range of alternatives in services, for example, in providing the patient's dietary preferences or health care beliefs [11, 13].

Communication barriers between nurses and their patients and families may arise because of cultural differences. It is important for nurses to recognize that caregiving within the family context may differ from their own interpretation and knowing how to integrate the family's health practices into the overall health care regimen will benefit both patient and family [14].

Nursing curricula must provide a foundation for the development of cultural competence that allows for acquisition of knowledge, skills, and attitudes. In addition, an examination of culturally diverse concepts stimulates commitment to moral and ethical values, while developing an appreciation for diverse cultural heritages. Acquisition of culturally competent concepts promotes an awareness of contemporary world issues and can be learned through multiple teaching strategies, including didactic and experiential methods [15–18].

In studies of cultural competence education in nursing, findings support that the addition of culturally competent content increases scores on culturally competence measures, as students gain experience during progression through the curricula [19–23]. A more recent review of the literature supports the findings of these studies [24]. Similarly, qualitative studies that examined cultural competence discovered emerging models for increasing cultural competence through education based on the patients' perspective, as well as that of nurse, and student nurses [25–29].

2. Purpose, Rationale, and Research Question of the Study

The purpose of this study was to determine if the self-perception of cultural competence in baccalaureate nursing students as a result of their education and experiences increased during the nursing program. As the curriculum committee members were examining the existing nursing curriculum and planning a major revision, this study was instrumental in informing the faculty of the perceived cultural competence of beginning and graduating nursing students. Data generated by this study allowed nurse educators a better understanding of student perceptions of cultural competence and informed the curriculum committee of the cultural competence gained throughout the nursing program. The research question which framed this study was as follows: is there a higher perception of cultural competence among graduating nursing students as compared to beginning nursing students?

For the purpose of this study, culture was defined as beliefs and values of a particular group that are learned and shared and are generally transmitted between generations and influence thinking, decisions, and actions [30]. Cultural competence was theoretically defined as a process by which nurses strive to achieve the ability and availability to work within a cultural context of a patient, family, or community [31]. Cultural competence was operationally defined by a total score on the Cultural Competence Assessment (CCA) tool [20]. A beginning nursing student was defined as a baccalaureate nursing student in the first clinical semester of the nursing curriculum. A graduating nursing student was defined as a baccalaureate nursing student in the last clinical semester of the nursing curriculum.

3. Theoretical Frameworks

The major focus of transcultural nursing is to focus on the humanistic and scientific study of individuals from different cultures with consideration to ways in which nurses can assist those individuals meet their health and living needs [32]. Leininger's Transcultural Nursing Theory posits that caring serves to improve human conditions through behaviors, techniques, processes, and patterns. In addition, caring behaviors such as comfort, compassion, concern, interest, tenderness, touching, and trust are illuminated as key concepts to providing quality care through the lens of culture. Culture is determined by one's personal life and worldviews. Caring and culture are linked to one another, and nursing care should be aimed at preserving, maintaining, accommodating, negotiating, and restructuring care patterns as these relate to the individual's cultural perspectives [33].

The 3-Dimensional Puzzle Model of Culturally Congruent Care was also chosen to guide this study. The four basic components of the cultural competence puzzle at the health care provider level include cultural diversity, cultural awareness, cultural sensitivity, and cultural competence [34]. The model is specifically operationalized using the CCA. This study tested quantitatively the fourth puzzle piece, cultural competence, using the CCA, as it measures perception to the actions taken in response to cultural diversity, cultural awareness, and cultural sensitivity.

4. Methods and Procedures

The Institutional Review Board (IRB) approved the research study. Guidelines set forth by the Family Educational Rights and Privacy Act (FERPA) were followed to protect the

TABLE 1: Subscale mean scores.

Student group	CAS subscale	CCB subscale	Marlowe-Crown Social Desirability Scale
Beginning student			
Mean	5.695	3.453	7.00
N	46	46	46
Standard deviation	4.544	1.210	2.477
Minimum score	4.454	0.000	1
Maximum score	6.545	6.000	13
Graduating student			
Mean	6.018	4.590	7.75
N	53	53	53
Standard deviation	5.295	1.132	2.336
Minimum score	4.727	2.142	3
Maximum score	7.000	6.785	12

privacy of student education records, and there was no identifying information collected. The design of this study was a comparative, descriptive design, testing for differences between beginning nursing students ($n = 46$) in the first clinical course and the last clinical course ($n = 53$) in a baccalaureate nursing program. Students were recruited during the first class meeting of the semester, and data were collected during the first week of classes using the CCA. The rationale for using a comparative design with data collection between two groups at one time instead of a longitudinal time frame allowed faculty to assess this concept in the current curriculum prior to a planned revision.

The CCA is a 43- item Likert scale and was administered to gather data about individual self-perceptions regarding culture competence. The CCA had demonstrated in a previously reported study test-retest reliability ($r = 0.85$, $P = .002$; [20]). The CCA is made up of three different subscales, including the Cultural Awareness and Sensitivity Subscale (CAS) consisting of an 11-question Likert scale; the Cultural Competence Behavior Subscale (CCB) consisting of a 14-question Likert scale; and the Marlowe-Crown Social Desirability Scale consisting of 13 questions that were answered with either true or false by the student participants. The CAS is scored using a range of 1 to 7, with a higher score indicating a greater cultural awareness and sensitivity. The CCB is also scored using a range of 1 to 7, with a higher score indicative of more cultural competence behaviors being demonstrated. The Marlowe-Crown Social Desirability Scale was added to the instrument as a check/balance for honesty on the CCB subscale. This scale is scored using a range of 0 to 13, with a higher score indicating more need for approval, which indicates that respondents answered the questions according to what they believed to be socially acceptable [20].

The data collected were analyzed using the independent t-test. This study measured perceived cultural competence as a total score upon which each groups' mean score was determined and subjected to independent t testing to determine differences between groups. The level of significance was set at $P < .05$. The data were analyzed using the Statistical Package for the Social Sciences (SPSS) 17.0 software.

5. Findings

There were a total of 99 nursing students, with an age range for the beginning nursing student participants of 19–35 years ($M = 22.54$) and an age range of the graduating nursing student participants of 21–65 years ($M = 27.53$). The average age of the graduating nursing students was statistically higher compared to the average age of the beginning nursing students ($t[\text{df} = 97] = -3.617$, $P = .000$). The racial/ethnic self-identification of the beginning nursing students included 24% Hispanic/Latino, 61% White/Caucasian, 4% Black/African American, and 11% Asian. The racial/ethnic self-identification of the graduating nursing students included 4% Hispanic/Latino, 72% White/Caucasian, 19% Black/African American, and 4% Asian.

The mean scores for the beginning and graduating nursing students are reported in Table 1. The graduating nursing students demonstrated a higher mean score for the CAS and the CCB (e.g., 6.018 and 4.590, resp.) as compared to the beginning nursing students (e.g., 5.695 and 3.453, resp.), indicating that the graduating nursing students have greater perceived cultural awareness and sensitivity and perceive that they demonstrate more culturally competent behaviors. However, it was noted that the beginning nursing students demonstrated a lower score on the Marlowe-Crown Social Desirability Scale as compared to the graduating nursing students (e.g., 7.00 and 7.75, resp.). This indicates that the beginning nursing students have a slightly less need for approval than do the graduating nursing students. Independent t-test findings demonstrated that perceptions of cultural diversity were significantly higher in the graduating nursing student group as compared with beginning nursing students ($t[\text{df} = 97] = -3.233$, $P = .002$).

One confounding variable encountered was age; the graduating nursing students' age was great, which was a statistically significant difference between groups. Therefore, a generalized linear model was conducted, using the CCA scores as the dependent variable and age as a predictor ($X^2[\text{df} = 23] = 22.47$, $P = .49$), which suggests that older age alone is not a sufficient variable for being culturally competent. Univariate analysis of variance on the dependent variable of the CCA scores with age held as the covariate was not statistically significant ($F = 0.60[\text{df} = 1]$, $P = .80$). The amount of variance in the dependent variable that is shared with age is 0.1% ($R^2 = .001$). Reliability statistics were completed on the CCA for this sample, which resulted in Cronbach's Alpha = .823.

6. Discussion

In examining the existing curriculum during a major revision, the concept of cultural competence was investigated for evidence of students' perception of their level of cultural competence. Extant research supports education, including a variety of teaching strategies in cultural diversity concepts, increases one's cultural competence. Study findings revealed a statistically significant difference in perceived level of cultural competence between the two groups, with graduating nursing students possessing a higher perceived level of cultural competence than the beginning nursing students. This indicates that graduating nursing students perceive that they have greater cultural awareness and sensitivity and have a greater understanding of what constitutes culturally competent behaviors. One assumption based on these results is that the role transition being experienced by the graduating nursing students may have influenced their answers. Oftentimes, there is a desire, on behalf of graduating nursing students, to be accepted in a Registered Nurse (RN) role rather than in a student role, and as such, graduating students may have answered the way they think an RN would have answered, as evidenced by their higher scores on the Marlowe-Crown Social Desirability Scale.

The findings of this study cannot be generalized beyond the geographical setting, as these were specific to the nursing population at this university. It is assumed that the findings of this study may not be similar to other nursing programs. All measures of cultural competence currently available are based on participant perceptions, which can be another limitation of the study. While the participants were chosen through convenience sampling, the entire student population of beginning and graduating students was invited to participate, and all who were present on the day of data collection did so. An additional limitation was that only two cohorts were examined in one measurement in time, whereas an ongoing analysis would provide stronger results.

7. Future Recommendations

There is an opportunity for nursing faculty at this university to use the information presented in this research study to develop additional culturally based student learning activities that will further increase the level of cultural competence in current and future baccalaureate nursing students. Specifically, based on the results of this study, additional activities have been added throughout the curriculum. It is recommended that all nursing courses address cultural competence in didactic activities as well as laboratory experiences, including simulation and clinical. It is recommended that a longitudinal study be utilized throughout all levels of baccalaureate nursing education to measure progress of cultural competence education as each student cohort progresses through the nursing program.

Although the findings in this study are specific to the nursing population at one university, other universities can use the same assessment tool to gather information about the perceptions of cultural competence of their students in order to evaluate processes that are currently in place or to gather information that will assist them in the development of new teaching methodologies.

References

[1] R. Bernstein, "Minority population tops 100 million," *U.S. Census Bureau News*, 2007, http://www.census.gov/Press-Release/www/releases/archives/population/010048.html.

[2] United States Census Bureau, "Census shows America's diversity," 2010, http://www.census.gov/newsroom/releases/archives/2010_census/cb11-cn125.html.

[3] United States Census Bureau, "US Census Bureau projections show a slower growing, older, more diverse nation a half century from now," 2013, http://www.census.gov/newsroom/releases/archives/population/cb12-243.html.

[4] R. Zoucha, "The keys to culturally sensitive care," *American Journal of Nursing*, vol. 100, no. 2, pp. 24GG–24II, 2000.

[5] Department of Health and Human Services, Office of Minority Health, Nursing Statistics, 2009, http://www.minoritynurse.com/minority-nursing-statistics.

[6] R. I. Gonzalez, M. B. Gooden, and C. P. Porter, "Eliminating racial and ethnic disparities in health care," *American Journal of Nursing*, vol. 100, no. 3, pp. 56–76, 2000.

[7] Institute of Medicine, "The future of nursing: leading change, advancing health," 2010, http://books.nap.edu/openbook.php?record_id=12956&page=R1.

[8] Texas Board of Nursing, "Continuing Education Requirements. Texas Administrative Code," Title 22, Part 11, Chapter 216, Rule 216.3, 2012, http://info.sos.state.tx.us/pls/pub.

[9] American Association of Colleges of Nursing, "Enhancing diversity in the nursing workforce," 2011, https://www.aacn.nche.edu/media-relations/fact-sheets/enhancing-diversity.

[10] A. Finkelman and C. Kenner, *Teaching IOM: Implications of the Institute of Medicine Reports for Nursing Education*, ANA, Silver Spring, Md, USA, 2007.

[11] The Joint Commission, *Advancing Effective Communication, Cultural Competence, and Patient- and Family-Centered Care: Roadmap for Hospitals*, The Joint Commission, Oakbrook Terrace, Ill, USA, 2010.

[12] American Nurses Association, "Discrimination and racism in health care," *ANA Nursing World*, 1998, http://nursingworld.org/readroom/position/ethics/etdisrac.htm.

[13] American Nurses Association, "Cultural diversity in nursing practice," *ANA Nursing World*, 1991, http://www.nursingworld.org/readroom/position/ethics/etcldv.htm.

[14] J. Wrubel, T. A. Richards, S. Folkman, and M. C. Acree, "Tacit definitions of informal caregiving," *Journal of Advanced Nursing*, vol. 33, no. 2, pp. 175–181, 2001.

[15] J. Campinha-Bacote, "Cultural competence in nursing curricula: how are we doing 20 years later?" *Journal of Nursing Education*, vol. 45, no. 7, pp. 243–244, 2006.

[16] J. Campinha-Bocote, "Delivering patient-centered care in the modst of a cultural conflict: the role of cultural competence," *The Online Journal of Issues in Nursing*, vol. 16, no. 2, article 5, 2011.

[17] S. Breier-Mackie, "Cultural competence and patient advocacy: the new challenge for nurses," *Gastroenterology Nursing*, vol. 30, no. 2, pp. 120–122, 2007.

[18] E. Calvillo, L. Clark, J. E. Ballantyne, D. Pacquiao, L. D. Purnell, and A. M. Villarruel, "Cultural competency in baccalaureate nursing education," *Journal of Transcultural Nursing*, vol. 20, no. 2, pp. 137–145, 2009.

[19] B. Majumdar, G. Browne, J. Roberts, and B. Carpio, "Effects of cultural sensitivity training on health care provider attitudes and patient outcomes," *Journal of Nursing Scholarship*, vol. 36, no. 2, pp. 161–166, 2004.

[20] A. Z. Doorenbos, S. M. Schim, R. Benkert, and N. N. Borse, "Psychometric evaluation of the cultural competence assessment instrument among healthcare providers," *Nursing Research*, vol. 54, no. 5, pp. 324–331, 2005.

[21] T. M. Lampley, K. E. Little, R. Beck-Little, and X. Yu, "Cultural competence of North Carolina nurses: a journey from novice to expert," *Home Health Care Management and Practice*, vol. 20, no. 6, pp. 454–461, 2008.

[22] A. M. W. Brennan and V. T. Cotter, "Student perceptions of cultural competence content in the curriculum," *Journal of Professional Nursing*, vol. 24, no. 3, pp. 155–160, 2008.

[23] G. M. Musolino, S. T. Burkhalter, B. Crookston et al., "Understanding and eliminating disparities in health care: development and assessment of cultural competence for interdisciplinary health professionals at The University of Utah-a 3-year investigation," *Journal of Physical Therapy Education*, vol. 24, no. 1, pp. 25–36, 2010.

[24] J. Allen, "Improving cross-cultural care and antiracism in nursing education: a literature review," *Nurse Education Today*, vol. 30, no. 4, pp. 314–320, 2010.

[25] J. S. Reeves and C. Fogg, "Perceptions of graduating nursing students regarding life experiences that promote culturally competent care," *Journal of Transcultural Nursing*, vol. 17, no. 2, pp. 171–178, 2006.

[26] J. Leishman, "Perspectives of cultural competence in health care," *Nursing Standard*, vol. 19, no. 11, pp. 33–38, 2004.

[27] M. J. Upvall and M. L. Bost, "Developing cultural competence in nursing students through their experiences with a refugee population," *Journal of Nursing Education*, vol. 46, no. 8, pp. 380–383, 2007.

[28] P. W. Garrett, H. G. Dickson, L. Young, A. K. Whelan, and R. Forero, "What do non-English-speaking patients value in acute care? Cultural competency from the patient's perspective: a qualitative study," *Ethnicity and Health*, vol. 13, no. 5, pp. 479–496, 2008.

[29] A. Wikberg and K. Eriksson, "Intercultural caring—an abductive model," *Scandinavian Journal of Caring Sciences*, vol. 22, no. 3, pp. 485–496, 2008.

[30] M. Leininger and M. R. McFarland, *Transcultural Nursing: Concepts, Theories, Research, and Practice*, McGraw-Hill, New York, NY, USA, 3rd edition, 2002.

[31] J. Campinha-Bacote, "Many faces: addressing diversity in health care," *Online Journal of Issues in Nursing*, vol. 8, no. 1, article 2, 2003.

[32] Leininger, *Transcultural Nursing: Concepts, Theories, and Practices*, John Wiley & Sons, New York, NY, USA, 1978.

[33] P. L. Chinn and M. K. Kramer, *Integrated Knowledge Development in Nursing*, Mosby, St. Louis, Mo, USA, 6th edition, 2004.

[34] S. M. Schim, A. Doorenbos, R. Benkert, and J. Miller, "Culturally congruent care: putting the puzzle together," *Journal of Transcultural Nursing*, vol. 18, no. 2, pp. 103–110, 2007.

18

The Value of Peer Learning in Undergraduate Nursing Education: A Systematic Review

Robyn Stone, Simon Cooper, and Robyn Cant

Monash University, School of Nursing and Midwifery, Berwick Campus, 100 Clyde Road, Berwick 3806, Australia

Correspondence should be addressed to Robyn Stone; rwstol@student.monash.edu

Academic Editors: L. H. Beebe and M. M. Funnell

The study examined various methods of peer learning and their effectiveness in undergraduate nursing education. Using a specifically developed search strategy, healthcare databases were systematically searched for peer-reviewed articles, with studies involving peer learning and students in undergraduate general nursing courses (in both clinical and theoretical settings) being included. The studies were published in English between 2001 and 2010. Both study selection and quality analysis were undertaken independently by two researchers using published guidelines and data was thematically analyzed to answer the research questions. Eighteen studies comprising various research methods were included. The variety of terms used for peer learning and variations between study designs and assessment measures affected the reliability of the study. The outcome measures showing improvement in either an objective effect or subjective assessment were considered a positive result with sixteen studies demonstrating positive aspects to peer learning including increased confidence, competence, and a decrease in anxiety. We conclude that peer learning is a rapidly developing aspect of nursing education which has been shown to develop students' skills in communication, critical thinking, and self-confidence. Peer learning was shown to be as effective as the conventional classroom lecture method in teaching undergraduate nursing students.

1. Introduction

Nursing education studies have often focused on traditional teaching methods such as classroom lecture learning, a behaviourism-based teaching method based on passive learning [1]. More effective student-centric learning methods are now being utilized to encourage active student participation and creative thinking [2–4]. One of these methods is peer learning, in which peers learn from one another, involving active student participation and where the student takes responsibility for their learning. Despite being used for many years, one of the barriers to advancement of peer learning is a lack of consistency in its definition [5]. It is known by different interchangeable titles such as "cooperative learning," "mentoring," "peer review learning," "peer coaching," "peer mentoring," "problem-based learning," and "team learning."

Peer learning has been used in education to address critical thinking, psychomotor skills, cognitive development, clinical skills, and academic gains [6–9]. One type of peer learning is problem-based learning (PBL) which is characterized by students learning from each other and from independently sourced information [10]. It is student centered, utilizing group work with the analysis of case studies as a means of learning. Alternatively "peer tutoring" involves individuals from similar settings helping others to learn, which may occur one-on-one or as small group sessions [11]. In nursing, high student numbers increase pressures [12] whilst varied and innovative teaching methods are beneficial [13] with peer learning offering a strategy that may be advantageous.

The Oxford Dictionary (2009) defines a "peer" as someone of the same age or someone who was attending the same university. The term "peer" can also refer to people who have equivalent skills or a commonality of experiences [14]. Both these definitions suit the concept of peer learning described here. The current study aimed to address the following research questions: (i) do undergraduate nursing students benefit from peer learning? and (ii) what approaches to peer learning are the most effective?

2. Methods

Operational terms as shown in Table 1 were developed after consulting several studies. Inclusion and exclusion criteria were defined. A search was conducted for peer-reviewed papers published in English between the years 2000 and 2010 that discussed any aspect of the curriculum for undergraduate or general nursing courses (e.g., clinical skills, communication, patient interaction, or theoretical knowledge).

The literature search was undertaken using the PICO algorithm of Participant, Intervention, Comparison, and Outcome and guidelines from The Cochrane Handbook [15]. For this study the following terms were used:

participant—undergraduate nursing students,

intervention—peer learning,

comparison—classroom lecture learning,

outcome—improvement in theory results or results of practical assessment or personal feelings relating to comfort, confidence, or competence.

A systematic literature search of multiple databases and search engines was undertaken using the keywords and the search strategy described in the following. The keywords used were student nurse, undergraduate nurse, peer learning, peer tutoring, peer mentoring, education, and opinion leaders. Also used were variations and truncations of these words, for example, peer education, nurse education, and problem-based learning. Each of the key words was searched for individually and then in combination with all others.

In addition, a number of key nursing journals such as Journal of Advanced Nursing and Journal of Nursing Education were hand-searched between the years 2000 and 2010. Snowballing, identifying suitable articles from the references of the selected studies, was then conducted to locate further studies.

Studies with all levels of evidence that met the criteria were included because studies in peer learning tended towards quasiexperimental, observational, or case study designs which are all lower on the hierarchy of evidence [16].

Two reviewers conducted a quality analysis of each study using quality criteria for qualitative and quantitative studies of the Critical Skills Appraisal Programme (CASP) [17]. They assessed methodology, validity, sample type, selection method, level of evidence, and any attrition rate and its effect (including biases), to determine selection. Consensus was reached through discussion. Data extraction and thematic analysis were undertaken to synthesize the data. Meta-analysis was not undertaken due to the inconsistent definition of "peer" and potential for bias if different methods of peer learning were combined. Although the primary review was conducted by a single researcher, inclusion and exclusion criteria were adhered to, using a transparent reporting process to allow the search to be reproduced.

Data were extracted and summarized in separate tables: quantitative studies (Table 2), qualitative studies (Table 3), and mixed method studies (Table 4). Drawing from this, data outcomes were collated into themes and subthemes; for example, the resources theme had three subthemes: faculty, students, and peers.

Table 1: Operational definitions.

Term	Definition
Peer	A person with a comparable or slightly higher level of knowledge and experience to the learner. A person of any age can be a peer, that is, a third year student tutoring a first year student but the peer must be an undergraduate nursing student.
Peer learning	Gaining, refining, or improving knowledge from interaction with a peer as defined previously.
Mentor	A peer, who supports, guides, and educates a learner.
Undergraduate nursing student	A nursing student at any stage of study prior to registration.

Sources: [10, 14, 45, 48–51].

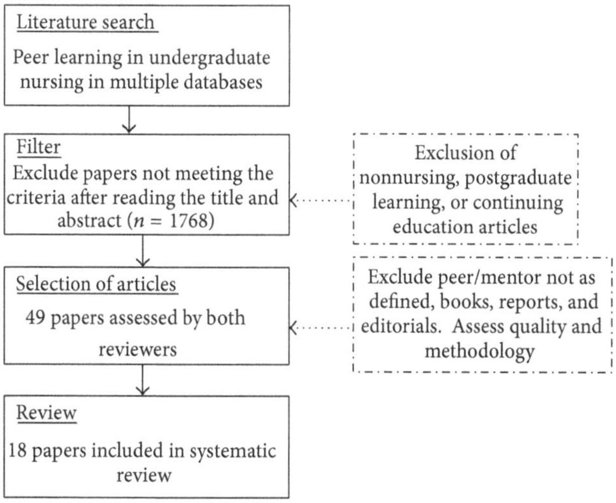

Figure 1: Flow chart of the systematic review selection process.

3. Results

Initially, 1813 studies were screened using the aforementioned criteria and 18 studies were selected for review. A flow chart (Figure 1) shows the selection process including number of studies excluded at each stage and the reason for exclusion.

3.1. Characteristics of Studies. Participants were undergraduate nursing students from first to final year. In line with nursing demography the majority of participants were females. Participant numbers and study duration varied, for example, 15 students over a three-year period [18] and 365 students over a two-year period [7]. A variety of peer learning terms and methods were used. These terms included "peer mentoring" [19], "peer tutoring" [7, 20–23], "peer coaching" [24], "inquiry-based learning" [25, 26], "problem-based learning" [27–31], and "team learning" [32].

Of these studies, eight used a qualitative method, six utilized a quantitative method, and four used mixed methods

Table 2: Summary of included studies.

Author	Design	Intervention and comparison	Country and setting
Broscious and Saunders (2001) [24]	Mixed method Group interview and questionnaire	Peer coaching	Junior and senior year students: Christopher Newport University in USA
Christiansen and Bell (2010) [19]	Qualitative Interpretive	Peer learning	UK University preregistration nursing course
Christiansen and Jensen (2008) [33]	Qualitative Ethnographic	Role playing	Third year student nurses in Norway
Cooke and Moyle (2002) [27]	Qualitative—case studies	PBL versus CLL	Second year students at university in Australia
Daley et al. (2008) [20]	Qualitative Observation, focus groups, and journaling	Peer tutoring	Ohio State University, College of Nursing Students
Feingold et al. (2008) [32]	Mixed methods Observation and interviews	Team learning	First year student nurses: university in South Western USA
Goldsmith et al. (2006) [7]	Mixed method Portfolios, clinical assessment, and questionnaires	Peer learning	First/third year students: Clinical Practice Unit (CPU) of a nursing school in Australia
Higgins (2004) [21]	Quantitative Quasiexperimental	Peer tutoring versus nonpeer tutored	Medical-surgical undergraduate nursing course: Texas, USA
Hughes et al. (2003) [35]	Quantitative Pretest/posttest crossover	Peer group experience versus nonpeer group experience	Baccalaureate school of nursing in USA
Horne et al. (2007) [25]	Qualitative Focus group interviews and use of fourth generation evaluation	Enquiry-based learning	Second year students at a higher education setting in the UK
Lin et al. (2010) [22]	Quantitative Experimental	Peer tutoring. PBL method in class versus CLL	Nursing ethics classes: university in Taiwan
Loke and Chow (2007) [23]	Qualitative Focus groups and individual interviews	Cooperative learning	Second/third year student nurses: university in Hong Kong
Morris and Turnbull (2004) [26]	Qualitative evaluation Focus group interviews, field notes	Peer tutoring	3-year undergraduate nursing course in the UK
Ozturk et al. (2008) [28]	Qualitative Descriptive, analytical	PBL versus CLL	Fourth year undergraduate student nurses from two universities in Izmir, Turkey
Rideout et al. (2002) [29]	Quantitative survey Cross-sectional analytical design	PBL versus CLL	Baccalaureate school of nursing and CLL programme in Canada
Roberts (2008) [18]	Qualitative Interpretive ethnographic	Informal peer learning	Undergraduate students over a three-year course in a range of acute settings including intensive care, general surgical, rehabilitation, and medical wards in the UK
Siu et al. (2005) [30]	Quantitative Descriptive, correlation survey design	PBL versus CLL	Two universities in Ontario, Canada
Tiwari et al. (2006) [31]	Mixed methods Random controlled trial and survey	PBL versus CLL	First year student nurses: university in Hong Kong

PBL: problem-based learning, CLL: classroom lecture learning.

(see Table 2). The quantitative studies favoured scaling and rating approaches (e.g., Likert scales), applying valid tools including the Californian Critical Thinking Disposition Inventory [28, 31], the Psychological Empowerment Scale [30], or the Nursing Ethical Discrimination Ability Scale [22] to collect data. The qualitative studies used a variety of collection methods such as participant observation [18], focus groups [19, 20, 25, 26, 33], individual interviews [23], and open ended short answer questions [27]. Combinations of these methods were used by the mixed method studies. In addition a variety of statistics software and applicable inferential statistics were used in the quantitative and mixed method studies, whilst the qualitative studies used applicable thematic approaches to analysis.

The analysis tools and tests used were presented (see Tables 1, 2, 3, 4, and 5) and considered as part of the quality analysis. Whilst quantitative studies give a definitive, measurable result, the use of qualitative studies in this paper

TABLE 3: Quantitative studies.

Author/year	Aims	Sample/method	Power calculation/software/analysis tool used	Outcomes	Generalization and confounding factors	Further research
Higgins (2004) [21]	To determine relationship between academic performance, retention, and participation in a peer-tutoring programme.	Purposive sample: 26 at-risk students were offered peer tutoring $n = 20$ peer tutored; $n = 6$ in nonpeer tutored group	(i) Power calculation not given. (ii) Fisher's exact test; a two by two bivariate frequency distribution.	Significant relationship between academic performance/retention and participation in a peer-tutoring programme. Attrition rate decreased from 12% to 3%.	Difficult to generalize—no randomization; those who sought peer tutoring may be more motivated to pass. Small sample limited the finding.	Other nursing programs should duplicate peer tutoring for at-risk students in their courses
Hughes et al. (2003) [35]	To investigate effect of an informal peer group experience on baccalaureate nursing students.	Convenience sampling Voluntary selection $N = 128$	Insufficient power to detect group differences; multiple tools assessed, anxiety, depression, professional socialization, and general self-efficacy.	No significant differences between groups, but increased depression (mean 0.83, SD 0.55) and anxiety (mean 2.40, SD 0.81).	Restricted to two universities. Not generalized. Anecdotal accounts: programme was beneficial maintaining contact with others from group, assisting coping skills.	Need for longitudinal study on nursing at varying stages in course
Lin et al. (2010) [22]	To compare the educational results of peer tutor problem-based learning and conventional teaching in nursing ethics education.	Convenience sampling Randomly assigned to control and intervention groups control = 70, intervention = 72	No power calculation done. Nursing Ethical Discrimination Ability Scale; Learning Satisfaction Survey. Internal consistency reached 0.8 and split-halves reliability was 0.76.	Both methods effective for teaching ethics with PBL ($P < 0.01$) slightly more effective than conventional lecture ($P = 0.020$).	Only one university. Limited training of peers, no evaluation of how peers did their job. Teaching materials/teachers may have influenced result. Students used to CLL may prefer this.	Method needs further validation.
Ozturk et al. (2008) [28]	To compare effects of PBL and traditional education on senior undergraduate nursing students' critical thinking dispositions.	Convenience sampling: PBL = 52, CLL = 95	Power calculation not given. California Critical Thinking Disposition Inventory. Independent t-tests for between-group differences.	PBL group showed higher levels of critical thinking than control group ($P < 0.01$); both groups in medium range for critical thinking (between 240 and 300 on CCTDI).	Two universities, voluntary participation, but good response rates. Generalization could be made with reservations as corroborate previous studies.	Alluded to development of a tool to measure critical thinking that is more specific to nursing.
Rideout et al. (2002) [29]	To compare graduate baccalaureate students in a PBL curriculum with others in a CLL programme.	Convenience sampling: PBL = 75, CLL = 52	No power calculation given. $P < 0.01$. t-tests, ANOVA for statistical analysis.	No differences in final exam results ($P = 0.21$) Passed: PBL 93% and CLL 98%)	Restricted to two universities.	Future studies to be longitudinal in design and relying less on self-report measures.
Siu et al. (2005) [30]	To evaluate if nursing students enrolled in PBL programme had higher perceptions of empowerment than those in conventional learning lecture (CLL).	Convenience sampling: PBL = 83, CLL = 70	No power calculation given. Conditions for Learning Effectiveness Questionnaire (CLEQ). Psychological Empowerment Scale, Teaching-Learning Strategies Questionnaire, Clinical Problem-Solving Scale. ANCOVA; Spearman's Rho applied.	PBL experienced greater structural empowerment ($P = 0.001$). Students taking responsibility for their own learning helped develop effective communication, listening, problem solving, and collaboration skills.	Sample from only two universities. Self-selection and self-reporting questionnaires were a potential problem.	Need for longitudinal investigation and replication with samples from several nursing programs.

Table 4: Qualitative studies.

Author/year	Aims	Participant selection	Assessment measures	Outcomes	Suggested research
Christiansen and Bell (2010) [19]	To explore impact of peer learning initiative to facilitate mutually supportive learning between student nurses.	Purposively selected. $N = 54$.	Focus group interviews. Narrative date analyzed thematically. Data collected over 18 months with 3 cohorts of students.	Active support from peers can reduce negative feelings experienced by first year student nurses. It assists coping and decreases attrition rates. Peers benefited by gaining confidence and increased readiness for registered practice.	Explore impact of peer learning on mentors in the workplace.
Christiansen and Jensen (2008) [33]	To explore classroom-based peer learning enabling students to cultivate their modes of expression.	Voluntary selection from 288 students doing third year communication course; 16 students took part in role play and 8 in focus group interview.	Observations and focus groups.	Provide tools that can be used in clinical practice. Students learnt from each other and appreciated being able to experience different roles.	Further study on students emotional learning during periods of clinical practice.
Cooke and Moyle (2002) [27]	To explore and evaluate the use of PBL over a one-month period in programme that uses CLL.	130 students—100 responded to questionnaire.	Open ended questionnaire.	Gave more control over learning and added responsibility, promoting independent, self-directed learning. PBL was enjoyable.	None mentioned.
Daley et al., (2008) [20]	To evaluate a peer-tutoring approach to teaching designed to meet needs of two different levels of students.	All first year and some senior students in a leadership and management course.	Observations, conferences, focus groups, and journals. Multiple levels of evaluation.	Assignment of higher acuity patients to first years. Confidence of weaker students increased. Better understanding of role of team member, improvement in cognitive and motor skills, increased comfort in asking questions/discussing concepts, and awareness of a future role as mentor.	Additional work and formal evaluation of programme.
Horne et al. (2007) [25]	To evaluate student and facilitator perspectives of hybrid model of problem-based learning.	All 121 second year students and 15 facilitators.	Focus group interviews and use of Fourth Generation Evaluation (nominal group technique).	PBL aided development of independent learning skills, self-awareness, and confidence skills. Improved interpersonal/communication skills but depended on group collaboration and concerns about teamwork and group dynamics.	Further study of effectiveness for large groups of students >100.
Loke and Chow (2007) [23]	To facilitate the development of "cooperative learning" among nursing students through peer tutoring.	Voluntary selection of 14 third year students as tutors and 16 second year-students as tutees.	Focus groups and individual interviews at half way and end of 10-week tutoring period.	Positives included enhancement of deep learning, critical thinking, problem solving, communication skills, confidence in own learning, and time management. Negatives included participants being late or feeling of not having adequate knowledge to share with one another and mismatched personalities.	Further studies to examine peer-tutoring effects on students in all years.
Morris and Turnbull (2004) [26]	To explore viability and value of using student nurses as teachers in inquiry-based nursing curriculum.	A purposive sample of 240 student nurses (36%) participated in interviews.	Focus group interviews, field notes, interviews audio-taped, transcribed, and analyzed using thematic analysis.	Student nurses were uncomfortable with this method and thought it mostly inappropriate, although it may be appropriate in some circumstances. Use of parallel resource sessions in a nonfacilitated forum is problematic. Participants did not think that skills were transferable.	Further research required on the use of students as teachers.
Roberts (2008) [18]	To explore if students learn from each other and how, when/where this takes place.	Voluntary selection of 15 students.	Audio-taped conversations of students and field notes; thematic analysis.	Friendships are important to learning. Peer learning in clinical practice is informal and considered part of the job. It helped students to ask questions and contribute to the ward. Students were approachable and had more time for teaching. Students valued peers in clinical setting helping each other to cope with demands of clinical practice.	Replicate study with other groups of students in different locations and branches of nursing.

Table 5: Mixed method studies.

Year/author/	Aims	Setting	Participant selection	Assessment measures	Outcomes	Generalizations and limitations	Suggested research
Broscious and Saunders (2001) [24]	To implement a strategy to reduce student anxiety during their first clinical experience.	Junior/senior year students in university in USA	20 senior students and 25 junior students. Convenience sample of all students in year.	Group interview and Likert scale survey: scale had statements presented as description of student experiences.	On 5-point Likert scale (only means reported) students reported decreased sense of anxiety (mean 4.29), increasing confidence (mean 4.08), improved organization (mean 3.91), and perception of being a member of the team (mean 3.83). Senior students practiced leadership skill (mean 4.53), established priorities (mean 4.4), and developed plan of care (4.4). Reiterated amount learnt by senior. Impact of coach decreased in subsequent clinical session.	Small sample and voluntary selection limits generalization.	Further study by modifying and different sites and larger sample.
Feingold et al. (2008) [32]	To evaluate student perception of team learning and effect on class interaction and engagement.	First year student nurses at a university in south-western USA	First year students in course. Convenience sample: for interview—10%, responses—21%.	Observation and interviews (Qualitative). STROBE classroom observation tool (Quantitative).	Team learning promoted student engagement and was predominantly interactive. Over 305 minutes, most students were engaged/on task for 84% of time, with 70% of time being learner to learner engagement and further 8% of time being used for self-engagement. Main behaviour was learner to learner engagement. Recognized benefit of discussion of problems.	The concept could be generalized. Small sample may not be representative of first year students (nonrandom, self-selected).	Further study to help refine team learning process and to guide implementation of interactive learning strategies.
Goldsmith et al. (2006) [7]	To explore impact of peer learning on anxiety of first year student nurses when undertaking clinical skills assessments.	First/3rd year students in Clinical Practice Unit (CPU) in Australia (Conducted over two years and two campuses)	First/3rd year students in 2-year time frame. First year cohort of 187; 3rd year: 178.	Portfolio submission as 3rd year, clinical skills assessment for first year students. Both groups completed questionnaires.	Learning enhanced by experience. Evaluation completed after 2 years; good representations of both campuses/years. Learning enhanced by experience. Positive answers to questions were given by a majority of both 1st/3rd years with 3rd years more likely to give positive responses.	Only two campuses of one university. Late development of assessment tool with not all students given opportunity to complete questionnaire. Voluntary completion of questionnaire which may not have been representative.	Not reported.
Tiwari et al. (2006) [31]	To compare effects of problem-based learning and lecturing approaches on development of students' critical thinking.	First year student nurses in one university in Hong Kong	All 79 students in first year randomly assigned to control and intervention groups. PBL = 40, CLL = 39. Selection by ballot.	Multivariate regression, 1 and 2 sample *t*-tests.	No significant difference between groups at initial testing ($P = 0.48$). 2nd and 3rd data collection points showed significant difference in overall CCDTI scores between PBL and control groups ($P = 0.0048$, $P = 0.0083$). The 4th collection point showed higher score on the CCDTI for PBL group but nonsignificant difference ($P = 0.1159$). PBL students found their course more enjoyable/inspiring than lecture group.	Only one university and a small sample. Results may have been influenced by how lectures were conducted. Use of self-reporting tool.	Monitoring of groups critical thinking in subsequent years.

examined how the participants felt about a different method of learning and how it impacted on them. These opinions would be important if peer learning was to gain acceptance from the students and peers. Qualitative studies had much smaller participant numbers and whilst larger numbers may have provided a more comprehensive sample, there were saturation and repetition of concepts even with the smaller samples.

Experimental studies with the highest level of evidence, that is, random controlled trials (RCTs), were not a common method of evaluating peer learning as they may not reproduce the true situation in an educational setting [34].

Eight studies used a comparison group [21, 22, 27–31, 35], and all except two [27, 31] were quantitative studies. Valid tools were used by 9 of the 10 quantitative or mixed method studies. It was concluded that valid tools measured what the authors intended, and hence data were an accurate representation of what had occurred and were credible. However, one study [21] failed to report the number of control and intervention group participants who passed their course. The qualitative studies documented the research process clearly, and the findings were consistent with the data provided. The details in description of the research process and findings varied between studies, whilst within individual studies, sample size, location, and the subjects taught were all potentially limiting; for example, small sample size, specific location, or subject may have caused a bias in the results, hence affecting the transferability of results [24, 31]. Publication bias was not evident as the included studies reported both the positive and negative results, for example, using comments from participants [26] or differences in means [35].

3.2. Effects of Peer Learning. Peer learning encouraged independent study, critical thinking, and problem solving skills. It could give students a sense of autonomy when they accepted responsibility for their own education. Peer learning was associated with increased levels of knowledge in a number of areas such as problem solving and communication [20, 25]. Tiwari et al. [31] showed that critical thinking was improved in students using PBL ($P = 0.0048$) whilst Daley et al. [20] reported that students showed improvement in cognitive and motor skills. An advantage of peer learning was that both groups learned and benefited from the interaction [23, 24]. The benefits differed between the students and peers with the peers gaining experience in communication and leadership, reinforcing their prior learning and discovering what they were capable of achieving in the mentoring/teaching fields [19, 24]. On the other hand, students gained confidence and experienced a decrease in anxiety when dealing with certain situations such as clinical placements. PBL was reported to be effective particularly in the theoretical learning component of education whilst peer tutoring, peer coaching, peer mentoring, and the use of role play as a form of peer learning were all effective, both in clinical and theoretical aspects of nursing education.

One negative aspect was related to anxiety levels. Group learning showed an increase in anxiety in both control and intervention groups [35], whilst other methods such as peer coaching showed a decrease in anxiety in the clinical setting [24]. The students indicated that having another person assist them decreased their anxiety levels which was pertinent when they were beginning their careers and were uncertain and anxious about what was expected of them [18]. Informal peer learning also benefited the students by providing them with "survival" skills that are not taught in lectures or text books, which in turn assisted in decreasing anxiety [18].

In addition to decreasing anxiety [24], many students showed an increase in satisfaction when peer learning was used [22, 29], appreciating having to think for themselves, problem-solve, and work as a team [20, 24, 27, 30]. The level of satisfaction is higher with peer learning [29] than the passive CLL method although some students still prefer CLL as it maybe better suited their individual learning style [22]. Whilst none of the studies in this paper directly investigated the link between course satisfaction and academic results, Higgins [21] noted a decrease in attrition rate but did not specify student satisfaction levels.

Four studies [20, 23–25] examined confidence in students when utilizing peer learning. They showed a subjective increase in confidence levels when completing clinical skills, problem solving, and critical thinking. In addition, 11 studies indicated that students appreciated interactive learning sessions and the emphasis on active participation, which encouraged them to take ownership and responsibility for their own learning.

3.3. Utilization. Peer learning was utilized in multiple situations from teaching ethics [22] and critical thinking [31] to helping students deal with emotional situations [19] with patients. In clinical situations peer learning was successful and improved integration into the ward situations [18] and students' confidence when dealing with actual patients rather than a simulator [20]. Further, a number of studies identified outcome measures showing an improvement in either an objective or subjective assessment.

4. Discussion

The purpose of this research was to ascertain whether undergraduate nursing students benefit from peer learning. Sixteen of eighteen studies demonstrated positive aspects to peer learning with outcome measures showing improvement in either an objective effect or a subjective assessment (such as a self-rated increase in student confidence). Furthermore, learning from peers was shown to be acceptable to most students. Much of the research into peer learning concentrated on formal peer learning with the evidence supporting the concept that peer learning may be an equally, if not more, effective method of delivering information in undergraduate nursing education.

Peer learning can be utilized to pass information to large groups of students with less faculty member involvement. At a time when there is pressure to train more nurses and minimize costs [12], peer learning could utilize resources more effectively with students teaching and supervising more junior students, thus decreasing the demand on the responsible faculty members. Therefore it may have cost benefits for managing some aspects of nursing education; however this theory requires further investigation as it was not the focus of any of the papers mentioned in this paper.

Regardless of any decrease in active involvement by lecturers, the need for student supervision remains important. If peers are not knowledgeable or do not have the appropriate skills, then they cannot accurately pass information onto another student. The learning of inaccurate information could potentially cause issues for students when these inaccuracies were demonstrated in exams and on clinical placements. Without supervision, learning may not be effective as shown in an earlier study by Parkin [4] who found that observation and supervision were required in all peer learning to ensure that correct and current information was being exchanged.

4.1. Advantages and Disadvantages. Peer learning may result in information being more readily accepted by a student as individuals often turn to others who have similar experiences, for advice and guidance. This could decrease anxiety associated with learning due to familiarity of the peer with the student's issues. As noted in the results, anxiety may occur when individuals are exposed to new concepts, whether they are novice or proficient learners [36]. In prior research [37], peer learning helped to decrease the student's anxiety and assisted them to fit into a ward situation and feel like part of the team. This sense of belonging has social implications particularly when it is known that learning occurs more effectively when there is socialization [38, 39].

Further, social interaction and collaboration between peer and student may have contributed to an increased learning curve and acquisition of further knowledge than would have occurred if students were studying independently. This was illustrated in this paper with students who had been in danger of failing and had received peer tutoring [21]. They gained additional knowledge and improved their academic result. This method may also allow junior students to problem-solve issues with their patients more independently and care for higher acuity patients, leading to an increase in their self-confidence. This concept was previously reported by Vygotsky [40], Aston and Molassiotis [41], and Secomb [5] who found that peer learning promoted self-confidence in junior students whilst assisting senior students with mentoring and teaching skills. Secomb [5] also showed that peer learning was an effective learning tool in clinical situations with both nursing and other health professionals. Peers perceived an increase in patient care competence when peer learning was utilized. Secomb [5] noted, however, that issues such as inappropriate pairing of students and peers should be addressed prior to the intervention.

Student satisfaction may play a part in scholastic achievement through acceptance of an active learning method such as peer learning. Four studies investigating this component [22, 28–30] discovered that students were satisfied with peer learning as the educational method. This may be because the student takes more responsibility and actively participates in their education, giving them a sense of autonomy. Whilst Ozturk et al. [28] reported a higher satisfaction level with PBL but no significant difference in academic scores, previous studies have shown a positive association between student satisfaction and grades achieved [42, 43].

Peer learning may also be more successful when peers are close in experience or stage of training as it provides a more relaxed, less intimidating, more "user friendly" learning experience than sessions conducted by registered nurses. Prior to the current study, El Ansari and Oskrochi [44], Eisen [45], and Secomb [5] also reported this finding whilst more recently Bensfield et al. [46] reported that first year students had comfortable learning with more experienced peers.

There is, however, a different perspective. Whilst peer learning has been used for years and might be becoming the norm, students may not be fully familiar with it and therefore be apprehensive about what it offers. Some students reported anxiety and apprehension when taking part in peer learning which was linked to feeling responsible for another's education [25, 26], being underprepared [23] or concerned that their own grades would be negatively affected by group work or dynamics [25, 26, 32]. Further, it was reported that enforcing the educational role of a peer may lead to resentment, particularly if the nurse felt unprepared or unwilling to undertake the role [26]. Previously Bensfield et al. [46] showed that whilst nurses have a responsibility to teach others, many are reluctant to do so as they feel unprepared for the role. Due to these issues, students who are familiar and comfortable with CLL may continue to prefer this learning method over peer learning.

4.2. Confusing Terminology Used in Peer Learning. Finally, this paper raises issues around the confusing terminology used to refer to peer learning. As mentioned, multiple terms such as peer teaching, peer mentoring, and peer coaching were used interchangeably with debate about whether they meant the same thing or referred to subtle differences in meaning. A clearer definition of each of the terms is needed to increase the rigor of nursing education research, as was also raised by Secomb [5], Eisen [45], and McKenna and French [47] who found a lack of clarity as to what peer education entailed due to the interchanging of terminology. We suggest amalgamation of some of the terms, for example, team learning and cooperative learning or peer mentoring and peer coaching and having distinct differences in definitions between other terms.

5. Limitations

Some limitations of this study were recognized. Only studies published in English were included. Despite a rigorous search strategy, some relevant articles may have been omitted owing to the search terms used. The mix of study designs and various methods of reporting meant that direct comparison between studies was limited. Some studies were location- or topic-specific, and some studies collected data using indirect outcome measures. However, the collection and review of the diverse papers that were selected offered the best option for determining the overall impact of peer learning in education of nursing students.

6. Conclusion

Peer learning: learning from others who possess a similar level of knowledge, is becoming a part of nursing education. This study showed that undergraduate nursing students could benefit from peer learning, with an increase in confidence and competence and a decrease in anxiety. Their peers also gained skills to prepare them for their role as a registered nurse. Conduct of peer learning within the curriculum was shown to require adequate academic supervision to be effective. It was difficult to ascertain the most effective learning methods because of the inherent variation between study methodologies, terminology, subjects, and settings. Inconsistency terminology was identified as a problem that should be addressed in order to provide clarity in future research.

7. Further Research

Further research is needed to fully investigate peer learning with the use of larger samples, various targeted curricula, courses, and locations to increase the validity of studies. The cost effectiveness of peer learning should be further investigated and compared to that of CLL to ascertain how this option could impact nursing education in terms of resources, time management, and effectiveness.

References

[1] C. L. Iwasiw, D. Goldenderg, and M. A. Andrusyszyn, *Curriculum Development in Nursing Education*, Jones & Bartlett, Boston, Mass, USA, 2nd edition, 2009.

[2] M. Banning, "Approaches to teaching: current opinions and related research," *Nurse Education Today*, vol. 25, no. 7, pp. 502–508, 2005.

[3] S. Paterson and R. Stone, "Educational leadership beyond behaviourism, the lessons we have learnt from art education," *Australian Art Education*, vol. 29, no. 1, pp. 76–83, 2006.

[4] V. Parkin, "Peer education: the nursing experience," *Journal of Continuing Education in Nursing*, vol. 37, no. 6, pp. 257–264, 2006.

[5] J. Secomb, "A systematic review of peer teaching and learning in clinical education," *Journal of Clinical Nursing*, vol. 17, no. 6, pp. 703–716, 2008.

[6] L. D. Owens and D. J. Walden, "Peer instruction in the learning laboratory: a strategy to decrease student anxiety," *Journal of Nursing Education*, vol. 40, no. 8, pp. 375–377, 2001.

[7] M. Goldsmith, L. Stewart, and L. Ferguson, "Peer learning partnership: an innovative strategy to enhance skill acquisition in nursing students," *Nurse Education Today*, vol. 26, no. 2, pp. 123–130, 2006.

[8] S. Blowers, P. Ramsey, C. Merriman, and J. Grooms, "Patterns of peer tutoring in nursing," *Journal of Nursing Education*, vol. 42, no. 5, pp. 204–211, 2003.

[9] H. Yuan, B. A. Williams, and L. Fan, "A systematic review of selected evidence on developing nursing students' critical thinking through problem-based learning," *Nurse Education Today*, vol. 28, no. 6, pp. 657–663, 2008.

[10] A. J. Neville, "Problem-based learning and medical education forty years on: a review of its effects on knowledge and clinical performance," *Medical Principles and Practice*, vol. 18, no. 1, pp. 1–9, 2008.

[11] D. Nestel and J. Kidd, "Peer tutoring in patient-centred interviewing skills: experience of a project for first-year students," *Medical Teacher*, vol. 25, no. 4, pp. 398–403, 2003.

[12] H. T. Allan, P. A. Smith, and M. Lorentzon, "Leadership for learning: a literature study of leadership for learning in clinical practice," *Journal of Nursing Management*, vol. 16, no. 5, pp. 545–555, 2008.

[13] D. Shipman and J. Hooten, "Without enough nurse educators there will be a continual decline in RNs and the quality of nursing care: contending with the faculty shortage," *Nurse Education Today*, vol. 28, no. 5, pp. 521–523, 2008.

[14] J. Green, "Peer education," *Promotion & Education*, vol. 8, no. 2, pp. 65–68, 2001.

[15] J. P. T. Higgins and S. Green, "Cochrane Handbook for systematic reviews of interventions: The Cochrane Collaboration," 2009, http://www.cochrane-handbook.org/ .

[16] The National Health and Medical Research Council, *NHMRC Additional Levels of Evidence and Grades for Recommendations for Developers of Guidelines. Stage 2 Consultation*, The Australian Government, Parkes ACT, Australia, 2009.

[17] Public Health Resource Unit, "Critical Appraisal Skills Programme Making sense of evidence, 10 questions to help you make sense of reviews," 2006, http://www.phru.nhs.uk/Doc_Links/S.Reviews%20Appraisal%20Tool.pdf.

[18] D. Roberts, "Learning in clinical practice: the importance of peers," *Nursing Standard*, vol. 23, no. 12, pp. 35–41, 2008.

[19] A. Christiansen and A. Bell, "Peer learning partnerships: exploring the experience of pre-registration nursing students," *Journal of Clinical Nursing*, vol. 19, no. 5-6, pp. 803–810, 2010.

[20] L. K. Daley, E. Menke, B. Kirkpatrick, and D. Sheets, "Partners in practice: a win-win model for clinical education," *Journal of Nursing Education*, vol. 47, no. 1, pp. 30–32, 2008.

[21] B. Higgins, "Relationship between retention and peer tutoring for at-risk students," *Journal of Nursing Education*, vol. 43, no. 7, pp. 319–321, 2004.

[22] C. F. Lin, M. S. Lu, C. C. Chung, and C. M. Yang, "A comparison of problem-based learning and conventional teaching in nursing ethics education," *Nursing Ethics*, vol. 17, no. 3, pp. 373–382, 2010.

[23] A. Y. Loke and F. L. W. Chow, "Learning partnership-the experience of peer tutoring among nursing students: a qualitative study," *International Journal of Nursing Studies*, vol. 44, no. 2, pp. 237–244, 2007.

[24] S. K. Broscious and D. J. Saunders, "Peer coaching," *Nurse Educator*, vol. 26, no. 5, pp. 212–214, 2001.

[25] M. Horne, K. Woodhead, L. Morgan, L. Smithies, D. Megson, and G. Lyte, "Using enquiry in learning: from vision to reality in higher education," *Nurse Education Today*, vol. 27, no. 2, pp. 103–112, 2007.

[26] D. Morris and P. Turnbull, "Using student nurses as teachers in inquiry-based learning," *Journal of Advanced Nursing*, vol. 45, no. 2, pp. 136–144, 2004.

[27] M. Cooke and K. Moyle, "Students' evaluation of problem-based learning," *Nurse Education Today*, vol. 22, no. 4, pp. 330–339, 2002.

[28] C. Ozturk, G. K. Muslu, and A. Dicle, "A comparison of problem-based and traditional education on nursing students' critical thinking dispositions," *Nurse Education Today*, vol. 28, no. 5, pp. 627–632, 2008.

[29] E. Rideout, V. England-Oxford, B. Brown et al., "A comparison of problem-based and conventional curricula in nursing education," *Advances in Health Sciences Education*, vol. 7, no. 1, pp. 3–17, 2002.

[30] H. M. Siu, H. K. Spence Laschinger, and E. Vingilis, "The effect of problem-based learning on nursing students' perceptions of empowerment," *Journal of Nursing Education*, vol. 44, no. 10, pp. 459–469, 2005.

[31] A. Tiwari, P. Lai, M. So, and K. Yuen, "A comparison of the effects of problem-based learning and lecturing on the development of students' critical thinking," *Medical Education*, vol. 40, no. 6, pp. 547–554, 2006.

[32] C. E. Feingold, M. D. Cobb, R. Hernandez Givens, J. Arnold, S. Joslin, and J. L. Keller, "Student perceptions of team learning in nursing education," *Journal of Nursing Education*, vol. 47, no. 5, pp. 214–222, 2008.

[33] B. Christiansen and K. Jensen, "Emotional learning within the framework of nursing education," *Nurse Education in Practice*, vol. 8, no. 5, pp. 328–334, 2008.

[34] B. Jolly, "Control and validity in medical educational research," *Medical Education*, vol. 35, no. 10, pp. 920–921, 2001.

[35] L. C. Hughes, P. Romick, M. K. Sandor et al., "Evaluation of an informal peer group experience on baccalaureate nursing students' emotional well-being and professional socialization," *Journal of Professional Nursing*, vol. 19, no. 1, pp. 38–48, 2003.

[36] L. T. Adams, "Nursing shortage solutions and America's economic recovery," *Nursing Education Perspectives*, vol. 30, no. 6, p. 349, 2009.

[37] P. Benner, "Using the dreyfus model of skill acquisition to describe and interpret skill acquisition and clinical judgment in nursing practice and education," *Bulletin of Science, Technology and Society*, vol. 24, no. 3, pp. 188–199, 2004.

[38] J. M. Parr and M. A. R. Townsend, "Environments, processes, and mechanisms in peer learning," *International Journal of Educational Research*, vol. 37, no. 5, pp. 403–423, 2002.

[39] I. A. G. Wilkinson, "Peer influences on learning: where are they?" *International Journal of Educational Research*, vol. 37, no. 5, pp. 395–401, 2002.

[40] L. S. Vygotsky, *Biological and Social Factors in Education. Educational Psychology*, St. Lucie Press, Boca Raton, Fla, USA, 1997.

[41] L. Aston and A. Molassiotis, "Supervising and supporting student nurses in clinical placements: the peer support initiative," *Nurse Education Today*, vol. 23, no. 3, pp. 202–210, 2003.

[42] B. Sinclair and K. Ferguson, "Integrating simulated teaching/learning strategies in undergraduate nursing education," *International Journal of Nursing Education Scholarship*, vol. 6, no. 1, p. 7, 2009.

[43] P. M. Casey, D. Magrane, and T. G. Lesnick, "Improved performance and student satisfaction after implementation of a problem-based preclinical obstetrics and gynecology curriculum," *American Journal of Obstetrics and Gynecology*, vol. 193, no. 5, pp. 1874–1878, 2005.

[44] W. El Ansari and R. Oskrochi, "What matters most? Predictors of student satisfaction in public health educational courses," *Public Health*, vol. 120, no. 5, pp. 462–473, 2006.

[45] M. J. Eisen, "Peer-based professional development viewed through the lens of transformative learning," *Holistic Nursing Practice*, vol. 16, no. 1, pp. 30–42, 2001.

[46] L. Bensfield, P. A. Solari-Twadell, and S. Sommer, "The use of peer leadership to teach fundamental nursing skills," *Nurse Educator*, vol. 33, no. 4, pp. 155–158, 2008.

[47] L. McKenna and J. French, "A step ahead: teaching undergraduate students to be peer teachers," *Nurse Education in Practice*, vol. 11, no. 2, pp. 141–145, 2011.

[48] D. Nestel and J. Kidd, "Peer assisted learning in patient-centred interviewing: the impact on student tutors," *Medical Teacher*, vol. 27, no. 5, pp. 439–444, 2005.

[49] R. Duggan, "A little help from your PALs," *Nursing Standard*, vol. 14, no. 38, p. 55, 2000.

[50] J. E. Duchscher, "Peer learning: a clinical teaching strategy to promote active learning," *Nurse Educator*, vol. 26, no. 2, pp. 59–60, 2001.

[51] S. Dennison, "Peer mentoring: untapped potential," *Journal of Nursing Education*, vol. 49, no. 6, pp. 340–342, 2010.

19

Nurse Managers' Perceptions Related to Their Leadership Styles, Knowledge, and Skills in These Areas—A Viewpoint: Case of Health Centre Wards in Finland

Soili Vesterinen,[1,2] Marjo Suhonen,[2] Arja Isola,[2] Leena Paasivaara,[2] and Helena Laukkala[2]

[1] *Lapland Hospital District, P.O. Box 8041, 96101 Rovaniemi, Finland*
[2] *Department of Health Sciences, University of Oulu, P.O. Box 5000, 90014 University of Oulu, Finland*

Correspondence should be addressed to Soili Vesterinen; soili.vesterinen@lshp.fi

Academic Editors: B. M. Andersen, K. Clark, and A. Kenny

The purpose of this study was to explore nurse managers' perceptions related to their leadership styles, knowledge, and their skills in these areas in health centre wards in Finland. The data were collected from nurse managers ($n = 252$) in health centre hospitals in Finland using a structured questionnaire (response rate 63%). Six leadership styles—visionary, coaching, affiliate, democratic, commanding, and isolating—were reflected on. Almost all respondents in every age group considered four leadership styles—visionary, coaching, affiliate, and democratic—to be very important or important. Nurse managers estimated their knowledge and skills in leadership styles to be essentially fairly sufficient or sufficient. Nurse managers' abilities to reflect, understand, and, if necessary, change their leadership style influence the work unit's success and employees' job satisfaction. Nurse managers, especially new nurse managers, need more theoretic, evidence-based education to cope with these expectations and to develop their professional abilities. Together with universities, health care organizations should start planning nurse manager education programmes that focus on strategic issues, leadership, job satisfaction, challenging situations in leadership, change management, work unit management (e.g., economy, efficiency, and resources), and how the nurse managers consider their own wellbeing.

1. Introduction

In many European countries, the public health care system is facing challenges, such as problems in recruiting professionals [1, 2] and staff retention [3]. The situation in Finland is similar. One of the major challenges in Finland is how to secure adequate, trained personnel. The proportion of persons aged over 65 in the Finnish population is estimated to rise from 17 percent to 27 percent by 2040 [4]. Shortage of staff is an imminent threat: 22.5 percent of the employees in social and health care will reach the age of 67 by 2020 at the latest. Most of them will retire at that time, or even earlier [5]. At the same time, 26 percent of young Finnish nurses have often thought of leaving their profession [6].

Nurses' work in health centre wards is physically and mentally burdensome; consequently, nurse manager's leadership skills have a key role in influencing nurses' job satisfaction and their staying on in a work unit [7, 8]. An essential part of leadership skills is the use of different leadership styles [9–11]. Leadership styles can be seen as different combinations of tasks and transaction behaviours that influence people in achieving goals [12].

This paper focuses on nurse managers' leadership styles in health centre hospital wards in Finland, because the Finnish health care system is a strong institution, where health care services are offered to all citizens and funded by taxes [13]. Health care services in Finland are of high quality [14]. It is important to explore nurse managers' leadership styles especially in this context.

The public health care sector in Finland is currently under changes. In June 2010, the government approved a proposal to amend the current health care law with the aim of strengthening primary health care, promoting welfare and health, and enhancing availability and effective production of health services [15]. Public health care system in Finland consists of primary health care and specialized medical care.

Primary care is offered in health centres, which often have a ward for inpatients.

Working in a health centre ward consists of shift work, evenings, nights, and weekends included. Most of the patients in health centre wards have many diseases and are old. In 2008, patients' average age was 75 years [16]. The importance of nurse managers' leadership skills is particularly emphasized in this work context. Essential nurse manager competencies for the future include among other things the ability to create an organization culture that combines high-quality health care and patient/employee safety and highly developed collaborative and team building skills [1]. One future challenge for nurse managers is to create a culture where nurses are not afraid of requiring an environment where they are recognized as invaluable partners in the organization [17]. Nurse managers' role is also essential for promoting evidence-based practice within organizations. Evidence-based practice is important for the professional practice of nursing for many reasons. Because nursing is a science and a profession, nursing practice should be grounded on the best available evidence, and the findings of nursing research should be translated into practice. Evidence-based nursing facilitates paying attention to efficiency (providing nursing care with the appropriate level of staffing) and effectiveness (achieving desired outcomes) in nursing [18]. All of these future challenges can be met with the help of using effective leadership styles [19]. Consequently, nurse managers' major challenges in Finnish health centre wards are related to leadership skills. A nurse manager with the readiness to observe his/her own behaviour and its effects on the work unit and employees can adjust to a better leadership style [12]. Goleman et al. [20] have described primal leadership, which consists of resonant and dissonant leadership styles, depending on the situation. It requires the leader to bring emotional intelligence (EI) to bear on his/her leadership. EI has been associated with positive empowerment processes as well as positive organizational results [21]. Resonant leadership styles have been identified as visionary, coaching, affiliate, and democratic styles, while dissonant leadership styles have been identified as pacesetting and commanding styles. Most leaders use both resonant and dissonant leadership styles [20].

In recent years, nurse manager's EI has been recognized as an important research area [22]. Nurse manager's EI leadership behaviour has a strong impact on nurses' empowerment and organizational commitment [23] as well as on team effectiveness and the quality of nursing care [24]. On the other hand, nurse managers with strong EI may not be able to empower their employees if their span of control is wide [25].

2. Materials and Methods

2.1. Aim and Objectives. This study is the fourth part of a larger investigation concerning nurse managers' leadership styles. The first part was a review of studies on nurse leaders' leadership styles in the years 1996–2006 [26]. In the second part the purpose of the study was to discover nurse managers' perceptions of their leadership styles and the factors influencing it [27]. The third part of the study consisted of exploring how nurses and superiors perceive nurse managers' leadership styles and the factors affected by leadership styles [28]. The aim of the present paper is to explore nurse managers' perceptions related to their leadership styles, knowledge, and their skills in these areas in health centre wards in Finland. The research questions are as follows.

(i) What is the prominent leadership style demonstrated by nurse managers as perceived by themselves in health centre wards?

(ii) How important do nurse managers consider different leadership styles?

(iii) How adequate do nurse managers consider their skills and knowledge in leadership styles? and how important do they consider these styles?

(iv) What are the associations between background variables (age, education, length of work experience as nurse manager, and updating education) and nurse managers' perceptions of the importance of different leadership styles and their knowledge and skills in leadership styles?

2.2. Questionnaire. The questionnaire used in the study is based on the primal leadership model 20 and earlier research of Vesterinen et al. [27, 28]. Once the questionnaire had been drawn up, its content was evaluated by an expert panel (n = 6). The expert panel consisted of nurse managers working in different types of hospital wards. Based on the results, the questionnaire was modified by making two statements more explicit and by revising the language.

In the final questionnaire, the leadership styles of the nurse managers were charted in the following three fields. Background information was asked for by 12 statements. To examine participants' prominent leadership style, they were asked to indicate how significant and important they considered the named factors in their work as nurse managers (36 statements). The response alternatives followed a 5-point Likert scale (1 = not at all important, 2 = rather unimportant, 3 = rather important, 4 = important, and 5 = very important).

Furthermore, the participants were asked to estimate how adequate their knowledge and skills were in different fields of management (34 statements). The response alternatives followed a 4-point Likert scale (1 = not at all sufficient, 2 = not quite sufficient, 3 = rather sufficient, and 4 = sufficient). In this 34-statement instrument, there were 18 statements concerning leadership styles. In this paper, we report on the basis of these statements the results of the respondents' perceptions regarding their knowledge and skills in different leadership styles.

2.3. Data Collection. The target population comprised all nurse managers in health centre hospitals in Finland. First, the number of all nurse managers in different health centres registered in the database of the National institute for Health and Welfare in Finland was enquired (n = 1,317). After that, different health centres were divided into five groups based on the number of nurse managers using stratified sampling: very small (1-2 nurse managers), small (3-4 nurse managers), medium sized (5–9 nurse managers), large (10–29 nurse managers), and very large (30–85 nurse managers). For the nationwide study, health centre organizations were chosen from these five groups using sampling proportional to size. After that, the nurse managers were chosen using systematic sampling until the number of 400 nurse managers was reached [29]. As the organizations had very differing numbers of nurse managers, a minimum of one and a maximum of 63 respondents were included in the study.

The data collection was conducted from November 2009 to April 2010. An application for a statement was submitted to the Local Research Ethics Committee. The administrations of the health centres were contacted via e-mail, and their willingness to participate in the study was enquired. Following approval from the administration of the health centre organizations (n = 108), the data for this study were collected using a mailed questionnaire. The respondents were reached via their work addresses or via a contact person. Questionnaires, information about the study, and return envelopes were mailed straight to the respondents or via the contact person who delivered the material further to the respondents. Participants were informed of the purpose of the study in the covering letter. They were told that their participation was voluntary and would be treated with confidentiality. The covering letter also included detailed contact information on how to reach the researcher. Returning the questionnaire to the researcher was organized by post, which ensured that the identity of the respondents remained unknown. The respondents had three weeks to respond to the questionnaire. The response rate of the study was 63%, which can be regarded as reasonable, considering that the questionnaire was sent by post. The nurse managers' background data are given in Table 1.

2.4. Data Analysis. The data were analysed using the SPSS 12.0 software (SPSS Inc., Chicago, IL, USA). Several variables were analysed using frequencies, mean scores, standard deviations, and descriptive statistics.

Some of the background data variables (age, education, work experience in health care, work experience as nurse manager, and number of employees) were classified before the calculation of frequency and percentage distributions. Some of the statements concerning visionary leadership style (n = 6), coaching leadership style (n = 6), affiliate leadership style (n = 6), democratic leadership style (n = 6), commanding leadership style (n = 6), and isolating leadership style (n = 6) variables were collapsed into sum variables (n = 6) and divided by the number of variables. Next, sum variables were rounded to full figures. The mean SD and minimum and maximum values were calculated for the new sum variables. The internal consistency of the sum variables was assessed with the coefficient Cronbach alpha; values varied from 0.6 to 0.7 [30]. Correlations between variables were analysed using cross-tabulation and chi-squared test. One-way analysis of variance was used to reveal differences in means of sum variables in background variable groups.

TABLE 1: The respondents' (n = 252) background data.

Background data	n	%
Gender (n = 252)		
Female	246	97.6
Male	6	2.4
Age (n = 248)		
32–45	56	22.6
46–50	69	27.8
51–55	56	22.6
56–65	67	27.0
Education (n = 245)		
Specialized nurse	151	61.6
Nurse	57	23.3
MSc	37	15.1
Work experience in health care (n = 249)		
<21	60	24.1
21–25	53	21.3
26–30	63	25.3
>30	73	29.3
Work experience as nurse manager (n = 252)		
<5	71	28.2
5–9	65	25.8
10–14	47	18.7
>14	69	27.3
Updating education in leadership (n = 252)		
Yes	237	94.0
No	15	6.0
Reading professional journals (n = 252)		
Yes	216	85.7
No	36	14.3
Reading scientific journals (n = 252)		
Yes	113	44.8
No	139	55.2
Searching information from internet (n = 252)		
Yes	173	68.7
No	79	31.3
Discussing with colleagues (n = 252)		
Yes	220	87.3
No	32	12.7
Consulting experts (n = 252)		
Yes	91	36.1
No	161	63.9
Number of employees (n = 247)		
<20	69	28.2
20–24	66	26.9
25–29	46	18.8
>29	64	26.1

TABLE 2: Nurse managers' leadership styles in health centre wards.

Leadership style	Mean	SD
Visionary	4.51	0.37
Coaching	4.45	0.38
Affiliate	4.33	0.39
Democratic	4.39	0.35
Commanding	2.97	0.55
Isolating	2.41	0.51

3. Results and Discussion

3.1. Participants' Background Data. Almost all participants were female (97.6%) with an average age of 50.50 years (SD = 7.096). Over half of the nurse managers (61.6%) were specialized nurses, and 15.1% had undertaken higher vocational training. The majority of the respondents (94.0%) had participated in updating education in leadership. The majority of the participants had worked in health care for more than 15 years (93.4%). They had an average of 26.31 years (SD = 7.715) of working experience in health care. The average duration of working experience as a nurse manager was 10.21 years (SD = 7.934). Most of the nurse managers (94%) had participated in updating education. Some nurse managers (13) reported that they led more than one health centre ward. The average number of patients was 34.96 (SD = 14.064), and the average number of employees was 25.58 (SD = 11.777).

3.2. Nurse Managers' Leadership Styles and Their Perceptions of the Importance of the Different Leadership Styles. All six leadership styles—visionary, coaching, affiliate, democratic, commanding, and isolating—were reflected on. The findings of the mean scores for the leadership styles as indicated in Table 2 revealed that visionary leadership style received the highest rating ($m = 4.51$), and isolating leadership style received the lowest rating ($m = 2.41$). The results of the nurse managers' perceptions of the importance of different leadership styles show that almost all respondents in every age group considered four leadership styles—visionary, coaching, affiliate, and democratic—as being very important or important (Table 3). The number of employees was not statistically significantly linked with any of the leadership styles.

Over half of the nurse managers (65.6%) reported that they considered visionary leadership style to be very important. The rest of the respondents reported visionary leadership to be important (33.6%) or rather important (0.8%). Regardless of respondents' education, over 60% reported that visionary leadership style is very important. 73.1% of nurse managers with more than 15 years of working experience considered visionary leadership style to be very important.

55.7% of the respondents reported coaching leadership style to be very important. It was most frequently reported to be very important by nurse managers over the age of 55 (69.7%) and least frequently by those aged 51 to 55 years (41.1%). Of the nurse managers with nurse education, 57.9% reported coaching leadership style to be very important. The importance of coaching leadership style was recognized more often by nurse managers who had participated in updating education in leadership ($P = 0.000$). 63% of the respondents with 10 to 15 years of work experience as a nurse manager considered coaching leadership style to be very important. Less than half of the nurse managers (43.1%) reported affiliate leadership style to be very important, while more than half (55.3%) in all age groups considered it important. Of the nurse managers with nurse education, 52.6% reported affiliate leadership style to be very important, while 35.1% of the nurse managers with M.S. education reported it to be very important. Regardless of respondents' length of work experience as nurse manager, 42.4% considered affiliate leadership style to be very important, while 56.0% considered it important.

A democratic leadership style was reported to be very important by half of the respondents (51.7%). It was most frequently (60%) reported to be very important by nurse managers under the age of 46 years and least frequently by those aged from 51 to 55 years (41.8%). 56.6% of the nurse managers with nurse education reported democratic leadership style to be very important, while 43.2% of nurse managers with M.S. education reported it to be very important. Regardless of respondents' length of work experience as nurse manager, 50.8% reported democratic leadership style to be very important and 48.8% to be important.

Over half of the nurse managers reported commanding leadership style to be rather important (61.1%), while 15.4% considered it rather unimportant. Regardless of respondents' education, almost 65% reported that commanding leadership style is rather important. 22.2% of the nurse managers with 5 to 9 years of work experience considered commanding leadership style not at all important. Regardless of respondents' age, education, or length of work experience as nurse manager, isolating leadership style was reported to be rather important by half of the respondents (53.9%) and rather unimportant by 43%.

3.3. Nurse Managers' Perceptions of Their Skills and Knowledge in Leadership Styles. Few nurse managers (7.2%) reported that they did not have at all sufficient skills and knowledge, while two-thirds of the nurse managers (64%) reported that they did not have quite sufficient skills and knowledge in visionary leadership style. Not quite sufficient skills and knowledge in this leadership style were reported by one in ten of the nurse managers aged from 32 to 45 years (9.1%), nurse managers with nurse education (10.7%), and nurse managers with less than 5 years of work experience as nurse manager (10.1%). Nurse managers' skills and knowledge in visionary leadership style became better with the increasing work experience ($P = 0.005$).

Two-thirds (64.8%) of the nurse managers thought they had rather sufficient skills and one-fourth thought (25.6%) they had sufficient skills and knowledge in coaching leadership style. One in every ten respondents (9.8%) reported that they did not have quite sufficient skills and knowledge in this leadership style, while 11.4% of the respondents

TABLE 3: Nurse managers' perceptions of the importance of different leadership styles.

Background data	Very important (%)	Important (%)	Rather important (%)	Rather little important (%)	Not at all important (%)
		Visionary leadership style			
Age					
32–45	72.7	25.5	1.8	0.0	0.0
46–50	63.8	34.8	1.4	0.0	0.0
51–55	55.6	44.4	0.0	0.0	0.0
56–65	69.8	30.2	0.0	0.0	0.0
		Coaching leadership style			
Age					
32–45	48.2	51.8	0.0	0.0	0.0
46–50	60.3	36.8	2.9	0.0	0.0
51–55	41.1	57.1	1.8	0.0	0.0
56–65	69.7	30.3	0.0	0.0	0.0
		Affiliate leadership style			
Age					
32–45	39.3	60.7	0.0	0.0	0.0
46–50	44.9	52.2	2.9	0.0	0.0
51–55	35.7	62.5	1.8	0.0	0.0
56–65	50.8	47.7	1.5	0.0	0.0
		Democratic leadership style			
Age					
32–45	60.0	40.0	0.0	0.0	0.0
46–50	55.2	43.3	1.5	0.0	0.0
51–55	41.8	58.2	0.0	0.0	0.0
56–65	49.2	50.8	0.0	0.0	0.0
		Commanding leadership style			
Age					
32–45	0.0	30.4	60.7	8.9	0.0
46–50	1.5	7.6	72.7	18.2	0.0
51–55	0.0	17.9	57.1	25.0	0.0
56–65	0.0	22.2	68.3	9.5	0.0
		Isolating leadership style			
Age					
32–45	0.0	0.0	49.0	51.0	0.0
46–50	0.0	3.0	38.8	58.2	0.0
51–55	0.0	1.9	38.9	59.3	0.0
56–65	0.0	5.2	46.6	46.6	1.7

with specialized nurse education reported this. It was most frequently reported by nurse managers who had less than 5 to 9 years of work experience as nurse managers (17.5%).

Regardless of age or education, some nurse managers reported that they (11.5%) had not quite sufficient, two-thirds that they (66.7%) had rather sufficient, and almost one-third (28.8%) that they had sufficient skills and knowledge in affiliate leadership style. Older nurse managers had better skills and knowledge in affiliate leadership style than younger nurse managers ($P = 0.005$). Every fifth (20.0%) of the respondents with 5 to 9 years of work experience as nurse manager reported that they did not have quite sufficient skills and knowledge in this style. Nurse managers with long-term work experience as managers had better skills and knowledge in affiliate leadership style than managers with shorter work experience ($P = 0.003$). Managers of big units with a large number of employees had less skills and knowledge in affiliate leadership style than managers of small units ($P = 0.003$).

Almost all of the nurse managers evaluated that they had rather sufficient (54.3%) or sufficient (42.4%) knowledge and skills in democratic leadership style. Nurse managers' updating education in leadership increased their skills and knowledge in democratic leadership style ($P = 0.005$). Having knowledge and skills in commanding leadership style was reported to be rather sufficient by 61.7% of the nurse managers and sufficient by 30%. One tenth (10.0%) of the nurse managers with specialized nurse education reported that they did not have quite sufficient skills and knowledge in this style. Nurse managers with shorter work experience as managers had less skills and knowledge in commanding leadership style than nurse managers with longer work experience ($P = 0.025$).

Over two-thirds (68.5%) of the nurse managers reported that they had sufficient skills in isolating leadership style. Nurse managers' participation in updating education increased their skills and knowledge in isolating leadership style ($P = 0.003$). A summary of the nurse managers' perceptions of their skills and knowledge in leadership styles, and the importance of these styles without background variables is presented in Table 4.

3.4. Discussion. Based on data from 246 nurse managers working in health centre wards, this study set out to explore nurse managers' leadership styles and their perceptions of the importance of the different leadership styles and their skills and knowledge in leadership styles. Today, nurse managers have to use leadership styles that are appropriate for the constantly changing and complex health care system [31]. The findings of this study suggest that nurse managers most often used visionary, coaching, affiliate, and democratic leadership styles. Commanding and isolating leadership styles were reported to be less frequently used. A previous study found affiliate and coaching leadership styles to be most common [32]. According to the results, regardless of respondents' length of work experience, over 70% considered visionary, coaching, and affiliate leadership styles to be important. It is remarkable that at the same time, approximately 25% of respondents with less than ten years of work experience as nurse managers reported that they had sufficient skills and knowledge in these leadership styles.

Considered as a challenge for nursing science and management, evidence-based practice could be seen as an ongoing desirable vision. A key question is how appropriate skills nurse managers have in utilising nursing research findings and translating them into practice [18]. According to earlier research findings, nurse managers wish for more time to articulate their vision [33], while nurses emphasize the importance of making the vision understandable by providing information about current issues [28]. These perceptions probably show a contradiction between the vision of the organization and the skills and resources available for its implementation.

Nurse managers' skills and knowledge in visionary leadership style improved with the increasing work experience. This is likely due to the fact that when nurse managers have worked longer in the organizations they have become acquainted with the strategy and vision of the organization and may have participated in creating the vision. It is important to bear in mind that especially new nurse managers need education in order to be better able to lead others toward the vision.

There is a generational shift going on among nurses, and young nurses have thoughts of giving up nursing. Their experience of job satisfaction and opportunities for development is poor [6]. Older nurses have their own expectations of work. In a Swedish study, informants described that leadership works when it is built on relationships that contribute to a well-functioning work unit, promoting a positive atmosphere [34]. Trust and job satisfaction have strong links with greater commitment and intent to stay on at work [35]. If nurse managers want to advance collaboration among generations, a positive and understanding attitude is needed. The most important thing is that nurses are committed to their patients, and nurse managers are committed to supporting these nurses, despite generational differences [36]. However, it is important to remember that creating harmony does not eliminate the fact that employees sometimes feel resentment and have different opinions [32].

Continuing education of the employees is one of the features of infrastructure the magnet hospital nurse managers emphasized because nurses were not able to keep up-to-date with their profession and newest treatment and care modalities [37]. However, even though attitudes towards a coaching leadership style were positive—almost all respondents considered it to be important or very important—one in ten respondents estimated their skills and knowledge to be insufficient. Health care organizations are undergoing changes, which puts pressure on nurse managers and employees to modify and develop their work, even though it provides opportunities for doing so. At the same time, nursing science and practice are fighting to maintain their position. Therefore, nurse managers with a coaching leadership style need strength and assertiveness in times of change to be able to lead employees in an environment where they are noticed as irreplaceable partners within the organization [17].

Nurse managers in Finland usually have nurse education, specialized nurse education, and/or academic education (M.S.). Nurse managers need updating education to develop their own professional abilities. Moreover, they need knowledge of nursing science and practice so as to be able to manage the work unit as a whole. Nurse managers should know how to argue decisions in order to get employees to commit to their work and changes. On the other hand, nurse managers need these skills also when they discuss evidence-based nursing in connection with efficiency (providing nursing care with the appropriate level of staff) and effectiveness (achieving desired outcomes) in nursing [18]. When the organization drafts a new strategy and vision for the future, including nursing practice, the nurse manager is the key person to examine nursing and its resources.

A democratic, participative leadership style allows nurses to become involved in decisions regarding patient care delivery and cooperation with other personnel groups [37]. This probably increases nurses' job satisfaction and commitment to work. On the contrary, it has been noted that some nurse managers do not stand out as leaders, but as team members. This means that the nurse manager's own tasks could be

Table 4: Nurse managers' perceptions of their skills and knowledge on leadership styles.

	How adequate are my knowledge and skills?			
	Not at all sufficient	Not quite sufficient	Rather Sufficient	sufficient
Visionary leadership style	7.2%	64.0%	28.8%	0.0%
Coaching leadership style	0.0%	9.6%	64.8%	25.6%
Affiliate leadership style	0.0%	11.5%	66.7%	28.8%
Democratic leadership style	0.0%	3.2%	54.2%	42.6%
Commanding leadership style	0.0%	8.8%	61.2%	30.0%
Isolating leadership style	0.4%	1.2%	29.9%	68.5%

of secondary importance [28]. However, it is important to remember that there are situations in which nurse managers have to make difficult decisions. Decision-making is facilitated by sufficient knowledge, work experience, and support from colleagues and supervisors.

In the future, well-motivated, professionally developing nurses are needed in health centre wards in Finland. At the same time, nurse managers will need skills and knowledge to lead their work units in a visionary manner. Work units, employees and situations differ, and it could be said that there is no one and only correct leadership style; the same result can be achieved in many ways. The behaviour of emotionally intelligent leaders stimulates the creativity of their employees [38]. Nurse manager's ability to reflect on their own behaviour makes it easier to regulate and estimate their leadership style with different employees in different situations. It is important to arrange enough updating education to support nurse managers in their leadership work.

3.5. Limitations. The questionnaire used in this study was based on the leadership styles presented by Goleman et al. [20] and earlier research of Vesterinen et al. [27, 28]. Goleman et al. [20] described primal leadership, which requires the leader to bring emotional intelligence (EI) to bear on his/her leadership. The complex phenomenon of emotional intelligence in nursing leadership is under the consideration of criticism. It is essential to have profound knowledge of EI and its scientific critique when integrating the concept into nursing research [39]. On the other hand, the content of the questionnaire was evaluated by an expert panel, which consisted of nurse managers working in different types of hospital wards. On the basis of this evaluation, the indicator used in this study can be considered valid in terms of the concepts used for studying nurse managers' leadership styles in health centre hospital wards. The value of Cronbach's alpha used to study the internal consistency between the six sum variables was between 0.6 and 0.7, which could be considered as sufficient [40]. The study has some limitations. The results achieved may not necessarily give a true picture of the nurse managers' skills and knowledge in the use of different leadership styles, as nurse managers' skills and knowledge were only estimated by the nurse managers themselves, not their employees or supervisors. In this study, the sample consisted of Finnish nurse managers; therefore, the results reflect only their perceptions of leadership styles.

4. Conclusions

Health care organizations are undergoing continuing changes, and vision should be present at all times. Employees need new skills and knowledge to be able to manage their work. At the same time, they hope that their individual needs are taken into account by the nurse managers. Nurse managers' abilities to reflect, understand, and, if necessary, change their leadership style influence a work unit's success and employees' job satisfaction. Nurse managers, especially new nurse managers, need more theoretic, evidence-based education to cope with these expectations and to develop their professional abilities.

Health care organizations should draw up visions of nursing leadership in the future. Together with universities, they should start planning nurse manager education programmes that focus on strategic issues, leadership, job satisfaction, challenging situations in leadership, change management, work unit management (e.g., economy, efficiency, and resources), and how nurse managers consider their own wellbeing. It is important that nurse managers have peer groups and mentors for helping them to develop as managers. It is health care organizations' responsibility to set up a clear vision and goals and make the successful nurse leadership possible as part of multiprofessional cooperation.

Acknowledgment

This research was financially supported by EVO funding from the Lapland Hospital District.

References

[1] C. Huston, "Preparing nurse leaders for 2020," *Journal of Nursing Management*, vol. 16, no. 8, pp. 905–911, 2008.

[2] M. Carney, "Leadership in nursing: current and future perspectives and challenges," *Journal of Nursing Management*, vol. 17, no. 4, pp. 411–414, 2009.

[3] H. K. Spence Laschinger, P. Wilk, J. Cho, and P. Greco, "Empowerment, engagement and perceived effectiveness in nursing work environments: does experience matter?" *Journal of Nursing Management*, vol. 17, no. 5, pp. 636–646, 2009.

[4] Statistics Finland, "*Population projection 2009-2060*," http://www.stat.fi/til/vaenn/2009/vaenn_2009_2009-09-30_tie_001_en.html.

[5] National Institute for Health and Welfare, "*Sosiaali-ja terveydenhuollon henkilöstö 2007*," Statistical report in Finland 7/2010, http://www.stakes.fi/tilastot/tilastotiedotteet/2010/Tr07_10.pdf.

[6] M. Flinkman, M. Laine, H. Leino-Kilpi, H. M. Hasselhorn, and S. Salanterä, "Explaining young registered Finnish nurses' intention to leave the profession: a questionnaire survey," *International Journal of Nursing Studies*, vol. 45, no. 5, pp. 727–739, 2008.

[7] D. C. Espinoza, A. Lopez-Saldana, and J. S. Stonestreet, "The pivotal role of the nurse manager in healthy workplaces: implications for training and development," *Critical Care Nursing Quarterly*, vol. 32, no. 4, pp. 327–334, 2009.

[8] T. Cowden, G. Cummings, and J. Profetto-Mcgrath, "Leadership practices and staff nurses' intent to stay: a systematic review," *Journal of Nursing Management*, vol. 19, no. 4, pp. 461–477, 2011.

[9] A. A. Farag, S. Tullai-Mcguinness, and M. K. Anthony, "Nurses' perception of their manager's leadership style and unit climate: are there generational differences?" *Journal of Nursing Management*, vol. 17, no. 1, pp. 26–34, 2009.

[10] A. M. Tomey, "Nursing leadership and management effects work environments," *Journal of Nursing Management*, vol. 17, no. 1, pp. 15–25, 2009.

[11] J. Casida and J. Parker, "Staff nurse perceptions of nurse manager leadership styles and outcomes," *Journal of Nursing Management*, vol. 19, no. 4, pp. 478–486, 2011.

[12] D. L. Huber, M. Maas, J. McCloskey, C. A. Scherb, C. J. Goode, and C. Watson, "Evaluating nursing administration instruments," *Journal of Nursing Administration*, vol. 30, no. 5, pp. 251–272, 2000.

[13] M. Suhonen and L. Paasivaara, "Shared human capital in project management: a systematic review of the literature," *Project Management Journal*, vol. 42, no. 2, pp. 4–16, 2011.

[14] J. Teperi, M. E. Porter, L. Vuorenkoski, and J. F. Baron, "The Finnish health care system: a value-based perspective," Sitra Reports 82, Edita Prima Ltd., Helsinki, Finland, 2009.

[15] Ministry of Social affairs and Health 2010, "*Terveydenhuoltolaki*," http://www.stm.fi/vireilla/lainsaadantohankkeet/sosiaali_ja_terveydenhuolto/terveydenhuoltolaki.

[16] National Institute for Health and Welfare, "*Terveyskeskusten perusterveydenhuollon vuodeosastohoito 2008*," Official statistics in Finland, 2010, http://www.stakes.fi/tilastot/tilastotiedotteet/2010/Tr01_10.pdf.

[17] S. Watters, "Shared leadership: taking flight," *Journal of Nursing Administration*, vol. 39, no. 1, pp. 26–29, 2009.

[18] R. P. Newhouse, "Creating infrastructure supportive of evidence-based nursing practice: leadership strategies," *Worldviews on Evidence-Based Nursing*, vol. 4, no. 1, pp. 21–29, 2007.

[19] D. Weberg, "Transformational leadership and staff retention: an evidence review with implications for healthcare systems," *Nursing Administration Quarterly*, vol. 34, no. 3, pp. 246–258, 2010.

[20] D. Goleman, R. Boyatzis, and A. McKee, *Primal Leadership Realizing the Power of Emotional Intelligence*, Harvard Business School Press, Boston, Mass, USA, 2002.

[21] K. Akerjordet and E. Severinsson, "Emotionally intelligent nurse leadership: a literature review study," *Journal of Nursing Management*, vol. 16, no. 5, pp. 565–577, 2008.

[22] R. Feather, "Emotional intelligence in relation to nursing leadership: does it matter?" *Journal of Nursing Management*, vol. 17, no. 3, pp. 376–382, 2009.

[23] C. Young-Ritchie, H. K. Spence Laschinger, and C. Wong, "The effects of emotionally intelligent leadership behaviour on emergency staff nurses' workplace empowerment and organizational commitment," *Nursing Leadership*, vol. 22, no. 1, pp. 70–85, 2009.

[24] A. McCallin and A. Bamford, "Interdisciplinary teamwork: is the influence of emotional intelligence fully appreciated?" *Journal of Nursing Management*, vol. 15, no. 4, pp. 386–391, 2007.

[25] V. Lucas, H. K. Spence Laschinger, and C. A. Wong, "The impact of emotional intelligent leadership on staff nurse empowerment: the moderating effect of span of control," *Journal of Nursing Management*, vol. 16, no. 8, pp. 964–973, 2008.

[26] S. Vesterinen, A. Isola, and L. Paasivaara, "Hoitotyön johtajien johtamistyylitutkimus vuosina 1994-2006," *Premissi*, no. 6, pp. 36–44, 2007 (Finnish).

[27] S. Vesterinen, A. Isola, and L. Paasivaara, "Leadership styles of Finnish nurse managers and factors influencing it," *Journal of Nursing Management*, vol. 17, no. 4, pp. 503–509, 2009.

[28] S. Vesterinen, M. Suhonen, A. Isola, and L. Paasivaara, "Nurse managers' leadership styles in Finland," *Nursing Research and Practice*, vol. 2012, Article ID 605379, 8 pages, 2012.

[29] N. Burns and S. K. Grove, *The Practise of Nursing Research*, W.B. Saunders Company, Philadelphia, Pa, USA, 4th edition, 2001.

[30] B. Munro, *Statistical Methods For the Health Care Research*, Lippincott, Philadelphia, Pa, USA, 4th edition, 2001.

[31] J. Casida and G. Pinto-Zipp, "Leadership-organizational culture relationship in nursing units of acute care hospitals," *Nursing Economics*, vol. 26, no. 1, pp. 7-15, 2008.

[32] P. Kenmore, "Exploring leadership styles," *Nursing Management*, vol. 15, no. 1, pp. 24–26, 2008.

[33] I. W. Graham and E. Jack, "Promoting leadership: the development of a nurse executive team in an acute hospital trust," *Journal of Nursing Management*, vol. 16, no. 8, pp. 955–963, 2008.

[34] K. Rosengren, E. Athlin, and K. Segesten, "Presence and availability: staff conceptions of nursing leadership on an intensive care unit," *Journal of Nursing Management*, vol. 15, no. 5, pp. 522–529, 2007.

[35] C. Way, D. Gregory, J. Davis et al., "The impact of organizational culture on clinical managers' organizational commitment and turnover intentions," *Journal of Nursing Administration*, vol. 37, no. 5, pp. 235–242, 2007.

[36] J. S. Mensik, "A view on generational differences from a generation X leader," *Journal of Nursing Administration*, vol. 37, no. 11, pp. 483–484, 2007.

[37] V. V. Upenieks, "What constitutes effective leadership?: perceptions of magnet and nonmagnet nurse leaders," *Journal of Nursing Administration*, vol. 33, no. 9, pp. 456–467, 2003.

[38] A. Rego, F. Sousa, M. Pina e Cunha, A. Correia, and I. Saur-Amaral, "Leader self-reported emotional intelligence and perceived employee creativity: an exploratory study," *Creativity and Management*, vol. 16, no. 3, pp. 250–264, 2007.

[39] K. Akerjordet and E. Severinsson, "The state of the science of emotional intelligence related to nursing leadership: an integrative review," *Journal of Nursing Management*, vol. 18, no. 4, pp. 363–382, 2010.

[40] D. Polit and B. Hungler, *Essentials of Nursing Research, Methods, Appraisal and Utilization*, Lippincott, Philadelphia, Pa, USA, 4th edition, 1997.

20

Gender, Work, and Health for Trans Health Providers: A Focus on Transmen

Judith A. MacDonnell[1] and Alisa Grigorovich[2]

[1] *School of Nursing, York University, Room 322, HNES Building, 4700 Keele Street, Toronto, ON, Canada M3J 1P3*
[2] *School of Women's Studies, York University, 206 Founders College, 4700 Keele Street, Toronto, ON, Canada M3J 1P3*

Correspondence should be addressed to Judith A. MacDonnell, jmacdonn@yorku.ca

Academic Editors: J. S. Lymn and M. Miyashita

Well-documented health research points to trans people's vulnerability to health inequities that are linked to deeply embedded structural and social determinants of health. Gender and work, as social determinants of health for trans people, both shape and are shaped by multiple factors such as support networks, social environments, income and social status, shelter, and personal health practices. There is a gap in the nursing literature in regards to research on work and health for diverse trans people and a virtual silence on the particular issues of trans-identified health providers. This qualitative study used comparative life history methodology and purposeful sampling to examine links among work, career, and health for transmen who are health providers. Semistructured interviews were completed with four Canadian transmen involved in health care professional and/or practice contexts with diverse professions, age, work, and transitioning experiences. Critical gender analysis showed that unique and gender-related critical events and influences shape continuities and discontinuities in their careerlives. This strength-based approach foregrounds how resilience and growth emerged through participants' articulation with everyday gender dynamics. These findings have implications for nursing research, education, and practice that include an understanding of how trans providers "do transgender work" and supporting them in that process.

... should it really matter? You know, should gender presentation, the way you dress... what you choose to talk about or not talk about...? Does it really disrupt... the workforce... in such profound ways?
(Transman (TM), page 7)

1. Introduction

Despite greater public and professional awareness of sexual and gender diversity and more positive work climates in recent years, lesbian, gay, bisexual, transgender, and queer (LGBTQ) people continue to encounter invisibility, overt and more subtle discrimination and violence, and other barriers to relevant, respectful care. According to the Registered Nurses Association of Ontario (RNAO), "Sexual diversity relates to sexual orientation (lesbian, gay, bisexual, and heterosexual) and gender diversity refers to gender identity (e.g., transgender) which refers to one's sense of being male and/or female or neither" [1]. This last decade has brought greater attention to transgender health, the "T" in LGBTQ, in health care and research has shown that ethnicity, race, geography, age, education, and other social categories across genders influence how particular trans-identified individuals experience and understand their health. Typically, transgender is used in the broadest sense to refer to people who transgress gender norms in some way [2]. In this paper, "...[*t*]*rans* refers to transgender, transsexual, gender nonconforming, and gender questioning (people)" [3] and transmen to those who identify with a masculine trans identity. Within trans communities, individuals express their gender and subscribe to identities in a variety of ways. These include transmen, transwomen, and genderqueer, and trans identities may shift over a lifetime [4]. Gender expression and/or transition processes can involve dress, electrolysis, and/or sex reassignment surgery.

Encounters with violence, transphobia, and discrimination related to sexuality and gender norms across home, community, work, and educational settings, and challenges to finding meaningful social support, shape trans people's disclosure with respect to trans issues and identities, their health status, and access to care [5–7]. Considerable hurdles also exist to locating sensitive and knowledgeable health providers, trans-positive services and obtaining hormone therapy or surgery if so desired, especially outside of large urban cities [6, 8]. All of these factors contribute to trans people's vulnerability to health inequities.

As social determinants of health, employment, and working conditions for trans people both shape and are shaped by multiple factors such as support networks, social environments, income and social status, shelter, and personal health practices [6, 7, 9, 10]. Decisions to transition in the workplace are informed by many factors that include underemployment, available support systems, and weighing the costs of job-loss or unpredictable discrimination that mark many environments for trans people [8, 9, 11]. Certainly income level and access to education are also relevant to trans individuals' capacity to enter the professions.

LGBTQ workplace issues have recently become high profile in North American media in relation to same-sex benefits, legal protections, and organizational policy and diversity education initiatives, and guides to support transition in the workplace are becoming increasingly visible [10, 12, 13]. Yet, workplace support for gender-variant individuals and those who self-identify on the trans spectrum remains highly politicized, even within LGBTQ communities. In Canada, inclusive policy change related to diversity is part of broader social policy and health professional advocacy for equity; nursing in particular has taken leadership in a Canadian context of the professions [1]. However, the policy context in which discrimination occurs for trans people is still fraught. In Ontario, Canada, findings from the Trans Pulse project [10] indicate that there is little known about trans people's work, although it is well documented that underemployment and barriers to education exist. Many are forced to leave education before completing high school due to experiences of harassment, bullying, and violence, yet there is some evidence that despite this, many are able to achieve some level of higher education [8, 10].

Narratives published in print, or online, offer insight into the dynamics of work and health and the complexities of diverse trans people's lived experiences of gender expression and transitioning in a Canadian context [14–16]. In 2008, the Canadian Professional Association for Transgender Health (CPATH) also emerged to offer resources and professional support for those involved in trans health provision, creating a community for trans-identified providers and allies to be visible in a professional context. However, few trans-identified members of the regulated health professions (e.g., nurses) are visible in the health sector and there is limited research that focuses on their work, and even less on their career trajectories, especially in the professional context (this includes both alternative and regulated health providers) (e.g., [17]).

Yet, gender and its intersections with race, sexuality, and other social categories inform a body of research on professionals and the nature of their work; dominant notions of masculinities and femininities as well as gender conformity have also been noted as relevant to LGBTQ health professionals' career/work dynamics (e.g., [18–20]). As a result, research that fosters an understanding of factors that influence the career, work, and health of diverse trans providers is needed to illustrate the complexities of their lives with the goal of creating supportive policies and practices.

In a nursing context, recent attention to the need to broaden understandings of culturally competent care in order to meet the diverse and holistic needs of patients and clients has pointed to the importance of addressing sexual diversity, and to some extent, transgender health [21–24]. Yet, when this is addressed, most health studies, including nursing research, focus on the context in which trans people are assumed to be patients or clients. By default, the assumption is that all care providers are not trans-identified, but cisgendered (a term used to describe people who are not transgendered [22]) and this has important consequences for the ways in which the health issues of diverse trans people are identified and articulated, and thus the practice strategies that are deemed relevant to supporting them. In fact, a search of the literature using CINAHL, PubMed, Social Science Abstracts, and Psychinfo databases using the terms "transgender" and/or "transsexual" and "work" in titles and abstracts yielded a handful of articles that focus on transgender or transsexual people and their workplace experiences. Typically across the health literature, transgender people and work get taken up in the context of sex work, sexual risk for HIV/AIDS [25] and/or in relation to how providers "work with" diverse clients in ways that often objectify them as "cases." A recent study suggests that such an approach erases the complexity of trans people's lives [22, 24]. A paucity of workplace-focused health literature exists that offers insight into trans people's workplaces in relation to experiences of transitioning, and/or relevant policy dynamics; in effect, their lives are equated with a patient context rather than a work context which has limitations to understanding health in a social determinants approach.

This paper foregrounds the experiences of health providers who themselves are trans-identified and illustrates the links in their work, careers and health and wellbeing, and the complex ways that gender is implicated in their lives. In particular, this paper focuses on how transmen who are health providers make meaning through their careerlives, that is, meaningful life activities encompassing work and personal endeavors, with implications for their health and wellbeing.

1.1. Purpose. This paper explores intersections of gender, health and work or career for transmen health providers in relation to their everyday lived realities. In particular, this paper explores two research questions.

(1) How do transmen who are health providers make meaning through their careerlives?

(2) What are the implications for their health and wellbeing?

2. Materials and Methods

2.1. Comparative Life History Methodology. This qualitative study used a comparative life history methodology design. Situating this study in the naturalistic and critical paradigms was appropriate for this exploratory study that examined sensitive dynamics of identity, work and career, and complex aspects of power. This life history approach attends to processes of narration, collaboration, and contextualization so that the researcher has an active role in situating participants' narratives in the larger sociocultural, political, economic, and historical contexts [26]. Critical gender analysis of career histories, within-case and cross-case analysis, can also identify critical incidents and influences, such as identity, that shape diverse professionals' careerlives [18]. In this approach to policy research, the goal is to generate understandings of policy and related processes and practices through the eyes of policy actors themselves in the field [27]. For trans professionals and health providers whose work lives are shaped by policy and whose work entails practices of implementing and creating policy, their lives as trans people are also inscribed by human rights and organizational policies that shape the ways in which trans people are variously included, marginalized, and/or legitimized in their work and larger social worlds [22, 28]. In this study, careers are conceptualized as moving beyond the organizational context to encompass meaningful life activities across the lifespan [29].

2.2. Sex/Gender-Based Analysis. Gender-based analysis in this paper, addresses both sex, biological differences between women and men, and gender, which takes into account the social dynamics or gender roles, identities, and norms which shape individuals' holistic health. Historically, sex has referred to biological characteristics that were used to determine discrete binary categories of female or male. However, trans people's attention to and experiences of gender variance and the ways that their biological characteristics are at odds with their sense of being male, female, and/or expressing their gender, blur the discrete boundaries of sex and gender. For transgender people, for example, binary categories of male and female are inadequate to represent the fluid and socially constructed nature of sex and gender. To understand their health requires simultaneous attention to the ways that gender norms influence gender expression and identities [22, 30]. Rather than an exclusive focus on health risks, a critical gender-based approach foregrounds trans people's agency, the ways that they negotiate their social worlds in particular times and places, and material and social dynamics characterizing their careerlives and the ways that gender intersects with work and other social determinants. It also encompasses how both material (e.g., physical embodiment) and social dimensions (e.g., identities, norms) are gendered. Although gender-based analysis has typically been used to examine how gender matters in the lives of cisgendered women and men, Johnson et al. [30] explain that it could be applied to understand transgender/transsexual issues, and more recently it has been taken up in health research on trans people [21, 22]. In this study, we incorporate this gender lens from the outset of the study [30], mindful of the ways that this methodology influences the way the study is conceptualized and questions asked, the data collection, analysis, and sharing of findings. As a type of feminist research, there is also an assumption that the research has political goals with an aim to improve the everyday lives of transgender people.

2.3. Procedures. Ethics approval from York University Research Ethics Board was received prior to commencing the study. At that point, a call for advisory group members for the study was sent out, and two trans-identified community members responded and provided feedback on the study materials and procedures. These two community members represented transwomen's and transmen's communities and had insight into health and social service delivery as providers in paid and/or volunteer roles; they opted not to be interviewed, instead showing their support for this study in this advisory capacity. Materials were revised with respect to the language used in the consent forms/recruitment material and the way that the researcher specified how she was situated with respect to the trans communities. The principal researcher, a health professional, conceptualized the study and was involved with recruitment, data collection, analysis and presentation of initial findings. The authors of this article, both of whom been involved with LGBTQ advocacy and research, collaborated on analysis and developed this article. The call out for participants was for individuals who self-identified as "trans health providers" working in the health and social services sector initially in Ontario; and at a later date, recruitment was expanded to include those working in Canada. Thus the study aimed to recruit both health and social service providers who were self-identified as trans (e.g., transgender, transsexual, Two-Spirited, genderqueer) and cisgendered providers who were involved in service delivery for trans communities and thus were key informants. This paper, however, reports on the trans-identified providers and specifically, trans providers who self-identified as transmen. Information about the study was posted through professional and LGBTQ networks in Canada. This included Rainbow Health Ontario and Rainbow Health Network online listserves which have broad reach to gender diverse communities and health providers throughout Canada, as well as the researcher's well-developed professional networks that included a focus on health equity-related research.

The interviews focused on career histories, everyday activities, experiences of health and work, as well as factors that shaped career and workplace decisions and practice dynamics. Interview questions were created for the study based on the literature and the principal researcher's engagement with issues that trans health communities had previously identified as relevant [6]. Interview questions focused on the everyday lived experiences and challenges shaping many trans people's worklives: gender presentation, transitioning, health concerns, discrimination, violence, underemployment, or unemployment, and social support. For example, the researcher asked about a typical day in their life as a trans-identified health provider, pivotal incidents, or key influences that played a part in their health, as well as workplace dynamics, policies, or issues that would contribute to trans providers' health and wellbeing and their vision for strategies that could improve practice environments for trans providers. The advisory group affirmed the focus of these questions in relation to the purpose and scope of the project.

Face-to-face or telephone semi-structured interviews were completed from April 2008 to April 2010 with four participants who self-identified as transmen. Probes were used to encourage participants to provide thick description and elaboration on the context of points raised [31]. These interviews lasted from 1 to 4 hours and were audiotaped and professionally transcribed. Participants were offered a small honorarium. Steps were taken to protect confidentiality and privacy. This was especially relevant given the small pool of "out" trans-identified people in professional positions whose identification could have enormous personal and professional implications, including career risks.

Conventional content analysis [31] was chosen as an inductive approach, a method that is appropriate for examining qualitative data for a study that is exploratory and whose aim is to describe a phenomenon which is not well understood. Analysis of descriptive data emerging from the interviews was guided by the gender-based analytical approach with its focus, for example, on social dynamics, gender norms, and experiences of gender variance. Both researchers independently coded the transcripts for themes and subthemes that were guided by an understanding of gender dynamics (e.g., the notion that both material and social factors are relevant to worklives). However, the researchers were also attuned to unexpected themes that emerged, such as some participants' experiences of congruence between their work interest and their social identities as members of trans communities. Transcripts were read as a whole for immersion in the data and then line-by-line coding was carried out in which key phrases were identified as initial themes and notations made with researchers' reflections on emerging codes, "allowing the categories and names for categories to flow from the data" ([31], page 1279). Where possible, verbatim phrases were used as codes. For example, we identified one code as "gender identity as career" based on one participant saying, "*being able to transcend the limits of um physicality... my gender identity is my career in a sense... or vice versa you know.... I see both of these unfolding more in the future.*" This code later became part of the theme "Fitting In". Under the theme of *Critical Influences*, we identified a subcategory: "*feminist work that influenced me most in terms of identifying as queer and coming out as queer.*" Researchers identified themes, codes, and subcategories which were later clustered in a coding scheme. The two researchers shared these initial themes, which were then validated using consensus process and were informed by the existing literature. When there was disagreement on emerging themes, discussion ensued with return to the transcripts until the researchers reached consensus. Thus the way gender-based analysis was used in this study considers the ways that gender normativity provides a reference point for understanding the experience of people who do not fit into the binary categories of male and female. As well, it affirms the unique experiences and identities of diverse trans people "who share the common experience of knowing themselves to be a gender that is not congruent with their birth sex" ([21], page 59).

2.4. Sample. In this paper, analysis focuses on the career histories of four health providers who self-identified as transmen. These participants, who ranged in age from their 20s to their 50s, had varied gender histories and experiences from those who had transitioned recently, to those who had done so over 10 years previously. All currently live and work in urban centers in Canada. The narratives represented experiences of students in professional and alternative health programs and providers with decades of work experience, some also with international experience. Professional work and/or education over their lifetimes included social work, medicine, nursing, midwifery, naturopathy, massage therapy, as well as other care work such as teaching. Because of the extremely small pool of openly trans-identified health providers and specifically those with professional credentials in a Canadian context, narrative excerpts and findings are reported in this paper in ways that will not identify participants; information such as age, profession, and place of work are omitted. TM identifies the participant as a transman, and a page number from the transcript is cited.

3. Results and Discussion

In this paper, we report on themes that represent how participants articulated gender identities in the context of work, their careerlives and larger lives, so that the focus is on meaning-making through gender/transition and "doing" gender in their work and other meaningful life activities. Themes relate to their engagement with their trans identities and careerlives with implications for fostering or challenging their health and wellbeing.

3.1. Gender(ed) Identities. All participants described themselves in ways that identified themselves as "transmen." Over their lifetimes however, they reported quite different identities, which, in part, shaped and were shaped by their particular engagement with gender identities, transition processes, and other ways in which gender factored into their social worlds. For instance, deeply entrenched homophobia, heterosexism, and biphobia contribute to gender norms and invisibility, lack of awareness, and transphobia as factors that hinder diverse trans people's ability to locate respectful, responsive, and meaningful health care in their lives [7, 22]. These narratives point to the ways that such dynamics can also influence their narratives of becoming aware of a masculine trans identity as relevant to their wellbeing. All four participants shared that their engagement with a trans identity occurred as adults, with three having also incorporated a same-sex identity for most, or part of their teenaged years. For instance, while coming out and exploring his bisexual and queer identities in his late teens, one of the participants noted that he

> "met a very different gendered world .... It was all really androgyny.... At first I didn't really want to do it, but it was very helpful in the end, because I didn't feel that pressure to conform to that gender world anymore, so I could come out and go out to something more myself in a different way." (TM, page 18).

Another described the initial "*trigger... not from becoming attracted to someone, which I think is not the usual way... just the access to those kinds of books, or the encouragement to read books that were exploring gender identities and sexuality*" (TM, page 9). For yet another participant, this awareness emerged in more gradual and complex ways:

> "Who am I really? And what choices can I make to be more at ease with myself? I don't want to be a woman like this anymore, because it's not working for me... people are rejecting me as I am and I'm being rejected by my partner and I can't be a mother in the way I want to because of my career. And I started to think, well maybe I was just made atypically, you know." (TM, page 26).

In each case, taking on a trans identity was incredibly affirming for these participants on a personal level, even as they encountered unpredictable challenges for disclosure and gender expression, which prompted both feelings of elation when things were working well and also at times, deeply wrenching emotional upheaval. Moreover, their narratives illustrated how their education into a profession and/or workplace context was linked to these dynamics.

3.2. Material and Social Factors Shaping a Career as a Health Care Provider. Several participants spoke of what drew them to health and care-related professions. As one noted, the journey of becoming queer-identified "led me into the health sector was...wanting to take care of my own health" (TM, page 4), while another suggested that trans people "definitely... have... a better chance of making it in health care or social services." He suggested that "it can be helpful for trans clients... Having a trans- [identified...] worker... would make sense for them, but you know that is not... common" (TM, page 14). In these ways, transmen in this study proposed that their careerlives and career choices represented a holistic, or spiritual component rooted in their gendered identities and their experiences of experiencing marginalization in social institutions.

Financial factors surfaced for some participants who acquired debts from education or weighed transition-related costs on top of living and/or education expenses. Working in contract positions or in alternative health contexts, which were not publicly funded, prompted some to take on heavy workloads and juggle several jobs—both in health or research and those that were not health-related. Such pressures exacerbated participants' everyday stresses.

3.3. Transitioning on the Job/School: Materiality of (Gender) Change. At times, the connection between work and identity was complicated by the material consequences of transitioning. Pressures to conform to rigid gendered expectations for roles and appearance carried over to their presentation in professional contexts and the unease that they experienced. As one participant shared, part of his transition included a gradual change in dress and appearance while working and this visibility in relation to his gender expression was an important step towards enhancing his psychological wellbeing:

> "So, I kind of on the one hand rejected traditional... womanhood I suppose... and I started to dress in a way that made me feel comfortable for the first time. I used to have long, long hair and I cut all my hair. I cut my hair and I started to feel much better" (TM, page 27).

Another participant pointed out some of the challenges of hormonally transitioning while working, indicating that he often avoided interactions with his peers because his voice was not yet low enough for him to feel confident that he wouldn't be singled out, noting, "I didn't want them to notice me, basically, and I definitely didn't want them to think poorly of me" (TM, page 40). Another related that while commuting to work during the transition period he experienced negative incidents riding the bus: "like... the bus driver being rude, you know, or interacting with someone who's being transphobic.... Sometimes I'd come in... demoralized before the day even started." (TM, page 12). Further, he added that while, "wearing pants to work was a blessing" when transitioning from female to male generally, but having to ride a bike to work to save money presented issues when binding his breasts. " I couldn't breathe... with all the hills.... I couldn't bind and ride my bicycle so .... I had to go into work and change ..." (TM, page 12).

Several participants also shared stories of the struggle to get registered as a working professional or to apply to a professional program. In each case, this professional context was a turning point for the provider. Working and transitioning, whether as a credentialed professional or professional-in-training, meant that these transmen had to worry about how to change their documentation and professional registration, in addition to dealing with the multiple decisions related to, and demands of, disclosing (or not) and living and working as a transman in various community and work contexts. As a result of this, application to professional schools and professional bodies was fraught. As one participant shared, "The struggle to get registered...

was like a warning of how hard it was going to be" (TM, page 25). Another participant justified the timing of changing his name at the beginning of his professional career having suddenly realized that, "you start meeting [colleagues] you'll be working with... people who... you'll want the support of for the rest of your career.... I should be ready to go as the person that I want to be for the rest of my life" (TM, page 15).

In terms of the work setting, another explained the complicated nature of having to determine how and when to disclose professional education and experiences obtained pretransition:

> "Before, I was, you know, passing when I was first transitioning.... What I struggled with was when to come out. Because if you put it on your cover letter you might not get called, but if you don't address it fairly on when you show up for the interview than they sort of look at you and they call your references.... And especially in social... health care... your reputation is, like, being able to verify your character is a very important part of people being able to hire you, right?" (TM, page 8).

In response to the question, "Why didn't you use your legal name?" by an administrator, one participant reported that he disclosed being trans, saying, "Well I've been like transitioning, not physically, but I'm in the process of questioning my gender identity and I feel more comfortable with [chosen name]" (TM, page 28). Although such processes were eventually resolved for this participant, disclosure of trans identity had significant negative impacts for other participants. Two participants reported that disclosure engendered larger questions about their credibility, mental health, maturity, and fit for the profession itself. One of the participants described that he

> "had a meeting with... support [staff...who] asked me if this was the right time for me to be in [professional] school... until I had sorted out my gender and like until I could pass as male, did I really think that this was the right time for me to be here?" (TM, page 53).

At times, the struggle to disclose or provide professional documentation was avoided by changing their legal name only and deferring gender transition until later. Participating transmen also reported having to move jobs and/or change careers to be able to work in their chosen genders. One participant further illustrated that even in a professional school environment that offered the potential of strong group support, disclosure and transition were not straightforward:

> "I was... coming out in my personal life in my second to last semester and so then in my last semester I was doing my practicum and I wasn't quite confident to share that with the whole school.... It seems like that was too much outing to deal with at once and I knew that they would have to process it because we were social workers." (TM, page 10).

3.4. Education and Work Environments. With few exceptions, trans-identified providers are invisible in health care. Those affiliated with mainstream education programs or work settings such as hospitals were thus likely to be the sole trans-identified provider in their workspaces. Professional isolation in particular, emerged in several career histories, with experiences of physical and mental distress as a result. This was a pervasive dynamic for at least one participant in several workplaces, exacerbated by the nature of the precarious work and related working conditions, and by the need to move to different job locations in order to find work and support the family: "It was just an incredible experience... just feeling utterly alone... through the whole year. Actually, professionally, I didn't really have any supports" (TM, page 21).

The experience of transitioning at work or in educational contexts meant that at times trans people's health suffered with the potential for adverse outcomes. One spoke of a long period of recovery after several spells of serious illness which made it impossible for him to work: With "no sick benefits [or] money... to tide me over... I was homeless for a period" (TM, page 28). Another shared,

> "It was very hard... I was coming up against the health care system and not being able to... get started with transition and then... being all stressed out at work... and obviously in my personal life as well going with lots of stuff at the beginning of transition.... I was underweight and coughing and didn't sleep well.... It was definitely impacting my mental health... my physical health too.... I was not thriving" (TM, page 7).

Participants spoke highly of allies they encountered in professional and educational contexts, who often, but not always, were members of LGBTQ communities. This played out in various ways, where individual mentors and champions advocated on their behalf, provided important emotional support, challenged systems to become more responsive to their needs and provided role modeling in clinical placements where they could engage with trans health. Participants in particular identified that being trans and working in health care meant that education and "coming out" were constant worries or struggles, and that employers who supported them through medical transition were highly valued. "I was very lucky... working in a health care agency.... They were very understanding that I needed to go to the doctor constantly" (TM, page 3).

At times, some of the participants could also tap into LGBTQ professional networks in their work and educational settings, which relived some of the isolation and marginalization that they felt:

> "It really kept it all together for me in... school because it can be overwhelming and it's isolating

> to feel like you're the only person who is like you. You know, there's no other trans people that I've encountered working.... So, going to [a LGBTQ-positive agency] really just re-energized me for the rest of the year." (TM, page 46).

Yet, their career histories showed that such support and resources were not always consistent, even within the same organization, and this created significant anxiety either throughout their experience, or at particular points. This prompted one participant to take action using a formal complaint process, despite having a supportive manager, remarking that his colleagues were "making inappropriate remarks towards me.... I'm getting upset and that's not fair" (TM, page 5). Transitioning at school, or living as a transman outside of work, also posed challenges in intensive programs where students were immersed in environments with professional colleagues and fellow students. Physical spaces also contributed to affirming or nonaffirming settings for individuals. As one participant shared, "There's just no space for me, you know, and the locker rooms... even us students... some of them are both genders but some of them are not" (TM, page 28).

Working in professions which were historically known for being female-dominated, or which had strong male roots, especially in institutional settings, prompted concerns more often than working in alternative health or small agencies that focused on the care of highly marginalized populations. One participant who worked in such a context noted that, "I was afraid I would have someone who would refuse to call me "he" or like... be ignorant or discriminatory, and, I just lucked out. These are the things that make people believe in, like, a higher power" (TM, page 45). Another participant, who had experienced workplace bullying and scapegoating, remarked that, "the more structured and hierarchical an organization is, the more you need to be just like a little cookie cutout... so everybody is comfortable... It's one less thing to worry about in the high stress situations, I guess..." (TM, page 7).

3.5. "Fitting In". Lack of fit within the profession surfaced as a theme for participants both before gender transition began, and afterward. At times "lack of fit" was also used by employers to discriminate against participants after they began to transition, and this influenced job opportunities and job security. As one participant explained:

> "'the glass ceiling'.... There's a point beyond which you can't reach and it's kind of invisible and you just kind of grind to a halt and there's no real explanation... you're nice, dependable... but there's something that just doesn't quite gel." (TM, page 6).

He recalled being stunned by employers' feedback. "They said, 'We just don't feel you're a good fit.' And I asked them to elaborate but they absolutely couldn't" (TM, page 23).

All of the narratives revealed instances of explicit work-related discrimination or challenges of "fitting in" that were insidious. One participant, who perceived discomfort from peers when he began a new job, questioned how much education his current coworkers had about working with trans people on a team: "I'm a tranny but no one seems to process that.... I don't know if they are totally blasé or nervous" (TM, page 8). Another participant received a clear message from several higher-ups that gender transition in the professional training context was a weakness. Their attitudes conveyed that "people need to give you a hard time about it until you're tough enough, you know, you're thick-skinned enough that it won't bother you" (TM, page 34).

On the other hand, fit was also associated with a positive change after transition consistent with processes that engendered participants' resilience and growth. For some, "fit" meant that how they did their job changed after transition because they identified a new niche for their practice, or a different way of doing gender that added a new element or a new community. One participant explained that he felt that he "does masculinity" differently than other men and that this is advantageous in his professional work with men who often have complex health concerns and who seek him out to discuss tough issues that they would not discuss with straight male or female providers. Another spoke of being "wowed" by the possibility of being able to weave together his trans and professional identities in ways that are valued in a health care context such as participating openly in LGBTQ-positive education, although he recognized that there is still much to be done before this is possible in all facets of his work as a provider: "So that was the beginning of... a new phase.... I'm beginning to integrate my identity with my health care provision" (TM, page 33).

For another participant, career choices involving alternative health care and health services research paralleled his emergent identity that for him were congruent, because both challenged the prevailing biomedical and binary discourses in health in ways that not only fostered the creation of trans-positive workplaces and professional practice, but also had profoundly positive consequences on a personal level. His narrative shows links between meaning-making in a career context and the process of coming to identify as trans:

> "My gender identity is my career in a sense... or vice versa you know.... I see both of these unfolding more in the future and yeah... I've, I feel that it is also significant that I have come to both of them at a similar time, like I feel like my life has really changed course as I've... um shifted as how I identify as both my sexual orientation and my gender identity...." (TM, pages 7-8)

Certainly, the opportunity to find supportive communities both within and beyond their workplaces where participants could validate their holistic lives and identities was enormously valuable for wellbeing. This was represented by one participant who shared, "I'm not going to go stealth. I don't want to erase my past as a female and I think that being trans gives me a unique position in the world and.... I want that to be known" (TM, page 75). Another spoke of connecting to "queer community [through] freelance writing and... through the gender expression performance"

(TM, page 9). Yet for another, his decision to disclose as a transman, which was sparked by professional concerns, prompted unexpected ripples of family support. "Well I'm thrilled... everyone is just okay with it" (TM, page 14). Finding community or re-reconnecting unexpectedly with colleagues or family surfaced as significant effects of the processes of expressing trans identities for all participants in some context, although support varied considerably among the narratives.

4. Discussion and Implications

This life history study, with its attention to analysis within and across narratives, points to critical events and influences that shape trans health providers' engagement with their identities as transmen and as health providers. Gender and sexuality are determinants of health that are relevant to diverse trans people, whose everyday lives reflect a continuum of femininities and masculinities in a context of cisnormativity. Cisnormativity, which is embedded in all social institutions and our everyday worlds [32], refers to the assumption that all people are cisgendered [22]. In these narratives, gender and work emerged as the most salient social determinants in trans people's career and worklives.

The findings of this study show that trans people have unique, and gender-related, critical events and influences that shape continuities and discontinuities in their careerlives. Examples of continuity are reflected in their decision to remain involved in health provision despite experiencing immense challenges brought on by experiences of discrimination, harassment, and ill health. Despite this, the narratives of the participants also reveal that at times their career trajectories were curtailed or limited by these challenges, and for some eventually necessitated an unanticipated shift in the scope of work or a change in health profession.

Both social and material factors figure in their gender articulations and in their careerlives. In fact, these narratives show how personal and professional identities, in conjunction with practices of gender expression, are intimately linked to professional socialization processes. As a result, this study adds to the necessity of expanding organizational and educational environments by bringing forth trans providers' narratives and experiences. As one participant indicated, it is particularly crucial to "bring [...] forth trans voices that have this reality made known to a wider audience" (TM, page 3) with a focus on gender fluidity and as opposed to sexuality, especially in a context of health care where transmen are often invisible.

The focus on ongoing transitions without an endpoint that was demonstrated in this study challenges the more dominant before/after transition models of trans people's lives with stages (e.g., [33]) and this is consistent with what we have foregrounded in this paper as a more fluid approach to gender and career/work transitions more broadly. The narratives revealed that both the professional and personal lives of trans providers reflect continuities and discontinuities that have particular consequences for their career and worklives. Although continuities between the personal and professional may be relevant to a variety of individuals, findings of this study suggest that these continuities and discontinuities also have health-related effects that are both health-promoting and health-depleting—in effect—deleterious.

In fact, the intersection of work, gender, and health are clearly depicted through these narratives, in terms of employment, working conditions, and professional culture, which all have implications for nursing. For instance, although it is crucially important for nurses to open spaces and contribute to the development of workplace policies that will foster transition processes for providers, as these findings suggest, ongoing workplace support of diverse colleagues encompasses a range of practices that move beyond the transition process. These include an awareness of the everyday challenges of living and working in one's chosen gender, the significance of one's chosen profession as it connects to one's trans identity, and the importance of interpersonal, organizational, and professional supports to enhance broader community and professional environments for trans people across their lifespan. Thus these findings bring to bear a complex understanding and novel way of exploring health for trans people as workers and in particular as health care workers.

While we appreciate that there is an assumption that LGBTQ health care providers experience similar workplace concerns in general, such as stigma, management of identity and social exclusion of minorities that factor into career trajectories and a range of workplace-related issues such as health, social support, and policy, we maintain that such literature is limited in its relation to our study's focus on the career/work context. In fact, some LGBTQ-focused literature on the workplace appears to address trans issues and focus on trans people; however in effect it actually elaborates on sexual orientation rather than gender identity. For example, Bell et al. [34], while offering important insights into workplace dynamics for sexually diverse groups, do not address the unique needs of trans people in comparison to LGB people, despite a title that espouses a focus on LGBTQ workplace concerns. In fact, Brewster et al. [35] call for the development of transgender-specific versions of vocational measures to study trans workplace experiences given the ways that LGBQ-focused measures are insufficient to capture the unique issues of trans people. As they note, "many of the issues discussed in LGB vocational scholarship may be pertinent to transgender people, but the unique manifestations of... experiences of workplace harassment and discrimination, workplace climate, and identity management... are shaped specifically by gender identity and presentation" ([35], page 61).

Thus, a key contribution of our paper is the juxtaposition of career, work, and health for trans-identified people who are health and social service providers, and in particular the gender-based analysis with its focus on transgender people is unique. This paper complements the main foci of health literature on trans people which assumes that they are clients, and the workplace literature which mainly addresses gender transition and related policies—important as they are to trans people's worklives (e.g., [10, 12, 17, 36]). The findings also extend the dearth of trans-focused literature in the counselling and vocational literature (e.g., [11, 33, 35–39]).

This study contributes to a small, but increasing, body of nursing and health professional studies on gender diversity in clinical care, cultural competence, and gender nonconformity in the professions (e.g., [19, 20, 23, 25, 28, 40–44]). The findings build on research on transmen and trans people's work experiences which address transition policies and practices, identities, disclosure, discrimination, and employment counseling (e.g., [17, 37, 45, 46]), and on LGBTQ-affirmative counselling and LGBTQ-positive climates in higher education (e.g., [39, 47]). The one nursing study that examines workplace experiences of LGBT-identified nurses in an American context [17] offers important survey data on three respondents who are trans-identified. Short narrative insights from these participants and same-sex-identified nurses as key informants indicate that trans nurses encounter challenging workplace dynamics with some positive support noted. Our contribution, a gender-based analysis of qualitative data, in-depth interviews with transmen whose lifetime careers represent a variety of health care professions, including nursing, offers new and unique insights. Given the significant gap—a silence—in the literature in relation to trans people who are health care providers and the gap in nursing publications in relation to trans issues in general, this study provides much needed information.

Without a doubt, making visible the career histories of these, often invisible, trans providers in ways that show resilience and complexity, provides not just stories of role modeling for other trans people and other marginalized people in the professions, but also acts as a counterpoint to the often grim evidence base that comprises trans health. Certainly, professional education and activism that aim to alter structural dynamics are needed to foster the creation of equitable spaces for diverse trans people to thrive as health providers (e.g., [7, 17, 47]).

These findings address the invisibility of trans people as health providers rather than as clients in ways that are strength-based and move beyond a focus on marginalization and mental health concerns. This qualitative research study provides thick description and illustrates the specific and multiple contexts of trans people's lives that show how challenging employment settings, poverty, ill health, and marginalization may be part of trans health professionals' life experiences. Yet, these are also positive narratives of people who are successful in their lives and careers and who recognize their privilege as trans people who can work and thrive in particular professional contexts. Certainly this small exploratory study of a selected group of trans providers who have had access to professional training and/or acquired professional credentials and who are working in the field reflects trans people with high social privilege and does not aim to represent all providers' or transmen's experiences, but instead aims for understanding. More research is needed to examine a range of trans people's careerlives that accounts for a diversity of identities, practice settings, and ethnoracial differences, for instance.

The findings show how work and career are mutually informing, and how work is meaning-making or community-finding—all of the participants talk about finding or establishing a community at some point. These narratives also point to the negotiation, compromise, and resistance that figure into their everyday decision-making in the education and workplace environments where they are doing this gender work. As they work within structures that are shaped by gender normativity and which prescribe "fit" within professional practice, they also often push the structures to change through their visibility when they are able. These are not client or patient narratives of transition or of being trans, but rather these are insider narratives of the health profession that expand the spaces for talking about gender and transgender in health care contexts [48, 49].

Meaning-making through work and career, and finding community through gendered practices, resilience, and lack of linear trajectory are about process rather than an endpoint. Such career experiences in a professional environment are characterized by both continuities and discontinuities, as noted earlier. The findings extend what is typically discussed about the physical and emotional upheaval that transition can bring. By foregrounding discontinuity we see multiple critical incidents and influences in trans people's personal and professional lives that complicate what is often represented as a linear trajectory of professional work and career decision-making in general, and for trans people more specifically [33, 46]. As transmen negotiate their work and identities, making meaning through their career paths, they are un/doing gender and doing transgender [46]. This work builds on the work of West and Zimmermen [50] on doing gender, and Connell's [46] extension of that in relation to the ways in which transgender people do "transgender work" by foregrounding the lived experiences of providers who are transmen who experience policy "on the ground" both as "clients" of health systems and as policy actors within health systems.

The focus on spiritual values [51, 52] in a professional context, which has often been in opposition to a medical model, is consistent with a holistic and hopeful framing of transgender that informs these participants' expression and articulation of their trans identities and practices as providers. This spirituality component in its focus on meaning-making is a unique contribution to the literature on gendered identities for trans people. Relating both to themes of continuity and "fitting in," for some of the participants, gender identity and transitioning have catalyzed an expanded meaningful and positive connection to their professional identity/role. In spite of discontinuities that they experience in relation to identities, and at times experiences of rejection in work and/or professional environments, there is a congruency in the ways they create career paths in relation to their practices as health providers [52]. They are working inside and outside the work context in political ways to challenge gender norms in the ways that they participate in professional, queer and/or trans community politics, connections and professional education; Connell [46] would suggest that this is doing transgender work. There are thus implications for nursing research, education, and practice in terms of understanding how trans providers "do transgender work" and supporting them in that process.

Certainly, research and educational strategies which make visible the lives of trans people as care providers in a nursing, and larger provider contexts, are important steps; trans-inclusive education and training for cultural competence to enhance individual nurses' awareness, as well as organizational support, are warranted in order to create positive working environments that support providers who are trans-identified. Such dynamics are intimately linked to nurses' capacity to practice in inclusive ways as advocates for sexual and gender minority clients and communities. As indicated in life history research with other diverse nurses, these work and practice links have health implications that point to fostering providers' wellbeing as well as their capacity to provide responsive care [19, 42]. In order to create trans-positive spaces, findings of this paper support the development of a working paper on the process of formally integrating trans providers into the professional context. This paper thus takes up the call by Eliason et al. [53] for emancipatory nursing research which examines more fully the complexity of diverse LGBTQ people's lives.

Conflict of Interests

There are no conflict of interests for the researchers to declare.

Acknowledgments

Earlier versions of this paper were presented to the Trans Provider Day, Philadelphia, Pennsylvania, USA, in May, 2008 and to the Rainbow Health Ontario conference in Ottawa, Ontario, Canada in March, 2012. The authors wish to thank the participants who shared their stories. They appreciated funding from the Faculty of Health, York University for this project.

References

[1] Registered Nurses Association of Ontario, "Respecting sexual orientation and gender identity, Position statement,," RNAO, Toronto, Canada, 2007, http://rnao.ca/policy/position-statements/sexual-orientation-gender-identity.

[2] S. Whittle, "Foreword," in *The Transgender Studies Reader*, S. Stryker and S. Whittle, Eds., pp. 11–16, Routledge, New York, NY, USA, 2006.

[3] LGBT Health Program, "Guidelines and protocols for comprehensive primary health care for trans clients," Sherbourne Health Centre, Toronto, Canada, 2009.

[4] T. Coleman, G. Bauer, K. Scanlon, R. Travers, M. Kaay, and M. Francino, "Challenging the binary: gender characteristics of Trans Ontarians," *Trans PULSE E-Bulletin*, vol. 2, no. 2, pp. 1–3, 2011.

[5] L. Dean, I. H. Meyer, K. Robinson et al., "Lesbian, gay, bisexual, and transgender health: findings and concerns," *Journal of the Gay and Lesbian Medical Association*, vol. 4, no. 3, pp. 101–151, 2000.

[6] S. Gapka, R. Raj, K. Chow, J. Clipsham, E. Hampson, J. MacDonnell et al., "The trans health project," Position Paper, Ontario Public Health Association, Toronto, Canada, 2003.

[7] N. J. Mulé, L. E. Ross, B. Deeprose et al., "Promoting LGBT health and wellbeing through inclusive policy development," *International Journal for Equity in Health*, vol. 8, article 18, 2009.

[8] J. M. Grant, L. M. Mottet, J. Tanis, J. Harrison, J. L. Herman, and M. Keisling, *Injustice at Every Turn: A Report of the National Transgender Discrimination Survey, Executive Summary*, National Center for Transgender Equality and National Gay & Lesbian Task Force, Washington, DC, USA, 2011, http://transequality.org/PDFs/Executive_Summary.pdf.

[9] W. Bockting, G. Knudson, and J. Goldberg, *Counselling and Mental Health Care of Transgender Adults and Loved Ones*, Vancouver Coastal Health, Transgender Health Program, Vancouver, Canada, 2006, http://transhealth.vch.ca/resources/careguidelines.html.

[10] G. R. Bauer, N. Nussbaum, R. Travers, L. Munro, J. Pyne, and N. Redman, "We've got work to do: workplace discrimination and employment challenges for trans people in Ontario," *Trans Pulse E-Bulletin*, vol. 2, no. 1, pp. 1–3, 2011.

[11] V. F. Sangganjanavanich and J. Cavazos, "Workplace aggression: toward social justice and advocacy in counseling for transgender individuals," *Journal of LGBT Issues in Counseling*, vol. 4, no. 3, pp. 187–201, 2010.

[12] C. Sheehy, *Transgender Issues in the Workplace: A Tool for Managers*, Human Rights Campaign Foundation, Washington, DC, USA, 2004.

[13] Public Health Alliance, *A Positive Space is a Healthy Place*, Ontario Public Health Association, Toronto, Canada, 2006.

[14] K. Cross, *The Trans Biography Project: Stories From the Lives of Eleven Trans People in BC*, Women/Trans Dialogue Planning Committee and Trans Alliance Society, Vancouver, Canada, 2001.

[15] K. Scott-Dixon, Ed., *Trans/Forming Feminisms: Trans-Feminist Voices Speak Out*, Sumach Press, Toronto, Canada, 2006.

[16] L. Merryfeather, "A personal epistemology: towards gender diversity," *Nursing Philosophy*, vol. 12, no. 2, pp. 139–149, 2011.

[17] M. J. Eliason, J. DeJoseph, S. Dibble, S. Deevey, and P. Chinn, "Lesbian, gay, bisexual, transgender, and queer/questioning nurses' experiences in the workplace," *Journal of Professional Nursing*, vol. 27, no. 4, pp. 237–244, 2011.

[18] N. Bascia, "Making sense of the life and work of racial minority immigrant teachers," in *Making a Difference about Difference: The Lives and Careers of Racial Minority Immigrant Teachers*, D. Thiessen, N. Bascia, and I. Goodson, Eds., pp. 1–14, Garamond Press, Toronto, Canada, 1996.

[19] L. S. Giddings, "Health disparities, social injustice, and the culture of nursing," *Nursing Research*, vol. 54, no. 5, pp. 304–312, 2005.

[20] J. Evans, "Men nurses and women physicians: exploring masculinities and gendered and sexed relations in nursing and medicine," in *The History of Nursing Ideas*, L. C. Andrist, P. K. Nicholas, and K. Wolf, Eds., pp. 35–44, Jones and Bartlett, Sudbury, Mass, USA, 2006.

[21] G. R. Bauer, "Making sure everyone counts: considerations for inclusion, identification and analysis of transgender and transsexual participants in health surveys," in *What a Difference Sex and Gender Make: A Gender, Sex and Health Research Casebook*, pp. 59–67, CIHR Institute of Gender and Health, Vancouver, Canada, 2012.

[22] G. R. Bauer, R. Hammond, R. Travers, M. Kaay, K. M. Hohenadel, and M. Boyce, ""I don't think this is theoretical;

this is our lives": how erasure impacts health care for transgender people," *Journal of the Association of Nurses in AIDS Care*, vol. 20, no. 5, pp. 348–361, 2009.
[23] R. Polly and J. Nicole, "Understanding the transsexual patient: culturally sensitive care in emergency nursing practice," *Advanced Emergency Nursing Journal*, vol. 33, no. 1, pp. 55–64, 2011.
[24] J. W. Snelgrove, A. M. Jasudavisius, B. W. Rowe, E. M. Head, and G. R. Bauer, "Completely out-at-sea" with, "two-gender medicine": a qualitative analysis of physician-sidebarriers to providing healthcare for transgender patients," *BMC Health Services Research*, vol. 12, article 110, 2012.
[25] M. Johnson, T. Smyer, and C. Yucha, "Methodological quality of quantitative lesbian, gay, bisexual, and transgender nursing research from 2000 to 2010," *Advances in Nursing Science*, vol. 35, no. 2, pp. 154–165, 2010.
[26] I. Goodson, "Scrutinizing life stories: storylines, scripts and social context, making a difference about difference," in *The Lives and Careers of Racial Minority Immigrant Teachers*, D. Thiessen, N. Bascia, and I. Goodson, Eds., pp. 123–137, Garamond Press, Toronto, Canada, 1996.
[27] J. Ozga, *Policy Research in Educational Settings: Contested Terrain*, Open University Press, Buckingham, UK, 2000.
[28] A. E. Daley and J. A. MacDonnell, "Gender, sexuality and the discursive representation of access and equity in health services literature: implications for LGBT communities," *International Journal For Equity in Health*, vol. 10, article 40, 2011.
[29] J. A. MacDonnell, "Gender, sexuality and the participatory dimensions of a comparative life history policy study," *Nursing Inquiry*, vol. 18, no. 4, pp. 313–324, 2011.
[30] J. L. Johnson, L. Greaves, and R. Repta, "Better science with sex and gender: facilitating the use of a sex and gender-based analysis in health research," *International Journal for Equity in Health*, vol. 8, article 14, 2009.
[31] H. F. Hsieh and S. E. Shannon, "Three approaches to qualitative content analysis," *Qualitative Health Research*, vol. 15, no. 9, pp. 1277–1288, 2005.
[32] C. McDonald, "Issues of gender and power: the significance attributed to nurses' work," in *Realities of Canadian Nursing: Professional, Practice, and Power Issues*, M. McIntyre, E. Thomlinson, and C. McDonald, Eds., pp. 334–347, Lippincott, Williams & Wilkins, Philadelphia, Pa, USA, 2006.
[33] S. L. Budge, E. N. Tebbe, and K. A. S. Howard, "The work experiences of transgender individuals: negotiating the transition and career decision-making processes," *Journal of Counseling Psychology*, vol. 57, no. 4, pp. 377–393, 2010.
[34] M. P. Bell, M. F. Özbilgin, T. A. Beauregard, and O. Sürgevil, "Voice, silence, and diversity in 21st century organizations: strategies for inclusion of gay, lesbian, bisexual, and transgender employees," *Human Resource Management*, vol. 50, no. 1, pp. 131–146, 2011.
[35] M. E. Brewster, B. Velez, C. DeBlaere, and B. Moradi, "Transgender individuals' workplace experiences: the applicability of sexual minority measures and models," *Journal of Counseling Psychology*, vol. 59, no. 1, pp. 60–70, 2012.
[36] C. L. Law, L. R. Martinez, E. N. Ruggs, M. R. Hebl, and E. Akers, "Trans-parency in the workplace: how the experiences of transsexual employees can be improved," *Journal of Vocational Behavior*, vol. 79, pp. 710–723, 2011.
[37] J. Kirk and R. Belovics, "Understanding and counseling transgender clients," *Journal of Employment Counseling*, vol. 45, no. 1, pp. 29–43, 2008.
[38] M. E. O'Neil, E. H. McWhirter, and A. Cerezo, "Transgender identities and gender variance in vocational psychology: recommendations for practice, social advocacy, and research," *Journal of Career Development*, vol. 34, no. 3, pp. 286–308, 2008.
[39] D. A. Scott, S. L. Belke, and H. G. Barfield, "Career development with transgender college students: implications for career and employment counselors," *Journal of Employment Counseling*, vol. 48, pp. 105–113, 2011.
[40] S. W. Morgan and P. E. Stevens, "Transgender identity development as represented by a group of female-to-male transgendered adults," *Issues in Mental Health Nursing*, vol. 29, no. 6, pp. 585–599, 2008.
[41] C. Hanssmann, D. Morrison, E. Russian, S. Shiu-Thornton, and D. Bowen, "A community-based program evaluation of community competency trainings," *Journal of the Association of Nurses in AIDS Care*, vol. 21, no. 3, pp. 240–255, 2010.
[42] C. O. Jenner, "Transsexual primary care," *Journal of the American Academy of Nurse Practitioners*, vol. 22, no. 8, pp. 403–408, 2010.
[43] C. A. Alegria, "Transgender identity and health care: implications for psychosocial and physical evaluation," *Journal of the American Academy of Nurse Practitioners*, vol. 23, no. 4, pp. 175–182, 2011.
[44] J. A. MacDonnell, "Comparative life histories of nurses who advocate for lesbian health in a Canadian context: sexual orientation as a factor in career and workplace dynamics," in *Sexual Orientation Discrimination: An International Perspective*, M. V. L. Badgett and J. Frank, Eds., pp. 118–135, Routledge, London, UK, 2007.
[45] K. Schilt, "Just one of the guys? How transmen make gender visible at work," *Gender and Society*, vol. 20, no. 4, pp. 465–490, 2006.
[46] C. Connell, "Doing, undoing, or redoing gender? Learning from the workplace experiences of transpeople," *Gender and Society*, vol. 24, no. 1, pp. 31–55, 2010.
[47] D. M. Keepnews, "LGBT health issues and nursing," *Policy, Politics and Nursing Practice*, vol. 12, no. 2, pp. 71–72, 2011.
[48] J. Savage, "Gestures of resistance: the nurse's body in contested space," *Nursing Inquiry*, vol. 4, no. 4, pp. 237–245, 1997.
[49] S. Halford and P. Leonard, "Space and place in the construction and performance of gendered nursing identities," *Journal of Advanced Nursing*, vol. 42, no. 2, pp. 201–208, 2003.
[50] C. West and D. H. Zimmerman, "Doing gender," *Gender & Society*, vol. 1, no. 2, pp. 125–151, 1987.
[51] G. H. Doane and C. Varcoe, *Family Nursing as Relational Inquiry: Developing Health-Promoting Practice*, Lippincott Williams & Wilkins, Philadelphia, Pa, USA, 2005.
[52] J. A. MacDonnell, "Exploring matrices of mothering and feminisms: life history methodology as a venue for understanding the complexities of mothering discourses for lesbian health advocates," *Journal of the Association for Research on Mothering*, vol. 1, no. 8, pp. 298–310, 2006.
[53] M. J. Eliason, S. Dibble, and J. DeJoseph, "Nursing's silence on lesbian, gay, bisexual, and transgender issues: the need for emancipatory efforts," *Advances in Nursing Science*, vol. 33, no. 3, pp. 206–218, 2010.

21

Understanding Race and Racism in Nursing: Insights from Aboriginal Nurses

Adele Vukic,[1] Charlotte Jesty,[2] Sr. Veronica Mathews,[3] and Josephine Etowa[4]

[1] *Dalhousie School of Nursing, Faculty of Health Professions, 1459 Oxford Street, Halifax, NS, Canada B3H 4R2*
[2] *Mijua'ji'j Aqq Ni'n, Unama'ki Maternal Child Health, 201 Churchill Drive, Membertou, NS, Canada*
[3] *Eskasoni Health Board, Eskasoni Community Health Center, Eskasoni, NS, Canada*
[4] *School of Nursing, Faculty of Health Sciences, University of Ottawa, Ottawa, ON, Canada K1H 8M5*

Correspondence should be addressed to Adele Vukic, adele.vukic@dal.ca

Academic Editors: R. C. Locsin and C. Winkelman

Purpose. Indigenous Peoples are underrepresented in the health professions. This paper examines indigenous identity and the quality and nature of nursing work-life. The knowledge generated should enhance strategies to increase representation of indigenous peoples in nursing to reduce health inequities. *Design.* Community-based participatory research employing Grounded Theory as the method was the design for this study. Theoretical sampling and constant comparison guided the data collection and analysis, and a number of validation strategies including member checks were employed to ensure rigor of the research process. *Sample.* Twenty-two Aboriginal nurses in Atlantic Canada. *Findings.* Six major themes emerged from the study: Cultural Context of Work-life, Becoming a Nurse, Navigating Nursing, Race Racism and Nursing, Socio-Political Context of Aboriginal Nursing, and Way Forward. Race and racism in nursing and related subthemes are the focus of this paper. *Implications.* The experiences of Aboriginal nurses as described in this paper illuminate the need to understand the interplay of race and racism in the health care system. Our paper concludes with Aboriginal nurses' suggestions for systemic change at various levels.

1. Introduction

Aboriginal people are significantly underrepresented in the health care professions. While statistics indicate that Aboriginal peoples comprise 3.8% of the Canadian population [1], currently less than 1% of Canadian nurses identify as having Aboriginal ancestry [2]. The relationship between Aboriginal Peoples and Western healthcare developed within a specific context of colonization and centralization in which medical professionals saw it as their role to help Aboriginal peoples "negotiate civilization," while ignoring the detrimental effects of interference [3]. The history of colonization has had a significant impact on the health of Aboriginal peoples. The inclusion of Aboriginal health care professionals in decisions affecting their lives would lead to more equitable decision making in the factors that influence Aboriginal health.

This paper presents the findings of a recent study that explored the work-life experiences of Aboriginal nurses in the Atlantic Provinces with the goal of strengthening current nursing recruitment and retention efforts. This paper was carried out with the recognition that efforts to diversify the nursing workforce must include an examination of the experiences of Aboriginal nurses already working within the system. Specifically, the research examined the nature of being an Aboriginal person in the nursing profession through the following research question: What are the work-life experiences of Aboriginal nurses working in health care systems in Atlantic Canada? Understanding Aboriginal nurses' work-life experiences informs how race, ethnicity, and culture intersect with nursing practice and education.

2. Literature Review

A number of initiatives have been implemented over the past few years to enhance Aboriginal peoples' participation in the health professions. For instance, in response to the problem of nursing shortage in Canada, the Federal Government in 2004 allocated \$100 M over 5 years to "create and implement strategies to increase the numbers of Aboriginal health professionals" [4]. Further, the Aboriginal Nurses Association of Canada (ANAC) has been involved in a number of initiatives. For example, ANAC met with nurses and stakeholders in May, 2006 to discuss ways of recruiting Aboriginal nurses, and equipping all nurses working with Aboriginal peoples with the tools necessary to provide culturally safe care [5]. ANAC [5] is currently partnering with a number of academic institutions to develop a mentoring program for Aboriginal nursing students. ANAC was formed in 1975 to "improve the health of Aboriginal people by supporting Aboriginal nurses and by promoting the development and practice of Aboriginal health nursing" ([6], page 34). According to ANAC, an increase in the number of practicing Aboriginal nurses is crucial to improving the health of Aboriginal communities overall [7]. The National Task Force on Recruitment and Retention Strategies [8] has identified the need for nursing leadership and support as a fundamental component of retaining practicing Aboriginal nurses in the profession. ANAC partnered with the Canadian Nursing Student Association (CNSA) in 2005 to cohost a strategic planning session designed to increase participation of Aboriginal nursing students in the CNSA and to develop a "framework supporting cultural diversity and safety in nursing education" ([9], page 10).

Several studies have examined the experiences of Aboriginal and minority nurses in Canada, Britain, and the United States ([10–20]). However, as Kulig and Grypma [21] note very little has been written about the history of Aboriginal nurses and despite their role in improving the health status of First Nations, Inuit, and Metis, very little research exists that explores the perspectives of Aboriginal nurses themselves. Kulig et al. [22] analyzed the results of a national survey of RNs working in rural and remote areas of Canada, in which 210 of the 3933 respondents self-identified as having Aboriginal or Metis ancestry. They found that 69.6% of Aboriginal nurses were originally from rural/remote communities, and that 66.7% chose to return to such areas because they wanted to work with their own people and raise families in smaller communities.

Motivated by difficulties in recruiting and retaining Aboriginal students into nursing programs, Martin and Kipling [18] interviewed Aboriginal nursing students, Aboriginal nurses, and nursing faculty members to explore what kinds of factors shaped students' experiences. Participants identified inadequate funding and lack of available childcare as significant challenges, and they identified personal issues, lack of social support, racism, and conflicts with teachers as negative factors affecting their experiences in nursing education. These authors highlighted the exclusion of Aboriginal ways of knowing within the curricula and the lack of attentiveness to Aboriginal health care issues. They also advocated for collaboration among Aboriginal students and teachers in curriculum development and instructional design. Currently, there is limited research that examines the experiences of Aboriginal nurses already working in the health care field. An in-depth understanding of the work-life issues of Aboriginal nurses already working in the health care system is necessary for the development of future

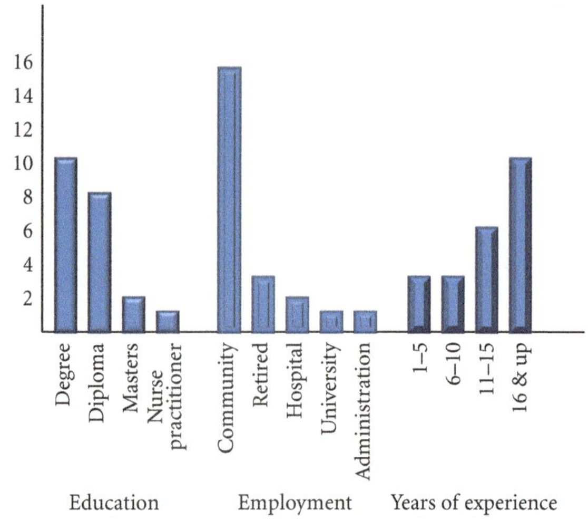

FIGURE 1: Atlantic Aboriginal nurses interviewed.

retention programs. The knowledge generated from our recent research on the work-life experiences of Aboriginal nurses in Atlantic Canada will inform the development of strategies to increase the representation of Aboriginal Peoples in nursing education, research, and practice.

3. Methodology

This qualitative study was based on Grounded Theory as described by Glaser and Strauss [23] informed by a Community-Based Participatory Research (CBPR) approach and the principles of Ownership, Control, Access, and Possession (OCAP). In keeping with the tenets of (CBPR), and the OCAP principles, Aboriginal Atlantic Canadians were an integral part of the research as team members; as coprincipal investigator, community partners, and coinvestigators. The project also had a capacity-building component, which facilitated the hiring and mentoring of a research assistant of Aboriginal ancestry who participated in all aspects of the research. Ethical approval was granted by the University Research Ethics Board and Mi'kmaq Ethics Watch. Data collection consisted of unstructured qualitative interviews with Aboriginal registered nurses who were working (or had worked previously) in the various parts of Atlantic Canada.

Participants were recruited through snowball sampling, an approach for selecting participants by asking well-situated people who to talk with and the list of interviewees increases as the research progresses [24]. Theoretical sampling technique guided the direction for further data collection and the achievement of data saturation. A total of 22 face to face interviews were conducted over a period of six months. Targeted effort was made to ensure maximum variation in the sample, thus study participants ranged from new graduates to retirees, young and more senior nurses who have held various nursing positions in the hospital, community, university; with education ranging from diploma, baccalaureate, nurse practitioner, and masters. See Figure 1 for details. All participants were female and the majority worked in a First Nations community. All interviews were conducted by one of the two academic members of the research team. The research assistant of Aboriginal ancestry accompanied some interviews to develop her Grounded Theory interviewing skills. In the interviews, participants were asked to respond to the following broad statement: "Tell me about your experience of being an Aboriginal nurse in the Atlantic Canadian health care system." Most interviews were 60 to 90 minutes long with participants sharing many stories from why they went into nursing, their nursing education experience, their day to day lived experiences, and their personal career development. Interviews were transcribed verbatim.

4. Data Analysis

Team members met to code and analyze the transcripts. Team members had data analysis meetings to code and analyze the information and Atlas-ti qualitative data software facilitated the management of this information. Data collection and analysis took place concurrently in keeping with the principles of Grounded Theory. Member-checks and peer-debriefing were used to evaluate the rigor of the research process and to enhance trustworthiness of the data.

5. Findings

Six major themes emerged from the study: Cultural Context of Work-life, Becoming a Nurse, Navigating Nursing, Race Racism and Nursing, Socio-Political Context of Aboriginal Nursing, and Way Forward. Racism was a major theme revealed in the study findings and is described as "Race, Racism, and Nursing." Participants talked about experiencing racism and of witnessing racism toward Aboriginal patients, and they shared some of the strategies they used to respond both to overt racism and to feelings of "otherness." Participants did not blame individuals and consistently referred to the need for increased awareness of issues and institutional commitment to respond to racism. Some participants found that being Aboriginal was advantageous in that it enabled them to gain the trust of Aboriginal patients and to provide culturally safe care in hospital and community settings. The nurses in this study also talked about the burden of having to educate their colleagues about Aboriginal issues and of the underrepresentation of Aboriginal people in nursing, especially in leadership positions. The theme of racism will be described under the following subthemes; Experiencing Otherness, Responding to Discrimination, Tokenism versus Competence, and Cultural Safety and Diversity.

6. Experiencing Otherness

The findings of this subtheme revealed a number of complex issues impacting on the work-life of Aboriginal nurses. Participants experienced personal discrimination from coworkers and patients, and several nurses interviewed also observed racism toward Aboriginal patients. One nurse asserted that racism toward Aboriginal patients in the hospital setting was more prominent than racism toward other minority patients,

> *"I've seen blatant racism in the hospital setting that shouldn't be allowed and a lot of it is; and as an Aboriginal person I see more centered around Aboriginal more so than Black people or Asian people or anything like that. When they come in the hospital they're like "oh, they're probably drunk" or things like that."*

This speaks to the lack of policies and resources to ensure that all nurses embrace cultural safety as an integral aspect of nursing care. Although another nurse felt angry and personally attacked when witnessing racism towards Aboriginal patients, both she and others feared that speaking up would put a strain on their relationships with coworkers. As one nurse remarked, *"I want to say more but I, I feel, I just don't know how to approach them without, without feeling like an outsider again."*

Though many participants identified experiences and observations of overt racism, some of the nurses expressed uncertainty around naming racism. As this statement explains, *"the comments can be very very subtle and you don't know whether you've just imagined a derogatory...tone, or if it was actually there."* This uncertainty often prevented participants from speaking up when they thought they had observed racism, as they did not want to confront someone or make accusations if they were unsure about what they had witnessed.

The nurses in this study talked about fitting in, belonging, and being accepted. While some participants struggled with feeling as though they did not "fit in" with their non-Aboriginal coworkers or fellow students, others experienced friendship and acceptance. Some nurses learned with Aboriginal students in their nursing courses, which allowed them to find a sense of belonging within their own group:

> *"I think because I had two other native students with me that we created our own sort of network of support. If I was by myself I might have had a different experience but I think having the other two nursing students together we could relate to each others' experiences yeah, and we could talk things out."*

Others chose to enroll in nursing partly because they knew of Aboriginal students in these programs. As one nurse explained, *"the only reason I went there is because...I knew somebody...They were 2 years ahead of me...So I [knew] I wouldn't be alone."*

Although some found acceptance with peers, others felt judged by instructors. One participant shared that instructors felt that she did not belong in higher education because she was Aboriginal, and that they even went so far as to tell her that *"You're not going to make a nurse, you'll never make a nurse, you're wasting your time."* The following quote captures how some Aboriginal nurses, as students, recognized that instructors may never have had the experience of being on the other end of comments that can be interpreted as racist, and how some try to apologize.

> *"And then when I walked back in the room, the instructor who had been in teaching the course tried to hug me in the, in the first thing, it was*

like one, you're invading my space, two just, just leave me be for a little while, just leave me be. And I think part of that was like not understanding the insult to begin with. And not being sensitive to, to having that experience."

In school, some felt that their personal learning style (the verbal learning and storytelling characteristic of Aboriginal culture) did not fit the norms of learning in the mainstream academic system and struggled with the written and concrete aspects of schoolwork.

Participants felt judged by other nurses working in the hospital but found solace in caring for Aboriginal patients:

"It was not a good experience. It wasn't like, I was alone. I felt I was alone, I was like, there was, especially around here, there's still racism eh? It was still here believe it or not. So when I worked in this hospital...there was only one person...one nurse that I got along with. I think she pitied me. But the other nurses I found, it was like, I don't know, I felt uncomfortable. I felt like they thought I didn't know anything. Or something like that. And my people were there, like the clients when they had native clients there like they were so glad to have a native nurse, like that made the difference...."

Others found it rewarding to work in an Aboriginal community and to experience in turn a sense of belonging to a community.

"Yes I worked seventy, eighty, ninety hours a week but I thrived on it. I, I, it made me feel whole to be able to help my community to help the people in my community. Part of that is the sense of belonging, the sense of being part of the community."

A few participants shared that they did not "fit in" to the mainstream nursing community partly due to the fact that English was their second language. Many pointed out that others sometimes misinterpreted their tone as bossy. Others found the transition from hospital nursing back to community nursing positive, in part due to language. As one nurse explained, *"here, I love it, I feel like I fit right in. I don't have to like hide the way I talk, like I'm not that good in English, like I kind of stutter a little and...they would say "You're not pronouncing that right." I'd be like "I can't help it."* Some participants confided that they would have felt more comfortable in nursing school as well as the hospital setting with a confidante who spoke Mi'kmaq.

The ability to speak a second language proved advantageous to the nurses who participated in this study. Participants commented how beneficial it was to be able to speak Mi'kmaq to Mi'kmaq patients. As one nurse explained, *"there's more of a bond between me and other Mi'kmaq patients...I can relate more to them."* Aboriginal nurses who worked in a community setting provided examples of instances in which they used their own language to discuss with patients the need to seek particular treatments and pointed out that patients are often more likely to open up to them when they share the same language.

7. Responding to Discrimination

This subtheme captured the ways in which the nurses responded to discrimination in their work as Aboriginal nurses. These include the use of both direct and indirect strategies, which varied depending on the individuals involved and on the particular situations they encountered. The strategies for responding to discrimination are categorized as; proving oneself, establishing credibility, educating others, passing as non Aboriginal and confronting the issue directly.

The nurses had to constantly prove themselves not only to the White community but also to their own people. In mainstream settings, establishing credibility meant proving one's competence. One nurse talked about being perceived as *that dumb girl*, and another talked about the need to prove oneself as follows:

"We've had to prove to other people that we're just as smart as they are. The racism as I said in the very beginning, the racism is slowly changing but [province] is still, racism is alive and well. And it's to prove that I'm just as good as anybody else, if not better." Another echoed a similar sentiment, stating, *"I find myself having to prove my skills and myself to, to them Like the, my experiences, I feel when I get down to nitty gritty, at times I feel that I'm not respected because I'm Aboriginal."*

As was the case for the nurses who worked in hospitals, the First Nations community nurses also had to prove their competence. As this comment explains:

"Always proving, proving, proving to people that you can do it right. So yeah and I think that um in our communities like when I worked as a community health nurse, when I came across that kind of attitude again and it was there with my own people that I would challenge it. And I'd sometimes say well you know, I think you really need to rethink about that because you know we are trained in the very same way those nurses are trained and actually we probably can even be better because we understand a lot of the cultural, the language and what you're going through. And so oftentimes I think over time you just didn't need to say it anymore."

Yet for these nurses, establishing credibility also meant proving not only their competence, but also their loyalty to Aboriginal people and practices. As this quote explains:

"Ok, so I am an Aboriginal nurse but I'm also a, you know, we also get educated in the mainstream so some of those ideas bringing into the community didn't go over quite as well. So when I first came either, well who does she think she is and yeah as if I was practicing as a mainstream nurse. Like you're supposed to be a native nurse why are you doing it that way."

These nurses had to prove that they would not abandon their communities, that they would remain loyal to their communities, and that they would remain true to Aboriginal culture and beliefs despite their mainstream schooling.

One of the ways in which participants responded to racism and discrimination was by educatingothers. Nurses spoke openly about personal experiences and observations of discrimination in order to educate many people about the fact that racism still occurs in hospitals and the need educate coworkers demonstrating racist behaviour by challenging stereotypes directly and by bringing to attention racial slurs.

While some participants actively took on the role of educating coworkers, others felt it should not be their responsibility. For example *"I'm just not taking on the role of educating people about it anymore...Especially in the workplace because it's not my job. It's not my job"*. Although some nurses did address racist remarks, they did not believe that individual nurses should be responsible for providing this kind of education: *"It shouldn't be. It shouldn't be but I don't see who else is going to do it, right? I don't see my manager or patient care leader out there educating you know, the nurses. They probably don't even know."* When confronting the issue of racism some participants reflected on the decision to speak up versus keep quiet in situations where one is confronting discrimination. Some participants felt comfortable addressing inappropriate language, but did not feel comfortable speaking up about broader issues. Some remained silent when overhearing discriminatory remarks in a hospital setting but defended personal racist attacks.

Participants spoke at length about fear of educating coworkers. Others did not feel comfortable verbally confronting those who made inappropriate comments and therefore chose to remain silent. Some identified "speaking up" as a critical skill that could assist Aboriginal people in fighting discrimination:

> *"I guess I haven't been taught the skills of conflict resolution or looking at a conflict. Um, maybe with more assertive skills or, or knowing how to address those things. I don't think we've ever been taught that. It's more if it happens it happens and you say nothing. Um, but maybe we need to start teaching people to speak up and say "I don't want to be spoken to that way" or "that's not how you should address me because I'm First Nations "you people"." You know, those little things that maybe we need to educate one person at a time, I don't know but um, I really don't know what the answer is to that."*

The issue of looking different versus passing as non-Aboriginal arose in the interviews. Some participants looked different from their coworkers, while others had a more fair skin tone and eye color and could "pass" as another race. One nurse decided against working in the hospital because she was sure she would have been the only nurse with dark skin. Numerous participants commented on being able to pass as non-Aboriginal. Many felt that passing was beneficial in terms of their fitting in to the workplace. As this quote explains:

> *"I think that was the first defense for me...See they didn't learn to know me as Mi'kmaq first, they learned to know me as a student nurse who is nice, would talk to you, give you a drink of water while you were you were you know, pleasant student. It helps when you don't have that barrier at first."*

Many chose not to identify publicly as Aboriginal during training unless asked directly. One nurse explains how she chose to stay away from Aboriginal groups on campus for fear she would experience discrimination.

> *"You know deep down I think that's why I never, because I didn't want anybody, you know...looking down on me because I was Aboriginal. As long as they didn't know I was Aboriginal, they treated me as equal. But I really felt that if they had known...once they know that, then it's different."*

On several occasions, participants encountered patients who preferred a White nurse because they assumed that White nurses had more training. Some participants were quick to challenge these assumptions and to point out that they had equal training. Some felt that being an Aboriginal nurse provided a certain level of authority when visiting and/or participating in professional development with other communities. Some felt that their voice was heard by non-Aboriginals specifically because they were Aboriginal.

Participants spoke of the high expectations communities had that they would be effective at *making the community better*. Many felt personal disappointment and the community's disappointment when positive changes did not occur immediately. Participants expressed that they felt very invested in their communities because they belonged to these communities in ways that extended beyond their nursing.

8. Tokenism versus Competence

This theme refers to the complacent attitude associated with a marginal representation of Aboriginal people in a given health care organization. It is seen as racism because when an employer hires one Aboriginal person who happens to be successful he or she often thinks that the problem of discrimination has been successfully addressed. One of the nurses referred to this as the "Token Indian." She went on to explain:

> *"Somebody that, oh, we should have this minority, this minority, oh yes, we should have First Nations here too. And that's what I mean by token Indian, so that they can make sure that the representation is from our community."*

Others chose to take advantage of this position as a "Token Indian" to seek out resources, programs, and services for the community. They also enjoyed the benefits of attending workshops and committees in order to connect to further resources.

Similarly, another nurse experienced tokenism when she first applied for a job in a hospital. Her interview was very short and she was awarded the job immediately. She stated that she believed this was because "*they wanted a native nurse at the hospital, because all our First Nations people were off loaded to that local hospital. So I was hired on.*" Some participants addressed the topic in reference to being hired to work for a particular organization, As one nurse concluded, this led her to "toil" over whether she had been hired because she was Aboriginal, or because of her experience.

9. Cultural Safety and Diversity

Cultural Safety takes us beyond cultural awareness and acknowledgement of differences to addressing inequities witnessed because of differences [5]. Many participants spoke about the lack of understanding they witnessed among non-Aboriginal coworkers in both hospital and community settings regarding how to work effectively across ethno-cultural boundaries. One participant defined:

> *"Cultural insensitivity to me, means that the nurses working in non Aboriginal clinic didn't really know too much about our culture and they were putting expectations on our people that they would expect from their own kind that were non Aboriginals. And I talked to them about it. I said, "You have to understand where these people are coming from.""*

Others commented on how unaccommodating hospitals are toward Aboriginal patients. These participants argued that hospitals needed to be more cooperative and flexible in respecting Aboriginal patients' culture, ideologies, and rituals. As an example, several participants addressed the practice exhibited by hospital personnel in restricting the number of visitors allowed at a patient's bedside at one time. One participant explains:

> *"A Mi'kmaq would never let a Mi'kmaq die alone. But you know with non-native there maybe just 2 people by that person's side when they're dying. But if it's a Mi'kmaq, maybe you're going to see maybe 50 to 100 people you're going to see at the hospital, and they have to realize like in [city], one of my friend's father-in-law just passed away and then they are all praying like, they wanted to do like a really traditional like sacred ceremonial, they were not allowed. They all wanted to go help him, like when you pray in Mi'kmaq you can help them get to heaven faster, to get to the spirit world faster. They were there too long they were saying, so the nurses they called security, security came up and they told them to stop and told them to invite only 2 people at a time. So they didn't realize like about our culture."*

Some participants asserted that allowances should be made for patients who wished to smoke a pipe to honor spirits. They concurred, not only should hospitals accommodate Aboriginal practices, but they should also attempt to understand the root of these practices: "*If an Aboriginal person wants to burn sweet grass how do you make those accommodations? Well if you don't understand why they're doing it then it's going to come, it's going to be a problem, you know?*" This nurse went on to say that many misunderstandings could be resolved if hospital staff were open to hearing and understanding where patients were coming from.

The study findings revealed that some Aboriginal patients often feign understanding to save face when in fact they require clearer instructions for collecting specimens, preparing for medical procedures, and so forth. To facilitate better communication between Aboriginal patients and non-Aboriginal hospital staff, some Aboriginal nurses took on the unofficial role of cultural interpreters. Participants suggested that non-Aboriginal community nurses need to be more aware of the importance of relationships with patients. They also emphasized the necessity of home visits in ensuring one's effectiveness as a community nurse.

The study finding also revealed the lack of formal diversity education in both education and workplace settings as a significant barrier to providing culturally safe care, some of the nurses recommended the integration of Aboriginal culture, customs, and ideologies in health professionals training curricula. Some nurses suggested that at times diversity education propagated generalizations and assumptions about Aboriginal culture. However, the nurses overall valued diversity in their education and some nurses took control of their own educatio because of this value. As this quote explains:

> *"I wanted to make sure that I could incorporate Aboriginal health within my education as much as I could, because it wasn't a course in itself or the theme throughout the four years. So I kind of had to create those opportunities for myself."*

Some participants observed a lack and in some cases absence of sufficient diversity education in the hospital workplace. As one participant described, "*And I know for like the non-Aboriginal nurse there's no cultural competency training or anything of the sort.*" Many participants provided suggestions on how to foster diversity in schools and workplace. Some recommended that Aboriginal nurses be invited into nursing classrooms to discuss cultural consciousness. As one participant commented "*I'd like to see that change. Maybe having guest speakers just who work in First Nations community nursing.*" Some advocated for an increase in the number of Aboriginal nursing teachers, while others also advocated for an increase in culturally safe instructors. Some asserted that a course focusing solely on Aboriginal health would benefit students. Others suggested that hospitals could incorporate cultural safety into their orientation processes, while others proposed that cultural safety be incorporated into "lunch and learn." sessions. One participant asserted that non-Aboriginal and administrative hospital staff should be more informed about issues pertaining to diversity. As she points out:

> *"I now realize the complexity of culture and racism and that it is an ongoing battle as each new generation comes to the fore. Being an Aboriginal*

nurse, I have firsthand experience of living the "other" and therefore feel that I have a degree of sensitivity in this area. However, I can have the "other" as well when it comes to non-Aboriginal people. In working with non-Aboriginals in my community, I find that I am, at times, teaching the way of life and dispelling the generalizations perceived by non-Aboriginals."

All of the nurses interviewed in this study indicated that an increase in the number of Aboriginal Peoples in schools, in the nursing workforce, and in administrative positions would be welcomed and would benefit them for numerous reasons. They expressed the need for more Aboriginal Peoples on committees concerned with Aboriginal health. As one participant explained "*There was this big Aboriginal committee, not one Aboriginal name! Not one Aboriginal person on that committee! And that is so upsetting and discouraging.*" Other participants also mentioned that, although there were some nurse practitioners and Masters prepared Aboriginal nurses, they would like to see an increase in the number of Aboriginal nurses seeking higher education such as a nurse practitioner or master's level degrees. Some participants also commented on the need for an increase of Aboriginal nurses filling administrative and leadership role. One participant explained with regard to a particularly influential organization; "*There's nobody in a leadership position that's of First Nations, which is really I mean, it's wrong. People you know should be making decisions about their own lives like self-determination.*" Others talked about the advantages of working in a clinic with other Aboriginal nurses. For example: "*I think because we go way back from the beginning that we have this and we're from this community that we have this real good bond and real good, we work well together because we understand each other.*"

Some participants offered explanations for the shortage of Aboriginal nurses in the workforce such as the underrepresentation of Aboriginal nurses in tertiary care settings. They suggest this may be part of the reason why many Aboriginal nurses choose to work in Aboriginal communities where they work with other Aboriginal nursing colleagues and are more comfortable. Some nurses suggested that many young Aboriginal people were more likely to choose careers such as teaching and business over nursing because the significance of the work of nurse is often invisible. To address this, they suggested that high school students should be encouraged to take science classes from a young age so that they will be qualified for nursing education and to have more role models discussing Aboriginal nursing in the high schools.

Other recommendations of the study include the use of innovative recruitment strategies such as facilitating summer camps in collaboration with Aboriginal communities, advertising in the field of Aboriginal nursing and promoting health fields through various venues, ensuring that Aboriginal nurses are represented at elementary and high school career days, and developing mentorship program for potential students who may be identified from career days or the summer camps. As one of the nurses asserted, Aboriginal nursing recruitment should focus on providing adequate support to students and on offering them a safe space in which to voice their concerns. She elaborated:

"If we want more Aboriginal nurses...then we have to try and understand them, and maybe look at their culture, they're different, very different, and you need to understand that, and you've got to have some resources there to assist them in those times, that they're going to be, you know, because like I said they're moving away from home, they're adjusting to a different culture."

10. Discussion

Racism was a common thread in the stories of these nurses. The various manifestations of racism described by these nurses demonstrate the painful reality of everyday experiences of discrimination in nursing and the magnitude of this systemic issue. While some participants spoke of subtle racism, others spoke of blatant racism, and while some spoke of personal experiences of racism, others spoke of witnessing other Aboriginal people especially patients being discriminated against. These everyday incidents of discrimination are rooted in systemic structures that perpetuate differential and culturally unsafe treatment of Aboriginal people. Although racism is manifested in a number of ways including individual and/or systemic actions (or inaction in the face of need), it is more deeply rooted at the systemic level because the power to make decisions, to take collective action, and to allocate resources resides at this level [25]. Systemic racism is supported by policy action and inaction regarding persistently compromised health outcomes of people in positions of disadvantage [26]. Racism at the systemic level manifests in material conditions and in access to power, including differential access to health care services [27].

The many faces of racism highlighted in this paper reveal the insidious nature of the problem of race and racism in nursing. The nurses shared how being Aboriginal was important to them as they were able to inform coworkers about Aboriginal culture and advocated on behalf of Aboriginal patients in the hospital and the community. They also shared how being Aboriginal was advantageous and how they felt welcomed by Aboriginal patients in the hospitals and in Aboriginal communities.

Participants offered innovative ideas for improving the system including specific suggestions for enhancing the recruitment and retention of Aboriginal nurses, such as summer camps, mentoring, role modeling, and increasing awareness of nursing as a career to high school students. An increase in the presence of Aboriginal nurses would create a greater support system and resources for Aboriginal nurses already working in hospitals and communities. The nurses in this study recommend that more Aboriginal nurses are needed in leadership positions to influence the policy and practices that affect Aboriginal Peoples. Currently only a few of the nurses in this study were in leadership positions. Senior leadership in the health care system should take some responsibility in ensuring the development and advancement of Aboriginal nurses into leadership positions and as Aboriginal nursing faculty. The time has come to support, recruit, and retain nurses in leadership positions so they are involved in influencing policy that affect Aboriginal people. Recruitment and retention is not simply a matter of more Aboriginal nurses to provide direct care.

While the majority of the Atlantic Aboriginal nurses in this study took it upon themselves to educate others in the context of their work environment they stressed the need for education on cultural safety with a concerted effort both in the nursing education and in hospitals. Nursing schools need to include cultural safety, conflict resolution, and negotiation skills in the curricula. Education of competent nurses capable of working effectively across ethno-racial boundaries should be everyone's problem. The study data highlights important insights into sensitive issues such as racism and discrimination, which are traditionally areas of discomfort. Nursing schools and workplace environments should have structures in place to address racism and promote diversity. These findings challenge nursing scholars to push the margins of nursing knowledge to explicate the complex social processes that influence human experience and consequently impact on health, especially the health of historically marginalized people. Some of their suggestions validate and reinforce current reports, research, and literature reviews on this topic. The literature supports the relevance of narrowing the gap between Aboriginal and non-Aboriginal health status by increasing involvement of Aboriginal Peoples in health delivery and policy-making [28, 29], and in recruitment of Aboriginal students into nursing programs and activities [9], as many of the participants in this study advocated.

A limitation to this study is that the majority of nurses participating in this study worked in the community as most of the Aboriginal nurses in the Atlantic Provinces are located in Aboriginal communities. A national study focusing on Aboriginal nurses in a variety of positions and in a variety of health care settings may provide further insights. Also, perspectives from non-Aboriginal nurses may constitute a broader analysis of race and racism in nursing.

11. Conclusion

This study provides some direction for improving the quality of work-life of Aboriginal nurses to advance the health and health care of Aboriginal Peoples. In summary, this paper has provided some insight into the work-life experiences of Aboriginal nurses in Atlantic Canada, particularly with the understandings of race and racism in nursing, and how these have influenced their practice and decisions. Clearly, the nurses in this study have identified priorities for action to address the complex and systemic issues influencing the health and health services delivery for Aboriginal Peoples. The nurses in this study are eager to be involved in the health care system to affect change that promotes equity. As one nurse in this study concurs it is all about, "*Knowing my history, knowing what's been before me, knowing the wrongs that have happened to our community and wanting to make a change.*"

Conflict of Interests

The authors acknowledge no conflict of interests in this paper.

Acknowledgment

Financial Assistance was provided by Atlantic Aboriginal Health Research Program funded by the IAPH-CIHR.

References

[1] Statistics Canada. Census of population, Statistics Canada catalogue no. 97-558-XCB2006010, 2006, http://www12.statcan.ca/census-recensement/2006/dp-pd/index-eng.cfm.

[2] L. M. Hunter, J. Logan, J. G. Goulet, and S. Barton, "Aboriginal healing: regaining balance and culture," *Journal of Transcultural Nursing*, vol. 17, no. 1, pp. 13–22, 2006.

[3] M. J. McCallum, "The last frontier: isolation and Aboriginal health," *Canadian Bulletin of Medical History*, vol. 22, no. 1, pp. 103–120, 2005.

[4] G. Hanson, "ANAC activities," *The Aboriginal Nurse*, 2006.

[5] Aboriginal Nursing Association of Canada, *Cultural Competence and Cultural Safety in Nursing Education*, Aboriginal Nursing Association of Canada, Ottawa, Canada, 2009.

[6] J. L. Dobbelsteyn, "Nursing in first nations and inuit communities in Atlantic Canada," *Canadian Nurse*, vol. 102, no. 4, pp. 32–35, 2006.

[7] F. H. Wasekeesikaw, "Challenges for the new millennium: nursing in the First Nations communities," in *Realities of Canadian Nursing: Professional, Practice and Power Issues*, M. McIntyre and E. Thomlinson, Eds., Lippincott Williams & Wilkins, Philadelphia, Pa, USA, 2003.

[8] National Task Force on Recruitment and Retention Strategies, *Against All Odds: Aboriginal Nursing*, Health Canada, Ottawa, Canada, 2002.

[9] K. McCulla, E. Smith, and R. Lonsdale, "Facilitating Aboriginal participation in Canadian Nursing Students Association activities," in *The Aboriginal Nurse*, E. McGibbon and J. Etowa, Eds., Anti-Racist Health Practice. Canadian Scholars Press, Toronto, Canada, 2005.

[10] H. Bessent, *Minority Nurses in the New Century: Characteristics and Workforce Utilization-A Survey*, American Nurses, Washington, DC, USA, 2002.

[11] A. Calliste, "Antiracism organizing and resistance in nursing: African Canadian women," *Canadian Review of Sociology and Anthropology*, vol. 33, no. 3, pp. 361–390, 1996.

[12] A. Calliste, "Women of "exceptional merit": immigration of Caribbean nurses to Canada," *Journal of Women and the Law*, vol. 6, no. 1, pp. 85–102, 1993.

[13] T. D. Das Gupta, *Racism and Paid Work*, Garmond Press, Toronto, Canada, 1996.

[14] D. Gregory, "Against the odds: an update on Aboriginal Nursing in Canada," A Research Report, Health Canada (First Nations and Inuit Health Branch, FNIHB), 2007.

[15] W. Head, "An exploratory study of attitudes and perceptions of minority and majority group health care workers," A Report Commissioned by the Race Relations Division of the Ontario Human Rights Commission, Toronto, Canada, 1986.

[16] Health Canada, "First Nations and Inuit Health Branch Nursing workforce survey," Final Report of a Survey of First Nations and Inuit Health Branch Nurses, EKOS Research Associates, Ottawa, Canada, 2006.

[17] J. Hezekiah, *Breaking the Glass Ceiling: The Stories of Three Caribbean Nurses*, The University of West Indies Press, Jamaica, 2001.
[18] D. E. Martin and A. Kipling, "Factors shaping Aboriginal nursing students' experiences," *Nurse Education Today*, vol. 26, no. 8, pp. 688–696, 2006.
[19] H. Stephen, "Shining through," *Nursing Standard*, vol. 13, no. 2, pp. 14–15, 1998.
[20] J. Vaughan, "Is there really racism in nursing?" *Journal of Nursing Education*, vol. 36, no. 3, pp. 135–139, 1997.
[21] J. Kulig and S. Grypma, "Breaking down racial barriers. Honouring pioneer Aboriginal nurses from the Blood Reserve," *Alberta RN*, vol. 62, no. 8, pp. 14–16, 2006.
[22] J. C. Kulig, N. J. Stewart, D. Morgan, M. E. Andrews, M. L. P. MacLeod, and J. R. Pitblado, "Insights from a national study," *Canadian Nurse*, vol. 102, no. 4, pp. 16–20, 2006.
[23] B. G. Glaser and A. L. Strauss, *The Discovery of Grounded Theory: Strategies for Qualitative Research*, Aldine, Chicago, Ill, USA, 1967.
[24] M. Patton, *Qualitative Research and Evaluation Methods*, Sage, Thousand Oaks, Calif, USA, 3rd edition, 2002.
[25] E. McGibbon and J. Etowa, *Anti-Racist Health Practice*, Canadian Scholars Press, Toronto, Canada, 2009.
[26] J. Etowa and B. Keddy, "Racism in Health Care: experiences of childbearing women of African descent," *International Journal of Diversity in Organization, Communities and Nations*, vol. 9, no. 2, pp. 17–34, 2009.
[27] J. Etowa, J. Wiens, W. T. Bernard, and B. Clow, "Determinants of black women's health in rural and remote communities," *Canadian Journal of Nursing Research*, vol. 39, no. 3, pp. 56–76, 2007.
[28] M. Adams, P. Aylward, N. Heyne et al., "Integrated support for Aboriginal tertiary students in health-related courses: the Pika Wiya Learning Centre," *Australian Health Review*, vol. 29, no. 4, pp. 482–488, 2005.
[29] D. Quantz and W. E. Thurston, "Representation strategies in public participation in health policy: the Aboriginal Community Health Council," *Health Policy*, vol. 75, no. 3, pp. 243–250, 2006.

Permissions

The contributors of this book come from diverse backgrounds, making this book a truly international effort. This book will bring forth new frontiers with its revolutionizing research information and detailed analysis of the nascent developments around the world.

We would like to thank all the contributing authors for lending their expertise to make the book truly unique. They have played a crucial role in the development of this book. Without their invaluable contributions this book wouldn't have been possible. They have made vital efforts to compile up to date information on the varied aspects of this subject to make this book a valuable addition to the collection of many professionals and students.

This book was conceptualized with the vision of imparting up-to-date information and advanced data in this field. To ensure the same, a matchless editorial board was set up. Every individual on the board went through rigorous rounds of assessment to prove their worth. After which they invested a large part of their time researching and compiling the most relevant data for our readers. Conferences and sessions were held from time to time between the editorial board and the contributing authors to present the data in the most comprehensible form. The editorial team has worked tirelessly to provide valuable and valid information to help people across the globe.

Every chapter published in this book has been scrutinized by our experts. Their significance has been extensively debated. The topics covered herein carry significant findings which will fuel the growth of the discipline. They may even be implemented as practical applications or may be referred to as a beginning point for another development. Chapters in this book were first published by Hindawi Publishing Corporation; hereby published with permission under the Creative Commons Attribution License or equivalent.

The editorial board has been involved in producing this book since its inception. They have spent rigorous hours researching and exploring the diverse topics which have resulted in the successful publishing of this book. They have passed on their knowledge of decades through this book. To expedite this challenging task, the publisher supported the team at every step. A small team of assistant editors was also appointed to further simplify the editing procedure and attain best results for the readers.

Our editorial team has been hand-picked from every corner of the world. Their multi-ethnicity adds dynamic inputs to the discussions which result in innovative outcomes. These outcomes are then further discussed with the researchers and contributors who give their valuable feedback and opinion regarding the same. The feedback is then collaborated with the researches and they are edited in a comprehensive manner to aid the understanding of the subject.

Apart from the editorial board, the designing team has also invested a significant amount of their time in understanding the subject and creating the most relevant covers. They scrutinized every image to scout for the most suitable representation of the subject and create an appropriate cover for the book.

The publishing team has been involved in this book since its early stages. They were actively engaged in every process, be it collecting the data, connecting with the contributors or procuring relevant information. The team has been an ardent support to the editorial, designing and production team. Their endless efforts to recruit the best for this project, has resulted in the accomplishment of this book. They are a veteran in the field of academics and their pool of knowledge is as vast as their experience in printing. Their expertise and guidance has proved useful at every step. Their uncompromising quality standards have made this book an exceptional effort. Their encouragement from time to time has been an inspiration for everyone.

The publisher and the editorial board hope that this book will prove to be a valuable piece of knowledge for researchers, students, practitioners and scholars across the globe.

List of Contributors

Hossein Karimi Moonaghi
Department of Medical-Surgical Nursing, Faculty of Nursing and Midwifery, Mashhad University of Medical Sciences, Mashhad 9137913199, Iran

Hossein Namdar Areshtanab
Department of Postgraduate, Faculty of Nursing and Midwifery, Mashhad University of Medical Sciences, Mashhad 9137913199, Iran

Leila Jouybari
Faculty of Nursing and Midwifery, Golestan University of Medical Sciences, Gorgan 49155568, Iran

Shuchang He and Junya Zhan
Department of Psychology, Peking University, No. 5 Yiheyuan Road, Haidian District, Beijing 100871, China

Yan Chen
Department of Psychology, Peking University, No. 5 Yiheyuan Road, Haidian District, Beijing 100871, China
Capital Institute of Pediatrics, Beijing 100020, China

Johnna Wu and Mark Opler
Department of Psychiatry, New York University School of Medicine, New York City, NY 10016, USA

Meng Zhao
College of Nursing and Health Sciences, Texas A&M University Corpus Christi, Island Hall 350E, 6300 Ocean Drive, Unit 5805, Corpus Christi, TX 78412, USA

Yingchun Ji
Asia Research Institute, National University of Singapore, 21 Lower Kent Ridge Road, Singapore 119077

Karyn Taplay and Lynn Martin
Department of Nursing, Faculty of Applied Health Sciences, Brock University, 500 Glenridge Drive, St. Catharines, ON, Canada

Susan M. Jack and Pamela Baxter
School of Nursing, Faculty of Health Sciences, McMaster University, 1280 Main Street West, Hamilton, ON, Canada

Kevin Eva
Centre for Health Education Scholarship, Faculty of Medicine, University of British Columbia, 950West 10th Avenue, Vancouver, BC, Canada

Mary Smith and Nazilla Khanlou
Queen's University, Kingston, ON, Canada
School of Nursing, Faculty of Health, York University, 4700 Keele Street, Toronto, ON, Canada

Meimanat Hosseini
Department of Community Health Nursing, Faculty of Nursing and Midwifery, Shahid Beheshti University of Medical Sciences, International Branch of Shahid Beheshti University of Medical Sciences, Tehran, Iran

Tahereh Ashk Torab
Department of Medical-Surgical, Faculty of Nursing and Midwifery, Shahid Beheshti University of Medical Sciences, Tehran, Iran

Mohammad Hossein Taghdisi
Department of Health Promotion, Faculty of Tehran University of Medical Sciences, Tehran, Iran

Safar Ali Esmaeili Vardanjani
Shahrekord University of Medical Science, Shahrekord, Iran

David E. Vance
School of Nursing, University of Alabama at Birmingham, Birmingham, AL 35222, USA

Alison P. Porter-Armstrong and May D. Stinson
The Institute of Nursing and Health Research, School of Health Sciences, University of Ulster, Newtownabbey BT37 0QB, UK

Catherine Adams
School of Health Sciences, Faculty of Life and Health Sciences, University of Ulster, Newtownabbey BT37 0QB, UK
School of Sociology, Social Policy & Social Work, Queen's University Belfast, Belfast BT7 1LP, UK

Anne S. Moorhead
School of Health Sciences, Faculty of Life and Health Sciences, University of Ulster, Newtownabbey BT37 0QB, UK
Institute for Research in Social Sciences, School of Communication, University of Ulster, Newtownabbey BT37 0QB, UK

Jeannie Donnelly
Tissue Viability, The Royal Hospital, Belfast Health and Social Care Trust, Belfast BT12 6BA, UK

Jane Nixon
Clinical Trials Research Unit, University of Leeds, Leeds LS2 9JT, UK

Daniel L. Bader
School of Engineering and Materials Science, Queen Mary University of London, London E1 4NS, UK
Faculty of Health Sciences, University of Southampton, Southampton SO17 1BJ, UK

Courtney Lyder
School of Nursing, University of California Los Angeles, Los Angeles, CA 90095, USA

Marika Poutiainen and Juha Holma
Department of Psychology, Psychotherapy Training and Research Center, University of Jyväskylä, P.O. Box 35, 40014 Jyväskylä, Finland

Susan M. Ludington-Hoe
Frances Payne School of Nursing, Case Western Reserve University, Cleveland, OH 44120, USA

Amel Abouelfettoh
Faculty of Nursing, Cairo University, Cairo, Egypt
College of Nursing, King Saud bin Abdulaziz University for Health Sciences, Al Ahsa 31982, Saudi Arabia

Gail Butt, Liza McGuinness and Terri Buller-Taylor
UBC/BCCDC, 655West 12th Avenue, Vancouver, BC, Canada

Sandi Mitchell
BC Centre for Disease Control, 655West 12th Avenue, Vancouver, BC, Canada

Bjørg Dale, Arne Leland and Jan Gunnar Dale
Faculty of Health and Sport Sciences, University of Agder, Postboks 509, 4898 Grimstad, Norway

Helga E. Breimaier and Christa Lohrmann
Institute of Nursing Science, Medical University of Graz, Billrothgaße 6, 8010 Graz, Austria

Ruud J. G. Halfens and Esther Meesterberends
Department of Health Services Research Focusing on Chronic Care and Ageing, Section of Nursing Science, Maastricht University, P.O. Box 616, 6200 MD Maastricht, The Netherlands

Doris Wilborn
Department of Nursing and Management, Faculty of Business & Social Sciences, Hamburg University of Applied Sciences, Alexanderstraße 1, 20099 Hamburg, Germany

Gunnar Haase Nielsen
Department of Nursing and Health Sciences, Protestant University of Applied Sciences, Zweifalltorweg 12, 64293 Darmstadt, Germany

Karen A. Monsen and Wendy S. Looman
University of Minnesota, Minneapolis, MN 55455, USA

Scott A. Elsbernd
Children's Hospitals and Clinics of Minnesota, Minneapolis-Saint Paul, MN 55404, USA

Maria Nardella, Linda Barnhart and Jacquie Stock
Children with Special Health Care Needs Program, Washington State Department of Health, Olympia, WA 98504, USA

Carla E. Prock
Benton-Franklin Health District, Kennewick, WA 98336, USA

Mohammadkarim Bahadori and Javad Smaeilnejad
Health Management Research Centre, Baqiyatallah University of Medical Sciences, Tehran, Iran

Ramin Ravangard
School of Management and Medical Information Sciences, Shiraz University of Medical Sciences, Shiraz, Iran

Amin Aghili, Jamil Sadeghifar and Mahdi Gharsi Manshadi
Students Scientific Research Center, School of Management and Medical Information, Tehran University of Medical Sciences, Tehran, Iran

Mervi Flinkman
Department of Nursing Science, University of Turku, 20014 Turku, Finland

Ulpukka Isopahkala-Bouret
Faculty of Behavioural Sciences, University of Helsinki, P.O. Box 9, 00014 Helsinki, Finland

Sanna Salanterä
Department of Nursing Science, University of Turku, 20014 Turku, Finland
Hospital District of Southwest Finland, Bureau of Administration, Turku University Hospital, P.O. Box 52, 20521 Turku, Finland

Helen Reyes, Lance Hadley and Deborah Davenport
Department of Nursing, West Texas A&M University, P.O. Box 60969, Canyon, TX 79016, USA

Robyn Stone, Simon Cooper and Robyn Cant
Monash University, School of Nursing and Midwifery, Berwick Campus, 100 Clyde Road, Berwick 3806, Australia

Soili Vesterinen
Lapland Hospital District, P.O. Box 8041, 96101 Rovaniemi, Finland
Department of Health Sciences, University of Oulu, P.O. Box 5000, 90014 University of Oulu, Finland

Marjo Suhonen, Arja Isola, Leena Paasivaara and Helena Laukkala
Department of Health Sciences, University of Oulu, P.O. Box 5000, 90014 University of Oulu, Finland

Judith A. MacDonnell
School of Nursing, York University, Room 322, HNES Building, 4700 Keele Street, Toronto, ON, Canada

Alisa Grigorovich
School of Women's Studies, York University, 206 Founders College, 4700 Keele Street, Toronto, ON, Canada

Adele Vukic
Dalhousie School of Nursing, Faculty of Health Professions, 1459 Oxford Street, Halifax, NS, Canada

Charlotte Jesty
Mijuajij Aqq Nin, Unamaki Maternal Child Health, 201 Churchill Drive, Membertou, NS, Canada

Sr. Veronica Mathews
Eskasoni Health Board, Eskasoni Community Health Center, Eskasoni, NS, Canada

Josephine Etowa
School of Nursing, Faculty of Health Sciences, University of Ottawa, Ottawa, ON, Canada